The Neuroscience of Human Movement

The Neuroscience of Human Movement

Charles T. Leonard, PT, PhD

Associate Professor
Director, Motor Control Research Laboratory
Physical Therapy Department
The University of Montana
Missoula, Montana

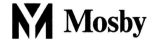

St. Louis   Baltimore   Boston   Carlsbad   Chicago   Minneapolis   New York   Philadelphia   Portland
London   Milan   Sydney   Tokyo   Toronto

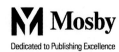
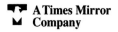

Mosby

Dedicated to Publishing Excellence

A Times Mirror Company

Executive Editor: Martha Sasser
Developmental Editor: Kellie F. White
Project Manager: Gayle Morris
Cover Designer: Dave Zielinski
Manufacturing Supervisor: Betty Mueller
Production Services: Ace Editorial Services, Inc.

Printed in the United States of America
Composition by Ace Editorial Services, Inc.
Printing/binding by R.R. Donnelly & Sons, Inc.

Mosby-Year Book, Inc.
11830 Westline Industrial Drive
St. Louis, Missouri 63146

International Standard Book Number 0-8151-5371-6

97 98 99 00 01 / 9 8 7 6 5 4 3 2 1

With love to
Jason and Hannah

Neuroscience is the study of the nervous system and how the 100 billion neurons that comprise the nervous system collectively contribute to function. *Function* is perhaps the key word to describe the contents of this book. Neuroanatomy textbooks typically provide a litany of structures and pathways. Neuroscience textbooks increasingly emphasize molecular biology. This book is an attempt to synthesize this information with the plethora of recent information on *human* motor control. The result is a text that confines itself to the neural basis of human movement. Pathways, structures, and neurophysiological principles are discussed but always in the context of human function and movement.

There were two primary audiences in mind during the writing of this book. The first is students involved in disciplines that involve the study of motor control and/or physical rehabilitation. I have been involved with teaching neuroscience courses to physical therapy, medical, and physical education students for the past decade. Two things have struck me during this time. One is the fact that the majority of the students do not have neurology as a career goal and will be entering fields more directly related to orthopedics or sports medicine. They tend to regard much of the detail inherent to a neuroscience course to be only marginally relevant to their future. In my teaching and in this book, I attempt to dispel this myth. By providing examples and anecdotes from sports and everyday activities, an attempt was made to create an essential connection between neuroscience and movement. Students also have a ten-dency to compartmentalize their education. They tend not to integrate their basic science courses with clinical courses such as therapeutic exercise, sport psychology, neurological rehabilitation, and motor learning. This book in intended to assist the student and professor in making this connection and is intended to be used as a crossover text between several courses.

The second intended audience is clinicians. I am occasionally asked to provide continuing education courses or lecture about my research to clinicians. Clinicians appear hungry to obtain recent neuroscience/motor control information that directly relates to the rehabilitation of their patents and clients. "Is there any text that will review and highlight neuroscience fundamentals or tell me how recent findings might relate to my work in the clinic?" The past 5 years have seen an explosion of information relating to the neural basis of human movement. Clinicians are well aware of this, but clinical duties typically make it impossible for them to acquire this information, which is dispersed throughout numerous journals. This book attempts to synthesize recent information with a review of basic neuroscience. Thus, the clinician does not need to undertake the dry drudgery of reading a basic neuroscience text or spend hours in search of research that relates to his or her clinical duties.

Rehabilitation techniques are under critical review from several fronts. Newer techniques, based on laboratory findings, have been developed, but have not been adequately disseminated to clinicians. This book, although not reviewing specific techniques, provides a scientific foundation from which clinicians can critically evaluate their methods. An understanding of the scientific basis of treatment is critical to clinical competence.

The book is written in a way that does not require cover-to-cover reading. In the neuroscience-related courses I teach to physical therapy students, I have used the chapters in the following way:

Chapter 1 is very introductory. The chapter reviews vocabulary and basic nervous system organization. It is an attempt to show that there is no need for the fear and loathing often associated with the study of neuroscience. For individuals who have not been exposed to this type of basic science information before, the reading of this chapter is probably essential to an understanding of subsequent chapters, which introduce more complex issues.

Chapter 2 reviews basic structures and neural connectivity that most directly relate to movement. It introduces nomenclature, establishes some foundations, and relates structure to function. I suggest that students read Chapters 1 and 2 *before* the start of the first year's neuroscience course. Students have informed me that they often refer back to Chapter 2 during the neuroscience course.

Chapter 3 stresses the relevance of basic neurophysiology to human motor control. For instance, what do flexor reflex afferents have to do with human ambulation and with the treatment of spasticity? What is the role of neural modulators and long-term potentiation in motor learning? Portions of this chapter have been used in first-year neuroscience courses. Other sections have been used as the first reading for second-year courses in motor control and neurological rehabilitation.

Chapter 4 introduces the fascinating and ever-changing role of the cerebral cortex in movement. Cerebral cortical nomenclature appears to change on a weekly basis. The reasons for this and an integration of older and newer terminologies are presented. Brain scanning techniques are also discussed. Most of this chapter, however, is devoted to the role of the cerebral cortex during various movements, clinical repercussions of damage to specific areas, and differences between right and left hemispheres wither regard to function. It is again useful as a crossover between first-year neuroscience courses and second-year courses in neurological rehabilitation, motor control, and higher cognitive function.

Chapters 5 and 6 present the neural basis of human locomotion, eye-hand coordination, and upper extremity control. Some of the concepts that were introduced in earlier chapters are presented again here, but in a more functional or practical context. As an educator, I have found that presenting similar information in different contexts aids learning. These chapters build on previously discussed concepts and moves the reader from the comfortable realm of fact to the more nebulous world of hypothesis and conjecture. These chapters meld basic and clinical sciences to bring the reader up-to-date on issues pertaining to important aspects of human movement.

Chapter 7 explores the neural basis of motor learning. It is perhaps the most theoretical of all the chapters, and requires the student to have a sound grasp of the neuroscientific principles discussed in previous chapters. In my teaching, I typically briefly present the information in Chapters 5, 6, and 7 in the first-year neuroscience course, but present the more detailed information within these chapters during the second-year clinical courses.

There is a serious temptation in a book of this sort either to make things too simplistic or to provide too much detail. If I have erred, it is toward presenting a traditional connectionist view of the nervous system. I consider this a necessary beginning to the understanding of the relationship between form and function. However, simple, hierarchical, connectionist constructs are no longer a tenable explanation for the wondrous workings of the human nervous system. I have therefore attempted to present, when appropriate and without introducing confusion, how integration of diverse systems contribute to human movement.

"The greater complex is never predicted by the parts of the lesser complex.
Therefore, I surmise that to learn anything you must start with the whole."

R. Buckminster Fuller

This is truly one of the greatest challenges facing teachers of the neurosciences. There is no
beginning and end to its study. The study of individual neural structures apart from an integration
with biomechanics, psychology, or biophysics
yields little toward an understanding of actual
function. And yet, an understanding of the whole
is not possible without an understanding of the
component parts.

I have written this book in a rather informal
voice and more than once present what I consider
to be humorous anecdotes and stories. I know I
run the risk of turning off some individuals with
this approach. After all, science is a serious business. I agree, but I also believe a sense of humor
is as essential to the successful completion of
neuroscience courses as are the other five senses.
As an educator, I believe we need to remove, as
much as possible, the intimidation inherent to the
study of neuroscience. We also need to make this
difficult subject as palatable and as relevant as
possible. We need to relay to our students the
wonder and fascination that initially drew us into
this field. By writing in an informal voice and
sharing some of myself in the writing, I have
attempted to do this.

In his book, "Over Our Heads: The Mental
Demands of Modern Life," Robert Kegan states
that the writing of his book won't be completed
until his readers do so. I share these same senti-
ments. This book won't be completed until I hear
from students, educators, and clinicians whether
or not I have come close to addressing your needs
and providing the information you seek. On a
final note, this book is intended to be a "primer."
Although I have been in this business for quite
some time, I must somewhat embarrassingly
admit, however, to learning a tremendous amount
as I researched and read material apart from my
increasingly esoteric island of specialized knowledge. My fascination and awe of the study of the
neural basis of behavior continues. It is my hope
that this sense of wonder is conveyed to you in the
subsequent pages.

Chuck Leonard, PT, PhD

■ ACKNOWLEDGMENTS

The writing of a book is never the result of a
singular effort. I am indebted to many individuals
for their contributions. I would like to start by
thanking the book's reviewers. Drs. Manuel
Hulliger, Stephen Lahr, and Mary Shall provided
excellent critical reviews. Dr. Hulliger, with his
Swiss-like precision and breadth of knowledge of
the neurosciences, was a guiding force throughout this process. He insisted that even though the
book is not intended as a treatise on the subject,
that nonetheless it not compromise on accuracy
and sufficient detail to describe neural processes
adequately. Dr. Stephen Lahr was ever vigilant
that the manuscript not drift into minutia but
rather maintain a focus on clinical and real-life
examples. His input regarding organization was
also much appreciated. Dr. Mary Shall combined
her talents as a neurophysiologist, physical therapist, and English literature undergraduate major
to greatly enhance this project in multiple ways.
She is an inspiration and a wonderful friend. I am
also indebted to Carolee Winstein for her review
of Chapter 7 and to several anonymous reviewers
who made valuable contributions. Ed Jenne, a
biologist whose illustrations bring to life the neuroscientific concepts and ideas discussed within

the text, remains a good friend despite the many occasions I asked him for multiple revisions of a drawing. I also would like to extend thanks to all of you who tolerated my late-night phone calls, E-mail messages, and faxes requesting information and references. I hesitate to name all of you individually for fear of omitting someone, but you know who you are and I am indebted to you.

This book would not have been written if it had not been for the insistence and persistence of several individuals at Mosby-Year Book, Inc. Klaus Gurgel and Martha Sasser initiated the process and Kellie White took over the reins and whip from them to ensure I attended to the book's completion. Emma Underdown of Ace Editorial Services, Inc. provided excellent copy editing skills. It is rare that one is given the opportunity publicly to thank others who have contributed to one's professional career and personal development. I would like to indulge in that opportunity. Foremost, I would like to acknowledge my parents and sister—my first mentors. They continue to be my compass and my strength. More recently, some very special people have entered and enriched my life. Jason and Hannah Leonard, my children and two favorite lab rats, literally since the time of their birth, have been poked and prodded as part of my research. Their mother, Paula Huston-Leonard, has added immeasurably to my life and is one of the strongest people I know.

I am indebted to Professor Robert Neeves, an exercise physiologist from The University of Delaware, who during my undergraduate education provided an inspiration to his students by showing, via example, that being an athlete and intellectual were not mutually exclusive domains. I am indebted to Professors Eleanor Branch and Emma Villanueva from Duke University, who were two of the best educators I was privileged to have as a physical therapy student. I am also thankful to Dr. Lorne Mendell, a neurophysiologist at Duke University when I was a student, who may or may not remember me as someone who occasionally showed up in his lab to observe and ask innumerable annoying questions. This experience, together with lectures from Dr. Talmage Peele and others during the infamous "12 days of Neuro," began my love affair with the neurosciences. It wasn't until several years later, after having worked as a clinical physical therapist and returning to school at The Medical College of Pennsylvania, however, that my real neuroscience education began. It arrived in the form of an extraordinary neuroscientist and human being named Dr. Michael Goldberger. Chapter 7 is dedicated to his memory and work.

My education continued with a postdoctoral fellowship at The Karolinska Institute in Stockholm, Sweden. This experience was enhanced by many people. I feel extremely privileged to have worked with individuals such as Hans Forssberg, Helga Hirschfeld, Sten Grillner, Johnny Nilsson, Lars Oddsson, Virgil Stokes, Eva Anderson, Per-Olof Astrand, Toshio Moritani, and Alf Thorstensson.

I would also like to thank the faculty at The University of Montana for their support and assistance. Two individuals in particular, Beth Ikeda and Dave Levison, both of whom are talented orthopedic/sports medicine therapists, have influenced many sections of this book with their clinical questions regarding motor control.

And finally, I would like to acknowledge the scientists referenced within this book. Their intellect and labor-intensive efforts have contributed much to our world. These people are my heroes.

CONTENTS

An Introduction to the Language of the Nervous System

What's in a Word?
The Peripheral Nervous System
Cells of the Central Nervous System
Neural Projections and Organization
The Tip of the Iceberg

W hy can someone sink 50 straight foul shots in basketball practice and go 0-for-October in game situations? Why does an individual's signature look the same, regardless whether it is written the size of a microchip or in large print on a billboard? Why do athletes lose their "feel" after relatively minor soft tissue injuries? How do firewalkers manage to do what they do? And, why does listening to Mozart improve memory and motor performance?

With a basic understanding of the divisions of the nervous system, a rudimentary vocabulary, a few basic directions (Fig. 1-1), and some measure of tenacity, you can begin to share in the exploration of these and other neuroscientific mysteries. A basic understanding is what Chapter 1 is all about. Subsequent chapters in this book introduce you to some of the neural complexities underlying human movement and assume a certain level of neural knowledge on your part. Chapter 1 was written for those individuals requiring a review of vocabulary and basic organization of the nervous system. So, if terms such as *corticospinal* and *cerebroreticulocerebellar* are already in your vocabulary and you know the difference between an interneuron and a sensory neuron, you can probably do without Chapter 1. If not, the reading of Chapter 1 and a review of the terms listed in the Glossary at the back of this book will greatly enhance your understanding of the remaining chapters.

■ WHAT'S IN A WORD?

Every profession develops its own vocabulary. Plumbers sweat joints, carpenters use 8-penny nails to frame out with two-by-fours, and dancers *ronde de jambe* and *plie*. Professions that involve the study of

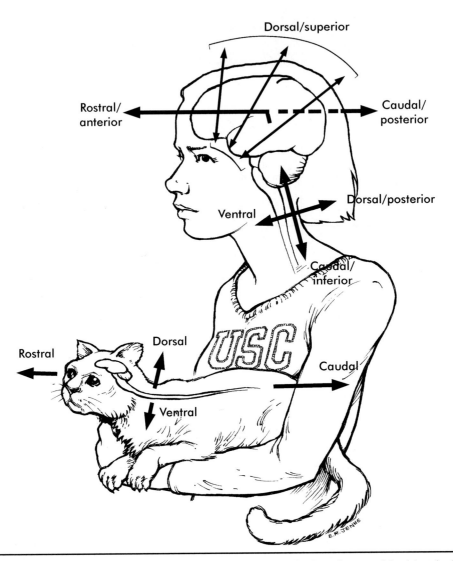

Fig. 1-1. Directional terms in the central nervous system are different between humans (bipeds) and other animals (quadrupeds).

neurology and motor control are no different. The vocabulary, however, tends toward the polysyllabic. Words such as cerebroreticulocerebellar, fastigioreticulovestibular, and, perhaps the grandaddy of them all, septopreopticohypothalamoparamedian are not exactly used in everyday conversation and do not roll off the tongue with ease even after 3 or 4 years of graduate school in the neurosciences. It is easy to be put off by such excessive letter usage, but do not be intimidated. Knowing the names and locations of a few anatomical structures allows even the most timid student to become at ease with the language of neu-

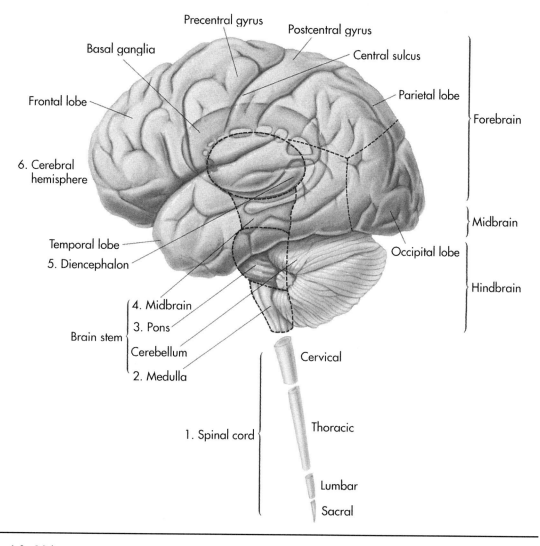

Precentral gyrus

Postcentral gyrus

Basal ganglia

Central sulcus

Frontal lobe

Parietal lobe

Forebrain

6. Cerebral
   hemisphere

Temporal lobe

Occipital lobe

5. Diencephalon

Midbrain

4. Midbrain

Hindbrain

3. Pons

Brain stem

Cerebellum

2. Medulla

Cervical

1. Spinal cord

Thoracic

Lumbar

Sacral

Fig. 1-2. Major components of the human CNS. (From Kandel ER, Schwartz JH, Jessell TM. Principles of neural science, 3rd ed. Norwalk, Conn: Appleton & Lange, 1991.)

rology. This is because 99% of neurological terms follow a logical sequence. Many words are, in fact, a type of road map. For instance, the words listed above indicate where a nerve cell is located and where it is sending its message. The name, therefore, merely indicates origins and destinations. Knowing the subdivisions of the central nervous system (CNS) (Fig. 1-2) allows you to make sense of even the most garbled mouthful of neurological syllables.

The CNS is subdivided into the brain and the spinal cord. The CNS can be further subdivided into seven anatomical regions:

1. the cerebral hemispheres,
2. the diencephalon (thalamus, hypothalamus),
3. the midbrain,
4. the cerebellum,
5. the pons,
6. the medulla, and
7. the spinal cord.

The medulla, pons, and midbrain are collectively referred to as the *brain stem*. Keeping these subdivisions in mind can greatly ease terminology angst.

If I wanted to name a group of nerves that were located in the spinal cord and projected to the cerebellum, I would list the point of origin first and its destination second. *Neurons (*the conducting cells of the nervous system) originating in the spinal cord and projecting to the cerebellum, therefore, become the *spinocerebellar* tract. *Corticospinal* refers to projections originating in the cerebral cortex (*cortico*) and terminating in the spinal cord (Fig. 1-3). Given this simple system, polysyllabic mouthfuls can be explained easily. The CNS is also comprised of many nuclei. *Nuclei* are groups of anatomically or topographically related and often densely packed neurons. Quite often these topographically related neurons are also functionally related. Unfortunately, each of the thousand or so nuclei within the CNS has its own name. For example, *fastigioreticularvestibular* refers to the fastigial nucleus of the cerebellum, which projects to reticular nuclei in the brain stem and then onto the vestibular nuclei in the medulla.

Admittedly, naming does get complex if you are inclined to memorize the infinite divisions and structures of the nervous system. Knowing how to dissect the parts of a cumbersome word, however, and armed with the Glossary at the end of this book, you can achieve a good understanding of the CNS without the pain, drudgery, and mental gymnastics of memorization.

■ THE PERIPHERAL NERVOUS SYSTEM

The CNS is not the sole component of the nervous system. The peripheral nervous system is the other component of the vertebrate nervous system. The *peripheral nervous system (PNS)* refers to *ganglia* (groups of functionally related neurons located outside the CNS) and peripheral nerves that are not contained within the brain and spinal cord. Peripheral nerves of sensory neurons convey sensory information to the CNS. Sensory neurons, therefore, are typically located in the PNS, but their projections to the spinal cord and higher brain centers are part of the CNS (Fig. 1-4). Motor neurons contained within the CNS project to the periphery via peripheral nerves. For instance, motor neurons contained within the spinal cord send projections to muscles. Their cell bodies are located in the CNS but their axonal projections are considered part of the PNS. Also considered part of the peripheral nervous system is the *autonomic system*. The actions and interactions of the autonomic nervous system are complex. Because the autonomic nervous system is not directly concerned with muscle contraction or sensory feedback about muscle or movement, one might be tempted to avoid the topic in a book devoted to the neuroscience of motor control. The autonomic nervous system, however, is comprised of the sympathetic and parasympathetic divisions—both of which are intimately connected to motor control mechanisms. One of the subdivisions of the autonomic nervous system, the enteric division, is concerned with gut motility, so we will skip that one. *Fight or flight* is a term often applied to the autonomic nervous system. The reason for this is that the sympathetic nervous system is primarily concerned with preparing the body to respond to stress, such as an incoming fist. The parasympathetic nervous system is more mellow and is primarily concerned with the *homeostasis,* or the maintenance, of bodily functions. The sympathetic and parasympathetic nervous systems, however, should not be thought of as being in opposition to one another. They both function together to provide us with the necessary degree of arousal to meet environmental demands. The perva-

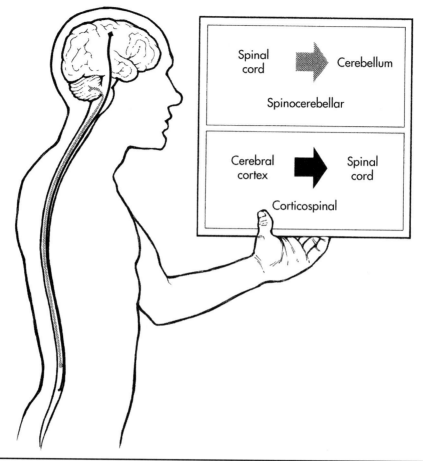

Fig. 1-3. The spinocerebellar tract is so named because the axon's cell of origin is located in the spinal cord and its terminal projection is in the cerebellum. The corticospinal tract originates with a cell in the cerebral cortex and projects to the spinal cord.

sive interconnectivity of the autonomic nervous system allows it to influence all bodily functions and behaviors, including motor behavior. Nervousness, a sympathetic response, can destroy an athlete's or musician's performance. The autonomic nervous system is also intimately connected with the immune system. Damage or dysfunction can dramatically alter an individual's response to stress, injury, and disease. Connectivity and interdependencies are pervasive in the human nervous system.

■ CELLS OF THE CENTRAL NERVOUS SYSTEM

The study of neurology and motor control involves the study of connections. Connectivity begins with a single nerve cell. Nerve cells, or *neurons*, are the cellular components of the nervous system that send messages. Neurons have projections known as axons and dendrites extending from their cell bodies.

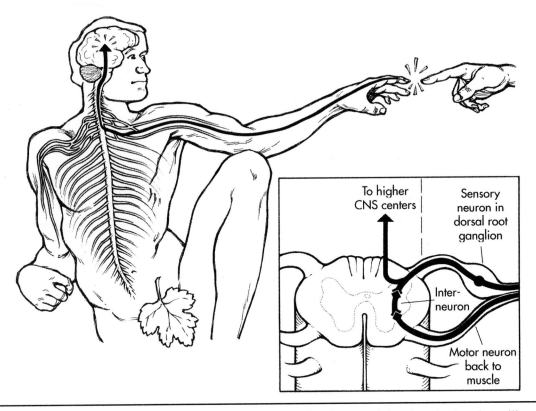

Fig. 1-4. A sensory neuron located in the dorsal root ganglion has a peripheral projection that will convey information back to the spinal cord from the receptor located at the tip of the finger. This projection is part of the peripheral nervous system. The dorsal root ganglion neuron will convey receptor information centrally into the spinal cord. This information might be used in a spinal reflex arc and elicit movement via activation of the motor neuron. The receptor's sensory information will also be conveyed to higher brain centers within the CNS.

Axons are the message-sending extension of the cell body. *Dendrites*, far more numerous than axons, are the message-receiving components of the neuron. With regard to motor control, if you are well connected, you are literally going places. Neurons have been the stars of the show. The supporting cast, known as *support* or *satellite cells*, are greater in number but have received less attention because they were not thought to be directly involved in neural transmission.

Satellite cells
Support cells, also termed *neuroglia*, are beginning to cast a shadow over the performing brilliance of the neurons. During development, support cells help guide neurons to their final destinations, provide nutrients to neurons, create protective barriers, secrete neuroprotective chemicals, and literally provide the glue and skeleton to hold the nervous system together. The promise of using fetal tissue transplants after

spinal cord injury to lessen paralysis or to treat diseases such as Parkinson's disease is attributable main-ly to the functioning of support cells and not the neurons themselves.

For simplicity's sake I will limit discussion solely to the 100 billion to 1 trillion neurons that comprise the human nervous system. Similar to snowflakes, every neuron is different both in terms of morphology and function. Luckily, neurons can be classified as sensory, motor, or interneurons. This taxonomy allows us to generalize and avoid the need for one trillion individual descriptions.

Sensory neurons

Sensory neurons for the body are located outside, but adjacent to, the spinal cord in a structure referred to as the *dorsal root ganglion* (Fig. 1-4). Sensory neurons for the face, head, and some aspects of parasym-pathetic visceral control are contained within ganglia adjacent to, or nuclei within, the brain stem. Sensory neurons respond to a wide range of stimuli, from a soft caressing touch to the pain of a slap in the face. These neurons keep us in touch with our world. At one end of a dorsal root ganglion sensory neuron is a receptor organ. The other end of this neuron projects into the spinal cord. We have sensory receptors for vision, smell, touch, hearing, cold, heat, pressure, pain, and detecting changes in movement. The nerve fibers that transmit the messages from the various sensory receptors are called *sensory afferent fibers*. Some sensory neurons connect with motor neurons in the spinal cord or brain stem nuclei to form reflex arcs. Spinal reflexes will be discussed in detail in a subsequent chapter. For now, suffice it to say that *reflexes* allow us to respond quickly and predictably to a sensory stimulus. You don't need to think a whole lot to realize stepping on a nail is painful and it is best to remove your foot from the situation. Sensory neurons not only form spinal reflex arcs, but they also project to higher brain centers such as the thala-mus and cerebral cortex (Fig. 1-5). It is in these higher brain centers that meaning is attached to sensory stimuli. Interpretations and perceptions of sensations are formed over course of our lifetime of involve-ment with the world.

Motor neurons

Motor neurons, with cell bodies located in the spinal cord or brain stem nuclei, send messages via their axons to muscles and muscle spindles. Their primary function is to control muscle contraction. Motor neurons receive their instructions from sensory neurons, interneurons, the cerebral cortex, and other ner-vous system structures. Motor neurons are the frontline troops that carry out CNS commands, that cause a muscle to contract and therefore generate movement. Many direct and indirect connections between sen-sory and motor neurons exist. The more direct the connection, the faster we can respond to the stimulus.

To illustrate the importance of the link between incoming sensory stimuli and movement, let's take a walk on the beach. You're looking and feeling good. You sense the eyes of admirers gazing in your direc-tion, so you break into a jog. No sooner do you start your jaunt, when a sharp shell finds its way into the soft, vulnerable flesh of the underside of your foot (Fig. 1-6). The jog instantly becomes a one-legged hop. The sensation of pain has an immediate effect on your movement, and this alteration in movement required no thought on your part. The sensation of pain caused a reflex response that involved lifting your leg away from the sharp stimulus. But think about this for a minute: You would not be able to lift your leg away from the painful source unless your opposite leg extended and muscles contracted so that you could stand on that one leg for a short period. Believe it or not, this rather complicated movement is part of a spinal reflex. Chances are, your face also turned red from embarrassment in having had your moment in the spotlight so abruptly halted. The perception of sensations, in this case embarrassment, has its own physiological consequences. But this discussion will be saved for our trek through higher brain centers (Chapter 4).

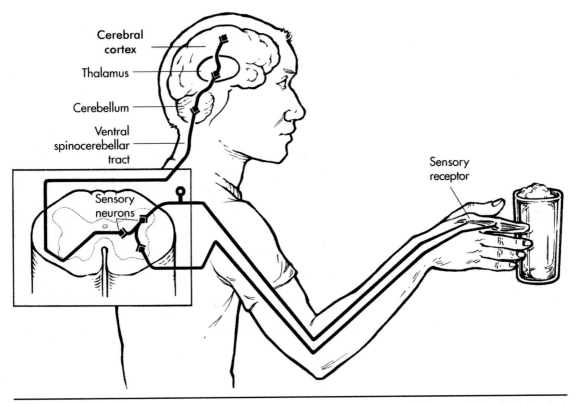

Fig. 1-5. Sensory neurons located within the gray matter of the spinal cord are typically not only involved in spinal cord reflex arcs, but will also convey sensory information to higher brain centers such as the cerebellum (spinocerebellar tracts) and directly or indirectly to the thalamus and cerebral cortex.

Interneurons

Interneurons, deeply imbedded within the spinal cord and other CNS structures, form connections between motor neurons, sensory neurons, and input coming down to the spinal cord from higher brain centers. To think of interneurons as merely one of the links in a reflex arc would be wrong. Rather, interneurons are responsible for integrating multifarious convergent input, processing these signals in some way, and sending their own unique signal to divergent locations. Of the more than 100 billion neurons in the human nervous system, only about 5 million are sensory neurons and only several hundred thousand are motor neurons. The remainder are interneurons. Interneurons, therefore, comprise more than 99.9% of the nervous system—yet we know less about these neurons than any others. Therefore, we know less than one tenth of what there is to know about the cells that comprise the nervous system. No wonder the complexities of the neural control of movement remain a mystery!

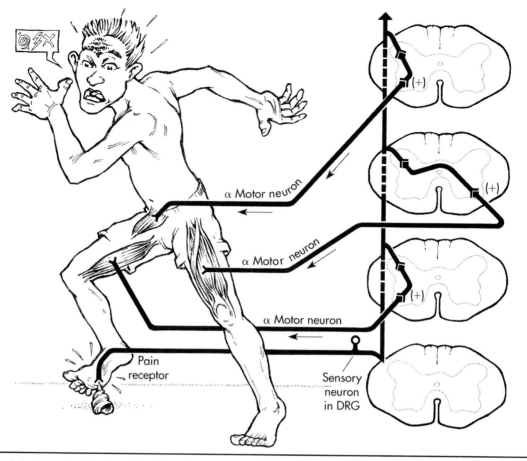

Fig. 1-6. Crossed extension reflex: Stepping on a sharp shell (or any painful stimulus) elicits a reflex that results in withdrawal of the foot and extremity away from the stimulus and a concomitant extension of the contralateral leg. The contralateral leg extends to provide postural stability while the other leg flexes. *DRG,* Dorsal root ganglion.

■ NEURAL PROJECTIONS AND ORGANIZATION
Dendrites and axons

Nerve cells receive and send electrochemical signals. The message-sending part of the nerve cell is called the *axon* and the message-receiving part is called the *dendrite.* Dendrites look a lot like furry little hair balls. The neuron's yearning for information causes dendrites to branch repeatedly as they search for as much incoming information as possible. A single neuron may receive thousands of inputs thanks to dendritic branching. The more dendrites a neuron has, the more information it can process. The shape of a neuron often takes on a treelike appearance, hence the term *dendritic arborization.* When we are born, most neurons have very few and poorly formed dendrites. As we grow, learn, and explore our world, the

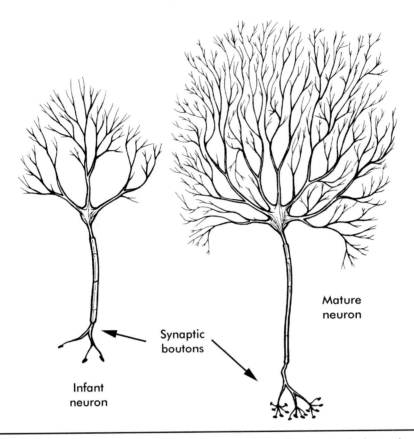

Fig. 1-7. Neural maturation includes increased dendritic arborization and an increase in the number of axonal synaptic boutons.

dendrites grow profusely (Fig. 1-7). This process continues, although in a more limited manner, throughout adulthood. Continue to learn and chances are you will continue to expand your brain—literally.

Processes of brain maturation can be altered during ontogenetic development. For example, alcohol has a devastating effect on dendritic growth and neural maturation in young animals, including humans. This is one of the potential effects of the *fetal alcohol syndrome*, a disorder that affects babies born to women who have ingested heavy quantities of alcohol during their pregnancy.

On a more optimistic note, experiments with rats, mice, and cats have shown that if newborn animals are exposed to an enriched physical environment with wheels, ramps, ladders, etc., they will develop more dendrites in areas of the brain devoted to motor activities than animals deprived of early movement experience.[2,6] Activity-dependent change in the CNS is apparently not limited to our furry brethren. Musicians, craftsmen, and highly educated individuals have enlarged cortical areas that are devoted to their area of specialty.[3,4] The earlier the individual received the training, the more enhanced the cortical representation.[1,5] The relative effects of nature versus nurture are complex and beyond the scope of this brief introduction to the human nervous system. It is becoming increasingly clear, however, that the nervous system, and the motor areas of the brain in particular, do not develop appropriately without adequate sensory input. Activity-dependent changes are not limited to dendritic formation. Synapses are strengthened with activity and weakened with inactivity.[5]

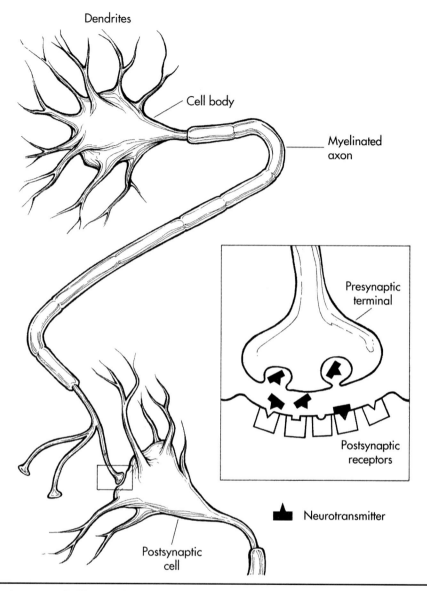

Fig. 1-8. An axosomatic synapse is illustrated. An action potential within the myelinated axon will cause neurotransmitter to be released by the presynaptic vesicle into the synaptic cleft. The neurotransmitter will bind to postsynaptic receptors, which will induce an ion flow across the postsynaptic membrane and the generation of a synaptic potential. (Adapted from Carey J. Brain facts. Washington, DC: Society for Neuroscience, 1990.)

Synapses

Where an axon meets a dendrite to convey its message is called a *synapse* (Fig. 1-8). Synapses are the connections between neurons that permit different parts of the nervous system to communicate and influence each other. Some synapses are purely electrical, but most use *neurotransmitters* (chemicals) to trans-

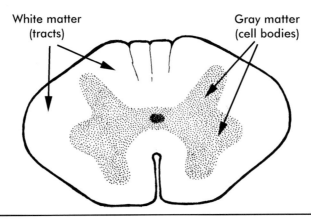

Fig. 1-9. A cross-section through one spinal cord segment. Gray matter represents the location of cell bodies. White matter represents various tract systems as they ascend and descend through the spinal cord. (Adapted from Carey J. Brain facts. Washington, DC: Society for Neuroscience, 1990.)

mit their messages. Santiago Ramon y Cajal, an early twentieth century Spanish physical educator-turned-neuroscientist, called synapses "protoplasmic kisses...the final ecstasy of an epic love story." Because of his pioneering contributions to neuroscience, he is known today as the father of neuroanatomy.

Gray and white matter
Nerve cells are not randomly distributed throughout the CNS. Rather, they congregate to specific areas. Typically, nerve cells form clusters within any given CNS structure (e.g., the spinal cord). Neuroscientists distinguish areas that are rich in neuronal cell bodies from areas that are dense with axonal projections, but contain few neurons, by assigning them colors. *Gray matter* refers to areas that are rich with nerve cell bodies and dendrites (Figs. 1-9 and 1-10). It is called gray matter because it has a pinkish gray color in living specimens. Within the gray matter are groupings of anatomically and functionally related neurons called *nuclei*. The *white matter* is comprised largely of axons, which, as you know, carry information from one part of the nervous system to another. And, yes, white matter does have a white appearance.

■ THE TIP OF THE ICEBERG
Molecular biologists, geneticists, computer modelers, biomechanists, neuroscientists, and engineers are working together to yield an exciting period in scientific history. It is a period as yet unsurpassed in its advances in the understanding of the human brain and nervous system. The United States Congress, not known for its scientific acumen, declared the 1990s the "Decade of the Brain." I predict the decade beginning in the year 2000 will be termed "The Tip of the Iceberg." The advances currently being made in the neurosciences are without historical precedent. Insights into the anatomy, physiology, biochemistry, and genetics of sensory-, motor-, and interneurons occur on an almost daily basis. These insights are revealing the personalities of each individual nerve cell. A personality, of course, does not exist in isolation. We are who we are not only because of our genetics, but also because of the experiences we have had and the influence of those around us.

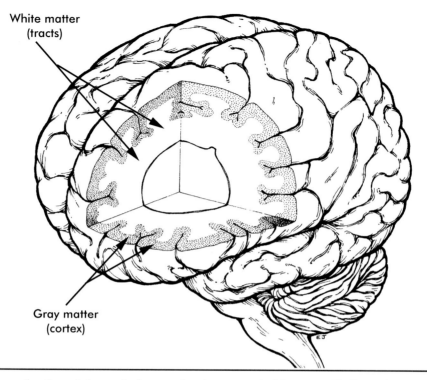

White matter (tracts)

Gray matter (cortex)

Fig. 1-10. Cross-section through the cerebral cortex showing gray and white matter. Similar to the spinal cord, gray matter (the outermost few millimeters) contains cell bodies. The remainder of the cerebral cortex is composed of white matter (axonal projections). Structures within the cerebral cortex, such as the basal ganglia and thalamus (not pictured), are areas rich in cell bodies.

"Talent is formed in stillness, character in the world's torrent."
—*Goethe*

SUGGESTED READINGS

Glial signalling: special issue. Trends Neurosci 1996;19(8):305-69.

Kandel ER, Schwartz JH, Jessell TM. Principles of neural science, 3rd ed. Norwalk, Conn: Appleton & Lange, 1991.

Nolte J. The human brain, third edition. St Louis: Mosby-Year Book, 1993.

Roland PE. Cortical organization of voluntary behavior in man. Human Neurobiol 1985;4:155-67.

Willis WD. Medical neurobiology. St Louis: Mosby-Year Book, 1977.

Wise SP, Evarts EV. The role of the cerebral cortex in movement. In: Evarts EV, Wise SP, Bousfield D, eds. The motor system in neurobiology. Amsterdam, The Netherlands: Elsevier, 1985:307-15.

REFERENCES

1. Elbert T, Pantev C, Wienbruch C, Rockstroh B, Taub E. Increased cortical representation of the fingers of the left hand in string players. Science 1995;270:305-7.

2. Pysh JJ, Weiss GM. Exercise during development induces an increase in Purkinje cell dendritic tree size. Science 1979;206:230-2.

3. Radestsky P. Experience and the brain. Brainwork 1992;2:3-4.

4. Schlaug G, Jancke L, Huang Y, Steinmetz H. In vivo evidence of structural brain asymmetry in musicians. Science 1995;267:699-701.

5. Singer W. Development and plasticity of cortical processing architectures. Science 1995;270:758-64.

6. Westerga J, Gramsbergen A. The effect of early movement restriction: an EMG study in the rat. Behav Brain Res 1993;59:205-9.

Glimpses of Organizational Form and Function

C an you imagine the hellacious and, needless to say, short existence of human life if we were given the responsibility of conscious control over our physiological processes? When is the last time you consciously thought about breathing? The complexity of this apparently simple task increases exponentially and beyond human imagining during exercise and exertion. Imagine if you had to decide, during a workout, in which muscles to increase blood flow and how to do it. You would have to decide whether to increase your respiratory rate or cardiac output. You would have to calculate how many beats per minute you should increase your heart rate as well as figure out how to increase the oxygen-carrying capacity of the blood, decrease the acidity of the blood, and dispose of the metabolic breakdown products of muscular contraction. Obviously the creator(s) of the universe knew we would have more important things on our minds than figuring out how to breathe. Luckily, similar to the mindless act of breathing, many aspects of movement do not require a lot of conscious attention. A great deal of movement, even learned movement, is highly automatic.

Move! Simple enough for most of us. Knowing the answer to your professor's question, you raise your hand and voice your thoughts. No sooner have you thought about it and it's accomplished—without a lot of conscious effort on your part. How it all happens, however, almost defies description and occupies a lot of conscious effort of some pretty smart people.

All movement occurs as a result of forces generated by muscular contraction. This is true regardless of whether the movement desired is the raising of an arm or the vibration of vocal cords. Your brain says move, and the muscles perform. Motor neurons within the spinal cord and brain stem control muscles and cause them to contract in an orderly, coordinated sequence. What, in turn, controls these neurons is where it gets interesting. The cerebral cortex has direct projections to spinal cord motor neurons, so one might be tempted to think that this is all that is required. My brain says "move," sends a message to the spinal cord, and the spinal cord relays the message to the muscles. Well, what happens if you pick up a pan of water only to find it's scalding hot? You drop it, right? No thought involved here—only reflex. You did not really "tell" your hand to let go. The sensation of pain was detected by sensory receptors in the skin and conveyed to spinal cord sensory neurons and interneurons. These neurons processed the incoming sensory information and then sent a message to motor neurons that, in turn, caused muscles to open your hand and drop the pan. In parallel, the signals from the sensory receptors were sent to higher centers where, much later, they gave rise to the conscious sensation of pain. If you had to rely on your brain to remove your hand from the painful stimulus, you would end up with a severely burned hand. Transmitting sensory messages to the brain is, in terms of neurotransmission, an extremely slow event.

Now, suppose you pick up this same pot of boiling water just as your 10-month-old infant comes crawling over to the stove. The conscious awareness of the consequences of dropping boiling water on your offspring might be sufficient to alter the course of your reactions, delaying by milliseconds the opening of your hand. This would allow you to return the pan to the stove without incident, except perhaps a hand that requires some medical attention. Obviously, awareness of your environment and situational context can change your reactions. The interactions between conscious thought and reflexes are some of the most intriguing aspects of the study of motor control.

■ AUTOMATIC VS. LESS AUTOMATIC MOVEMENT: STORIES OF REFLEXIVE BEHAVIOR

Reflexes are largely automatic, consistent, and predictable reactions to sensory stimuli. Reflexes are often thought of as being "hard-wired." But not even reflexes involving just a single synapse are entirely immutable. Reflex responses can be modulated or "tuned," a feature that adds greatly to the nervous system's ability to adjust to a changing environment. The first example of dropping the hot pan is an example of a reflex. Given a certain sensory stimulation, a predictable motor response is elicited. A physician taps her patient's knee and the leg extends. This is an example of a very simple reflex: the stretch reflex. The tap stretches the muscle. This stretch is detected by a sensory receptor, the muscle spindle, and is conveyed directly to a motor neuron. Only one synapse is involved: a sensory afferent to motor neuron. The term *monosynaptic* is, therefore, typically used to describe the stretch reflex (Fig. 2-1). Although the stretch reflex is termed monosynaptic, the sensory afferent from the spindle also contacts interneurons, sensory neurons, and neurons that send ascending projections to higher centers such as the thalamus. From there, processed messages return to the motor neurons, closing a longer parallel reflex arc. The stretch reflex, therefore, also has *polysynaptic* components (i.e., involving more than one synapse).

All reflexes, no matter how simple, can be modified by signals from the brain. Not dropping the hot pan on your infant is an example of the brain modifying a reflex. Let's consider another real-life experience as an example of a complex movement that does not directly require the brain.

I have attended numerous backyard barbecues and campfire cookouts in my lifetime. I have yet to see anyone accidently step on a hot coal with a bare foot and not respond by quickly withdrawing the foot and hopping around so that the painful foot does not again make contact with the offending piece of charcoal. This entire response—the withdrawal of the foot and the extension of the opposite leg to provide the

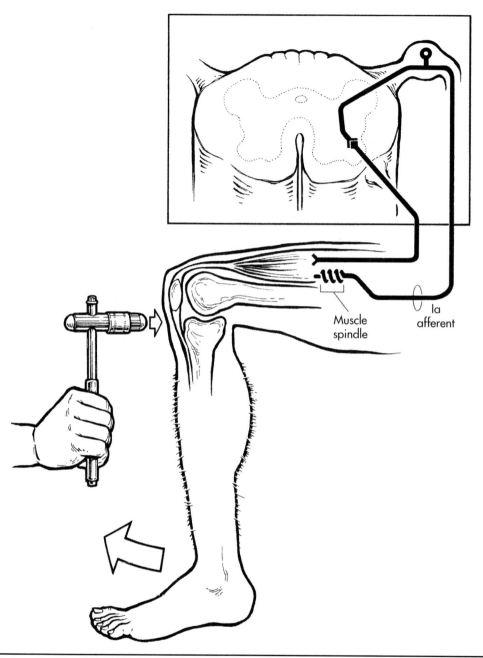

Fig 2-1. Stretch reflex: Stretching the quadriceps muscle by striking it with a reflex hammer will stimulate muscle spindles within the muscle. The spindles convey this information via Ia afferents that will synapse directly on alpha motor neurons that, in turn, will cause quadriceps muscle contraction.

ability to hop on one leg—is a reflex. The subsequent verbal tirade that often follows this reflex is not. It is, however, a good indication that the pain message has been received by the brain. This universal summertime experience brings to mind an interesting neurological phenomenon that might involve integration of reflexive pathways and the brain. Consider the following scenario a neural behavioral mystery to be solved.

We have all heard stories or seen films of individuals who are capable of willfully walking over a bed of hot coals and not reflexively removing themselves from the situation. How this is accomplished has been a matter of speculation and debate among scientists. One theory, proposed by a physicist, suggests that anxiousness causes excess sweating of the soles of the feet, and this sweat layer provides a protective evaporative barrier. This is perhaps true, but I have seen very few anxious fire walkers; the film footage I have seen indicates fire walkers are a pretty calm bunch. I, a neuroscientist, have a slightly different interpretation. I would explain the fire walker's performance as the ability consciously to ignore any pain signals arriving from the feet. This is most likely accomplished by a neurohormonal reaction that involves the release of endorphins. *Endorphins* are the body's naturally occurring pain killers. Their release is controlled by the sympathetic nervous system. When stimulated, the sympathetic nervous system, the "fight or flight" system, causes the release of endorphins. Interestingly, stimulation of the sympathetic nervous system also causes excess sweating. Hmmm, perhaps the sweating contributes to a protective evaporative barrier and prevents any blistering of the skin and the endorphins block pain. Physicists may not be so far off the mark after all. Being a neuroscientist, I am biased to look for neurological solutions. The physicist, with a different set of educational tools, looks elsewhere. As it is often said, "If a man's only tool is a hammer, everything starts to look like a nail." Biophysics and endocrinology are two disciplines intricately interwoven with neuroscience.

There are limitations of the extent to which the brain can modify reflex activity. Consider the childhood game, "Dizzy-Izzy." Here is an activity even the bravest fire walker would not dare attempt. The game consists of running 25 yards or so to a designated spot. The participant then runs in a circle with his head placed down on an upright bat for 20 revolutions. Once the self-imposed dizziness is sufficient, the astronaut-in-training tries to find his way back to the starting line. No amount of conscious effort can keep the individual upright for the return voyage. In fact, many mothers' carefully prepared lunches are likely to find themselves unceremoniously making a reappearance during this game. Some behaviors can be controlled by the brain, and others cannot.

The point with the above anecdotes is to illustrate that there is more to motor control than the command "go" from the cerebral cortex to spinal motor neurons. There are times when conscious intervention is needed and times when it is just a hindrance. There are times when movement is purely a reflex and other times when conscious control can alter reflex activity. A multitude of neural pathways originating from the cerebral cortex, brain stem, cerebellum, inner ear, visual system, spinal cord, and the muscles themselves have vital roles to play during movement. Those roles often depend on the context in which the movement is to occur. It is also becoming increasingly evident that initial body position, motivation, knowledge of desired motor output, the type of afferent stimuli involved in the movement, and biomechanical constraints all contribute to the response. But before any of this can begin to make sense, you must understand the functions of the various components of the nervous system.

The remainder of this chapter will discuss, in brief, the major components contributing to motor control. Discussion will begin with the muscles and their receptors and progress to the cerebral cortex. Just as knowing the individual characteristics and abilities of every player on a team contributes to a coach's winning season, knowledge of the components of the nervous system and their interactions will contribute to an understanding of how humans put it together to move with grace and efficiency.

■ MUSCLE

All humans, regardless whether they are couch potatoes or elite athletes, depend on muscles for their own particular styles and methods of movement. Muscle, an engineering and molecular biological marvel,

Motor unit

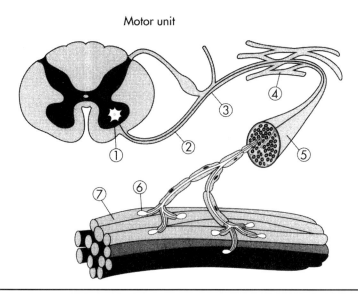

Fig. 2-2. The motor unit consists of an alpha motor neuron and all muscle fibers that it innervates. *1*, Anterior horn cell; *2*, nerve root; *3*, spinal nerve; *4*, plexus; *5*, peripheral nerve, *6*, neuromuscular junction; *7*, muscle fiber. (From Dumitru D. Electrodiagnostic medicine. Philadelphia: Hanley & Belfus, 1995.)

converts chemical energy into mechanical work far more efficiently than anything yet designed by man. The degree to which an individual can master, organize, and isolate muscular contraction into efficient patterns of movement determines, for the most part, the level of physical skill and grace that can be achieved. The classic anatomy text, *Gray's Anatomy*,[21] lists more than 326 muscles for the human animal—and this listing doesn't include smooth muscles that line blood vessels and the intestinal tract, cardiac muscles, or individual multipennate muscles. Each muscle, in turn, is composed of hundreds to thousands of muscle fibers. A muscle fiber is a single cylindrical cell.

Skeletal muscles are muscles that we can control voluntarily. Every muscle fiber, or muscle cell, receives its own innervation from a spinal cord motor neuron. Neurons that innervate skeletal muscle (also called striated or voluntary muscle) are called *alpha motor neurons*. Because the axons from their nerve fibers branch, one neuron might innervate several muscle fibers (also termed *extrafusal fibers*). The alpha motor neuron and the muscle fibers it innervates are collectively referred to as a *motor unit* (Fig. 2-2). Each muscle is typically composed of multiple motor units. The ratio of nerve fibers to muscle fibers varies with the degree of movement precision that is required. Eye movement, which needs to be very precise and finely tuned, is controlled by extraocular muscles that have a nerve-to-muscle fiber ratio ranging from 1:10 to 1:50. That is, one motor axon innervates from ten to fifty muscle fibers. The ratio for the laryngeal muscles (partially responsible for talking, swallowing, and spitting) is slightly larger. The hand is in the 1:100 range and in the large muscles of the leg, one motor nerve fiber might innervate from 200 to 2,000 muscle fibers.

All movement requires muscle contraction. Different movements, however, require varying amounts of contractile force. Somehow, humans have evolved into having the ability to lift considerable weight, without sacrificing the ability to contract muscles in a very controlled and precise manner, so as to perform dexterous tasks such as typing, microscopic surgery, playing a musical instrument, and threading a needle.

These different motor skills require vastly different degrees of control and muscle contractile force. The amount of force that can be generated by a muscle depends on the number of motor units recruited, the type of muscle fibers involved, and the firing rate of motor neurons. The gradation of force by varying the number of active motor units is referred to as *motor unit recruitment*. Although some exceptions appear to exist that depend on the type of muscle and type of muscle contraction (i.e., concentric, eccentric, isometric), most motor units are recruited in a predictable sequence. Recruitment often, but not always, follows the *size principle*: alpha motor neurons with the smallest cell bodies (they innervate slow, fatigue-resistant muscle fibers) generally have the lowest threshold for synaptic activation and are therefore recruited first, followed by recruitment of larger alpha motor neurons (they innervate fast, fatiguable muscle fibers capable of more force generation). As more force is required for a task, more motor units are recruited.

A second method by which muscles can vary force production is *rate modulation*. A motor neuron can vary the number of action potentials it sends to the neuromuscular junction. The higher the action potential firing rate, the greater the force production.

How the nervous system knows how hard to contract a muscle remains a bit of a mystery, but the discovery of tiny sensory receptors embedded within each muscle or muscular tendon has shed some light on the issue. Within each muscle fiber are receptors called *muscle spindles*. Spindles are special sensors that respond to the stretch of a muscle. Another specialized receptor is the *Golgi tendon organ (GTO)*. GTOs are specialized receptor organs located primarily in the musculotendinous junction. GTOs provide information regarding the amount of force, or tension, being generated within the muscle. The functioning of these peripheral receptors is absolutely essential to the control of muscle contraction. GTOs will be discussed later in this chapter. Our present discussion will focus on muscle spindle functioning.

■ MUSCLE SPINDLES

Spindles provide information to the nervous system regarding the absolute length of the muscle and the rate of change of the length (velocity) of the muscle. An example of their function can be illustrated by considering that dreaded of all stretching exercises: the hamstring stretch. Athletes of all types, but especially those involved in sports that require explosive power such as football, volleyball, and sprinting, are aware of the importance of stretching the hamstrings. If you have tight hamstrings and attempt to extend the leg quickly, as in a jump or sprint, you have a very good chance of experiencing a painful and debilitating injury known as a hamstring pull. For this reason, most athletes work on stretching and increasing hamstring flexibility. If you are lying on your back and someone tries to raise your extended leg quickly, you will notice your leg reflexively counters the movement. The quick, passive movement of your leg causes a stretch of the hamstrings, which elicits a stretch reflex. The result is a contraction of the hamstrings. This is the muscle spindle, or more specifically the *primary spindle afferents* or *spindle Ia afferents*, at work detecting the rate of change of the muscle's length. Obviously, to have the muscle you are trying to stretch contract during the stretching is counterproductive. This is why it is thought that all stretches should be done slowly. A slow stretch is likely to diminish the influence of one type of muscle spindle sensory afferent and allows for greater movement and flexibility of the leg. Notice that a quick stretch primarily engages only one type of spindle sensory fiber, the large-diameter and rapidly conducting Ia afferent.

Muscle spindles are composed of intrafusal fibers, sensory endings, and motor axons. Each spindle contains several muscle fibers and sensory endings and is innervated by specialized motor neurons. The specialized motor neurons are often referred to as *fusimotor neurons*. Presently, three types of intrafusal muscle fibers have been identified: *nuclear bag1*, *nuclear bag2*, and *nuclear chain*. Other nomenclature refers to these intrafusal fibers as dynamic nuclear bag, static nuclear bag, and nuclear chain.

Two types of sensory afferent endings convey muscle spindle information: a primary ending and a secondary ending. The primary ending is connected to a large-diameter Ia afferent axon. The secondary ending connects with a smaller diameter group II afferent axon. The larger the diameter of a nerve fiber, the more rapidly it conducts action potentials. Thus, Ia afferents are fast conducting, whereas group II afferents are relatively slower.

Primary afferent endings are particularly responsive to the rate of change in muscle length and are, therefore, velocity sensitive. They respond very quickly to changes in stretch and must be equally sensitive in shortened positions as well as in lengthened positions of the muscle. They tend to increase the rate of their firing at the beginning of a muscle stretch. Because the body needs to be informed quickly about dynamic changes in muscle length, primary ending information needs to be conveyed by a fast afferent system. Group I afferents, the largest and therefore the quickest sensory afferents, convey nuclear bag fiber spindle information back to the spinal cord.

Static nuclear bag2 and nuclear chain fibers are responsible for detecting the absolute length of a muscle. Sensory information from these fibers is conveyed by group II afferents, which are slightly slower than the larger group I afferents. Because Ia afferents also have primary endings on these fibers, the Ia afferent provides information not only about velocity, but also contributes to position sense or absolute muscle length (Fig. 2-3).

One of the most interesting attributes of muscle spindles, and a property that puts them in a very select group of peripheral receptors, is the fact that they receive neural input from the central nervous system (CNS). The sensitivity of spindles is under central control and is therefore modifiable. The neural input comes from fusimotor neurons located in the spinal cord. The main function of fusimotor neurons is to control the sensitivity of spindle afferents to dynamic stretches. Fusimotor efferents are mostly small gamma motor neurons. These innervate intrafusal muscle fibers exclusively. Some fusimotor neurons (beta motor neurons) innervate both extrafusal and intrafusal muscle fibers. Functionally, fusimotor efferents (both gamma and beta) are classified as either dynamic efferents or static efferents.

Dynamic fusimotor neurons control only primary (Ia) afferents and strongly sensitize them to dynamic stretch. *Static fusimotor neurons* act on both primary and secondary afferents (Fig. 2-3). They regulate background Ia discharge, reducing the sensitivity of the primary afferents to dynamic stretch, and they stabilize secondary afferents.

You, no doubt, are a bit puzzled by all this. You are not alone. The physiology of the muscle spindle is an ongoing story. It is a complex area of study and the references and suggested readings listed at the end of the chapter provide a more detailed analysis.

The spindle sends its messages to the spinal cord, cerebellum, reticular activating system in the brain stem, and the motor cortex. Spindle functioning is essential for our awareness of limb position (*proprioception*) because the degree to which a muscle is stretched indicates angular joint changes. Spindles not only detect movement, but they also contribute to the presetting and regulation of muscle stiffness (tone).

Tone is determined by the level of excitability of the pool of motor neurons controlling a muscle, the intrinsic stiffness (spring-like qualities) of extrafusal muscle fibers, and the level of sensitivity of the reflexes. Tone is assessed clinically by determining the degree to which a muscle resists being lengthened. Tone can be divided into a velocity-dependent (dynamic) and a length-dependent (static) component.

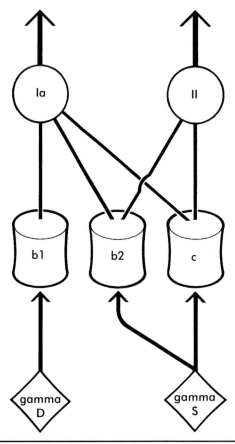

Fig. 2-3. The relationship between fusimotor drive from gamma motor neurons to muscle spindles and the afferents conveying the information from the spindles. Ia primary afferents convey information to the CNS from all three types of muscle spindles. Secondary afferents convey information from bag2 and nuclear chain spindles. *gamma D*, dynamic motor neuron; *gamma S*, static motor neuron; *b1*, nuclear bag1 muscle spindle; *b2*, nuclear bag2 muscle spindle; *C*, nuclear chain muscle spindle; *Ia*, primary afferent; *II*, secondary afferent. (Concept for diagram courtesy of Dr. Manuel Hulliger.)

Increased static tone is characterized by abnormal tonic activation of motor neurons. Increased dynamic tone manifests itself in exaggerated dynamic stretch reflexes.[37] It is important to realize that "tone" is a clinical concept. For several reasons, the clinical assessment of tone is less precise than desirable. First, alterations in tone are ascribed to altered motor neuron excitability or reflex sensitivity, but it is assessed by observing a mechanical property of muscle (i.e., resistance to stretch). Secondly, increased reflex responses may be due to increased motor neuron excitability (increased sensitivity to synaptic inputs) or to exaggerated fusimotor drive. Common clinical testing procedures do not allow for the determination of these important distinctions. Thirdly, tone can be altered in pathological conditions. A number of changes in neural properties can contribute to this alteration in tone, yet current clinical testing procedures do not lend themselves to these types of determinations. Lastly, there is nothing to suggest that abnormalities in muscle tone after CNS injury or disease are restricted solely to exaggerated stretch reflex pathways. Other reflex pathways might be equally affected, yet are not typically assessed clinically.

A certain amount of tone is needed even for the most sedentary of activities. For instance, it is muscle tone that allows you to maintain a sitting or semireclined position as you read this book. Some activities require considerable increases in tone. The tone required in the legs and trunk while walking over an icy street is considerably different from that required of the same individual during a choreographed dance routine. An individual walking across an icy street needs to be prepared for a slip and sudden unexpected loss of balance occurring at any time. For this reason, muscle spindles hypothetically should be in a state of heightened awareness to detect quickly stretches coming from any direction. Input from dynamic fusimotor neurons would have to be increased so that the spindles would be sensitive to the smallest change in muscle length. According to this view, spindle activity would increase and thus increase muscle tone.

In contrast to this scenario, it can be proposed that a dance routine requires presetting tone to a different degree. A choreographed dance routine has required hundreds of hours of practice devoted to specific movements. Elongation is a key concept for dancers. Typically, they want to achieve the appearance of maximal muscle length. To achieve maximal leg extension, for instance, the dancer will want minimum resistance from the hamstrings. The tone, therefore, will be set higher in the quadriceps than in the hamstrings. Spindle sensitivity and tone in the hamstrings should be lessened. These changes reflect motor learning. Although direct testing of this concept remains to be done, the fusimotor system actually seems to learn to anticipate the most advantageous muscle tone required for each movement. *Alpha-gamma coactivation*, *servo-assistance theory*, and *fusimotor set* are terms and theories related to the fusimotor system's situationally appropriate presetting of spindle sensitivity and muscle tone and its coordination of these parameters with voluntary activation of extrafusal muscle fibers. The contribution of spindles to muscle tone and proprioception are not their only functions.[29,54] Even though spindles have been studied extensively since the 1800s, scientists are still discovering new aspects of these intriguing organs and still argue about their exact function.

Of importance for motor control, spindles also have an important role to play in coordinating and smoothing out muscle contraction. For instance, as you reach across a table to pick up a glass of liquid refreshment, one set of muscles contracts so that you can perform the reaching movement. Just as importantly, any muscles that would oppose the movement (*antagonist muscles*) will relax. This allows for smooth movement. Changes in muscle spindle activity are likely to contribute to your ability to do this. At any moment in time, the nervous system and brain are being bombarded by information. Input needs to be prioritized. Depending on the situation and the desired task, certain sensory information is more important than others. At times, information can actually be contradictory in nature. If the divergent messages are not integrated properly, the resulting movement will be less than efficient. Fusimotor neurons that control the spindles appear well positioned to integrate the various signals coming from the brain, brain stem, and other peripheral sensory receptors to provide the necessary and situationally appropriate muscle tone for the movement desired. This provides considerable contribution to the attainment of smooth movement and motor control (Fig. 2-4).

Spindles provide ongoing feedback to the nervous system about the changing conditions of muscle length. They probably help to correct movement and ensure that the movement is appropriate for the desired task. Without muscle spindles, movement would be ataxic and lacking in an ability to compensate appropriately for disturbances. Spindles also contribute to optimization of motor skills in other ways.

For a moment, think about shopping during the holidays. Let's say you need to go to your local mall on Christmas Eve. Human nature being what it is, you are not alone and are forced to park about 2 miles away. Several hours later, you return to the parking lot with your arms loaded with packages. At some

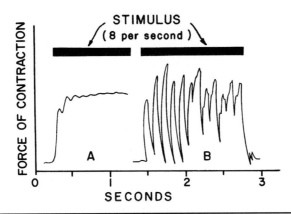

Fig. 2-4. The effect of muscle spindles on smoothing muscle contraction force. Graph A shows a normally innervated muscle. Graph B shows a muscle that has been denervated of muscle spindle input. (From Guyton AC. Textbook of medical physiology. Philadelphia: WB Saunders Co., 1981.)

point during the trek across the parking lot, your arm muscles will fatigue and the packages' load will begin to be greater than your biceps' ability to continue to hold their weight. Unable to maintain elbow flexion, the biceps muscle will begin to stretch even though it is still maximally contracting. The stretching activates muscle spindles, which elicits a stretch reflex. The reflex activation will further excite the skeletal muscle and cause it to increase the force of its contraction. In this way, the muscle spindle, independent of input from the brain, might compensate somewhat for muscle fatigue by eliciting a reflex stimulus to create a stronger contraction. This type of reflex compensation has a limit. Motivation also plays a role and the brain becomes increasingly involved. "The wall" is not just a marathon runner's phenomenon. Now, consider yourself as an overly laden, fatigued shopper trekking across an *icy* parking lot... You get the picture. Spindles are wondrously complex structures whose demur size (about 5 mm) belie their monstrous duties. We have many more millimeters to cover before we can begin to understand the magic of these receptors and that of the human nervous system.

At this point you may be wondering if it is possible consciously to control fusimotor drive and the stretch reflex. For a long time, conventional scientific thought was that the regulation of spindle sensitivity was not under conscious control. However, it now appears that this is not true. It appears that humans can regulate the sensitivity of the stretch reflex.

In a series of elegant and labor-intensive studies, Dr. Jonathan Wolpaw, a neurologist from Albany, N.Y., and his colleagues have proven that monkeys have the ability, via conditioning and electromyographic biofeedback, to alter the gain of the stretch reflex.[12,63] Dr. Wolpaw hypothesized that if monkeys were given the correct incentive, they could be trained either to increase or to decrease the excitability of motor neurons. He was right. Monkeys, using biofeedback, learned to increase or decrease motor neuron excitability to receive a food reward.[62] Their studies have progressed to identifying pre- and postsynaptic membrane changes associated with this type of learning. It appears that motor learning involves *plasticity* (changes or conformability) of neural connections, neural membranes, and transmitter storage and release throughout the nervous system.[11]

Humans have a considerable advantage over the monkey. Alpha and gamma motor neurons in humans receive more direct, and theoretically stronger, innervation from the cerebral cortex than other mammals, including the monkey. This difference implies that humans have evolved increased capabilities in regulating muscle contraction and postural tone than other less cerebral species. Indeed, Drs. Steven Wolf and Richard Segal from Emory University have demonstrated that humans have the ability consciously to alter stretch reflexes. Using electromyographic biofeedback, human volunteers learned, in a shorter amount of time than Dr. Wolpaw's monkeys, to regulate the stretch reflex.[16,58,61] The ability to control reflex activity might, in the future, play a role in rehabilitation of patients with CNS injury.

The cerebral cortex appears to be vitally important to spindle and muscle functioning. After a stroke, the involved muscle becomes *paretic* (partially paralyzed). Fast-twitch motor units are lost and motor unit recruitment is compromised (i.e., disruption of motor unit rate modulation). These findings cannot solely be attributed to disuse and appear to reflect the importance of higher centers, such as the cerebral cortex, in the modulation of muscle activity.

Human use of the stretch reflex has already made it out of the laboratory. A training technique has been developed that uses quick muscle stretch to increase force output. *Plyometrics* is a sports training technique that emphasizes quick stretch to a muscle before initiating a voluntary contraction. Preliminary studies have shown that strength gains occur faster with this technique than with other more traditional exercise methods. The technique hypothetically involves the stretch reflex and, in all probability, takes advantage of certain biomechanical muscle and tendon tissue properties. This technique has actually been adapted from a procedure physical therapists have used for quite some time for the treatment of patients with various neurological disorders. Physical therapists often use a quick stretch to a paretic muscle to increase the force of a voluntary contraction.

The nervous system's ability to modulate fusimotor drive and spindle activity depends on receiving afferent feedback from the spindle and other peripheral receptors. Without appropriate feedback, the regulation of muscle force is disrupted and compensatory mechanisms designed to lessen the effects of muscle fatigue are compromised.[18,42]

These results give hope to athletes, therapists, and patients that additional control can be gained over various parameters of muscle contraction. If, as it now appears, muscle spindles preset the background activity of muscle tone in preparation for a movement, and if we can somehow gain increased conscious control over this process, then we have given ourselves an edge in that we can change the gain of muscular stretch reflexes depending on situational demands. Patients with *spasticity* (a neurological condition that results in increased tone, such as from stroke, cerebral palsy, or spinal cord injury) might be able to alter alpha motor neuron and fusimotor neuron activity, thereby lessening the effects of movement-impairing spasticity.

As more becomes known about the projections from other portions of the nervous system onto motor neurons, an intriguing story is emerging that sheds light as to why some of us move with grace and others lack any semblance of coordination; why emotion has such a direct influence on athletic performance; and why certain techniques hold great promise for enhancing rehabilitation efforts.

Muscle spindles are only one type of receptor that provides information necessary for movement. Control of posture and movement requires monitoring not only of muscle length, but also of muscle tension.

■ GOLGI TENDON ORGANS AND IB AFFERENTS

As mentioned earlier in this chapter, GTOs respond to muscle tension. The source of the tension can either be a stretch to the muscle or muscle tension generated by muscle contraction. A single GTO has many muscle fibers from different motor units associated with it, typically 10 to 15. Within a given motor unit only one muscle fiber acts on the GTO (Fig. 2-5). A single GTO, therefore, receives one muscle fiber from 10 to 15 different motor units. GTOs, therefore, appear to monitor whole muscle tension (or more specif-

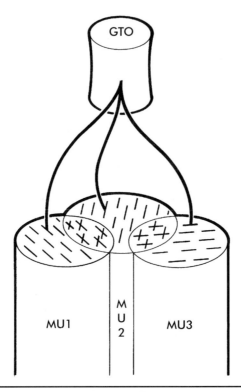

Fig. 2-5. A single GTO detects changes in muscle tension from several motor units (*MUs*). A GTO will only monitor changes of a single fiber from each MU. (Concept for diagram courtesy of Dr. Manuel Hulliger.)

ically, a fraction of whole muscle tension) rather than individual muscle fiber tension.[30] It appears that the CNS probably relies on aggregate information provided by an ensemble of GTOs from each muscle to extract information about whole muscle force.

GTOs have a low threshold (i.e., they tend to respond to small changes) to contraction-induced changes in muscle tension, and a higher threshold to stretch-induced tension. In fact, muscle stretch does not always activate GTOs, whereas muscle contraction will always activate these receptors. Some researchers have reported that GTOs are more sensitive to *concentric* (shortening) contractions than they are to *eccentric* (lengthening) contractions or passive lengthening. Others have reported increased GTO activity during eccentric contractions.[29] Fusimotor drive has been reported to be increased over resting levels during both concentric and eccentric muscle actions.[9] The sensory information detected by the GTO receptor is conveyed via *Group Ib* sensory afferents.

Group Ib afferents from GTOs mediate *nonreciprocal inhibition*. Nonreciprocal inhibition, also termed *autogenic inhibition*, refers to inhibitory input to an *agonist muscle* (i.e., the prime mover) and its synergists concomitant with an excitatory input to opposing (antagonist) muscles (Fig. 2-6). The inhibition of agonist motor neuron pools and the excitation of antagonist motor neurons is accomplished by Ib interneurons. GTOs are activated by muscle tension. This tension signal is conveyed by Ib afferents to Ib interneurons, which in turn synapse on agonist and antagonist alpha motor neurons to cause either inhibition or excitation. Ib interneurons can be either facilitatory or inhibitory. Therefore, GTO activation

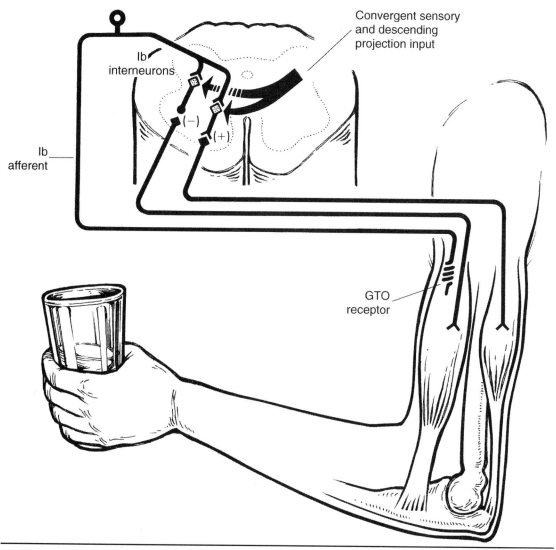

Fig. 2-6. Nonreciprocal (autogenic) inhibition. GTO receptors detect changes in muscle force. Ib afferent fibers convey this information to Ib interneurons that inhibit the contracting muscle and excite its antagonists.

results in many other responses in addition to nonreciprocal inhibition. Inhibition of an agonist muscle during tension development was one of the first functions attributed to GTOs and their Ib afferents and led to some false assumptions.

It was once thought that GTOs were responsible for a reflex that protected the contracting or lengthening muscle from generating tensions that exceeded the muscle's mechanical capabilities. Once tension reached a threatening level, GTOs were thought to initiate neural inhibition to the muscle to prevent injury. The *clasp-knife reflex* was also attributed to GTO functioning. This abnormal reflex is seen in some patients with spasticity and is generally a sign of damage to the corticospinal tract. The clasp-knife reflex

TABLE 2-1	Classification of the sensory receptors	
Afferent	**Receptor**	**Conduction velocity (msec)**
Ia	Muscle spindle primary endings	70-120
Ib	Golgi tendon organs	70-120
II	Encapsulated endings: spindle secondary endings, Meissner, Merkel receptors	30-70
III	Hair, visceral, cold, and pain receptors	5-30
IV	Primarily nociceptors (pain), postganglionic autonomic efferents, visceral and mechano-receptors	0.5-2

Adapted from Nolte J. The human brain, 3rd ed. St. Louis: Mosby-Year Book, 1993.

manifests by muscle resistance to passive stretch that suddenly gives way, similar to the blade of a jack-knife. Given the role of GTOs and Ib afferents in monitoring muscle tension and their ability to inhibit an agonist's muscle alpha motor neuron pool, it is easy to understand why scientists and clinicians hypothesized that they caused muscle relaxation and unloading in response to excess tension development. It now appears, however, that free nerve endings, mainly small-diameter group III and IV afferents, are more involved than GTOs in protective responses to elicit unloading of muscle tension. This is not to say that GTOs are not involved. In fact, the rich convergent input that Ib interneurons receive from supraspinal and multisensorial peripheral afferent pathways in addition to GTO input suggests that GTOs and Ib afferents contribute to a wide array of reflexive and nonreflexive sensorimotor behaviors in addition to non-reciprocal inhibition.

Ib interneurons receive afferent input from Ia afferents (spindle afferents), Ib afferents from different muscles, cutaneous and joint afferents, and group III and IV afferents. Table 2-1 lists sensory receptor types and associated afferent fiber types. This afferent input is not limited to homonymous motor neurons or afferents from a single joint. Multisensorial input from the entire limb impacts the Ib pathway. Ib interneurons receive supraspinal input from the rubrospinal, vestibulospinal, and corticospinal tracts as well as from cerebellar nuclei (fastigial), the anterior cerebellar cortex, and various brain stem areas. Input from supraspinal centers probably modulates activity of the Ib pathway and encodes muscle forces that are situationally appropriate. Lending support to this idea is the fact that Ib afferents project not only to spinal interneurons to mediate reflexive regulation of muscle force, but also to cells of spinocerebellar tract origin. The information conveyed in this pathway, and others, ultimately arrives at the cerebral cortex and probably contributes to conscious perception of muscle tension.

Consider the following potentially unfortunate personal incident as an example of a motor behavior possibly controlled by GTOs and Ib afferents. The other day I reached across my desk to pick up a glass that I distinctly remembered as being filled to the brim. In my absent-mindedness, or optimism, I had forgotten it was only half full and, therefore, it was considerably lighter than I expected. My brain was encoding a message to my muscles that I needed to exert a strong pincer grasp and a sizable force in my elbow flexors to lift the glass. Muscle receptors, among them the GTOs and spindles, were saying, "Hey, this ain't so heavy—lighten up!" The force that was generated in the elbow flexors exceeded that required for the task. One can presume that GTO activity responded to this discrepancy by eliciting a reflexive response that inhibited the elbow flexors to a more appropriate level. The spindles within the antagonist elbow extensors, in all probability, also contributed to the response by informing the CNS that an unexpected quick stretch was occurring because of the unopposed contraction of the elbow flexors. If it were not for the quick response of GTO and muscle spindles, I would have continued to exert a force that was greater than necessary and ended up with the glass in my face and the drink in my lap.

Although the theory has not yet been tested directly, GTOs and spindles must be active during tasks such as a reach and grasp. Some very interesting studies have examined reach and grasp tasks. Reaching and grasping form an upper extremity synergy that appears to be a learned task.[17,20] With experience we actually begin to establish a grip force that is appropriate to the size and perceived weight of the object to be lifted before we ever complete the reaching part of the task. This learning has to involve presetting of muscle receptors.

Muscle contraction involves a series of options that must be decided on by the CNS. These include which muscles to activate for any given situation, which type and quantity of motor unit(s) to activate, and the duration of motor unit activity and muscle contraction. GTOs are actively engaged in these processes. These receptors, however, must act in concert with other receptors to monitor and control motor output. For instance, Ib and Ia afferents converge onto some of the same interneurons. There is also a close relationship, with some apparent exceptions such as the hands, between the number of spindles and GTOs within any given muscle. These findings indicate that muscle length and force are not controlled as separate entities. Rather, parallel signal processing and feedback of Ia and Ib afferents must be occurring, as well as parallel processing of other sensory afferents, similar to that necessary for proprioception. Part of the role of supraspinal input onto Ib interneurons might be to filter incoming stimuli to allow one type of receptor to increase or decrease its input onto the interneuronal milieu depending on situational demands such as muscle fatigue.[10,25,42,44,53,57] Many statements regarding GTOs are conjectural because their exact function is not yet known. For technical reasons, studying GTO function is very difficult. Many misconceptions remain, but as new techniques are developed, neuroscientists continue to decipher their complexity. We now know that GTOs are more numerous in antigravity muscles (the extensor muscles of the legs, back, and neck). These muscles, especially the more proximal ones, also receive a rich input from vestibular nuclei. Perhaps, therefore, GTOs monitor muscle tension in relation to gravity and combine with vestibular input to orient the position of the body and head in space. One caveat to bear in mind, however, is that GTOs have been most extensively studied in the hindlimbs of cats. This might pose a problem because the antigravity muscles of a cat (a quadruped) are different from the antigravity muscles of humans (bipeds). Neuroscientists and other scientists actively engaged in motor control research are increasingly finding that CNS functioning is species specific.

In summary, data are compatible with the view that GTO receptors provide input to the spinal cord for reflexive regulation of motor output, especially of parameters associated with muscle force. GTO input is also transmitted to supraspinal centers, where it is presumably used for intentional force adjustments. GTOs appear to contribute to the modulation and smoothing out of muscle contraction. Rather than controlling individual muscle fibers, GTOs and the integration of their input with other sensory afferents provide for tuning of forces among different muscles within a limb to fit the requirements of the movement. GTO discharge does not increase linearly with force. If GTO force feedback inhibition increased proportionally with force, we would experience greater difficulty in motor unit recruitment with increasing effort (i.e., with increasing force of contraction would come more nonreciprocal inhibition via Ib afferents, therefore making activation of more motor units difficult as more force is required to lift a certain load). The relationship between motor unit or whole muscle contractile forces and GTO receptor discharge rate during human movement has not yet been determined. Some other GTO-related questions or mysteries for you to ponder: Do Ib afferents influence gamma motor neurons, and therefore spindle sensitivity, because they converge with Ia afferents onto some of the same interneurons? If GTOs monitor force, why is there a paucity of receptors in hand and jaw muscles, where the precise control of muscle force is essential to function? For every question that is being answered regarding GTO receptor functioning, three more take its place. Come to think of it, the same could be said for every structure associated with the human nervous system. Are you beginning to see why its study is so addictive?

■ THE SPINAL CORD

Muscles and muscle receptors are often considered the machinery of movement. Let's now examine how we control this machine. The spinal cord can be considered a highway through which signals from the brain and from the peripheral receptors travel. It is not, however, merely a thruway. The spinal cord, independent of input from higher brain centers, contains all the necessary circuitry for reflex reactions and rhythmic patterns of movement. And, as research has elucidated, it may contain circuitry for even complex activities such as walking and running.

The spinal cord and brain stem are the only places that house motor neurons that innervate muscles. The spinal cord also contains efferents of the autonomic nervous system. The spinal cord receives multisensorial input from every part of the body. The processing of sensory input begins in the spinal cord and brain stem. This processing is poorly understood and involves linear signal summation and nonlinear mechanisms such as gating and modulation of transmission along certain pathways. These mechanisms are sometimes loosely defined as *integration*. This sensorimotor integration is essential for coordinated movement. The spinal cord maintains considerable autonomous control in changing motor output based on the afferent input it receives at any given moment. In addition to integrating peripheral sensory input, it must also convey this sensory input to higher centers such as the cerebellum, brain stem, and cerebral cortex for further integration. In turn, it conveys messages from these centers to the spinal cord circuitry. The spinal cord does so via relatively simple physiological mechanisms. Its exquisite complexity and control, which is manifest by our broad movement repertoire, are derived by its apparent infinite connectivity, the plasticity of these connections, and its ability to cause immediate changes in function to match situational demands.

The grey and white matter of the spinal cord are topographically organized. The gray matter contains mainly cell bodies and the white matter contains axons that form the ascending and descending tract systems. Cells within the gray matter are organized, with specific cells located in fairly well-defined areas (Fig. 2-7).

Tract systems are also organized (Fig. 2-8). For instance, the corticospinal tract occupies a specific location in the lateral funiculus of the spinal cord white matter, whereas the spinothalamic tract occupies a more ventral zone (Fig. 2-8). Although most tracts form fairly distinct bundles, considerable overlap exists. Within each tract, laminations form such that arm representation is located separate from trunk and leg regions. This is referred to as *somatotopic* organization. This organization will not be detailed in this chapter; for more detail, consult a basic neuroanatomy text such as ones listed at the end of the chapter. The topographic organization within the spinal cord is not a trivial matter, especially for those interested in clinical work or neuropathology. The location of damage to the spinal cord dictates the signs, symptoms, and disability that result. The remainder of this section will describe briefly the types of cells located in the spinal cord and their function. Knowledge of the spinal cord cellular makeup is a necessary first step toward understanding its circuitry and functions.

The grey matter of the spinal cord can be divided into a dorsal horn, an intermediate zone, and a ventral horn. Each of these sections are further subdivided into laminae numbered I-X (see Fig. 2-7). Within the dorsal horn are interneurons and neurons of origin for some ascending sensory tracts. The intermediate zone is the black hole of the spinal cord, comprising an infinite array of known and (almost certainly) as yet undiscovered interneurons. The ventral horn contains primarily motor neurons.

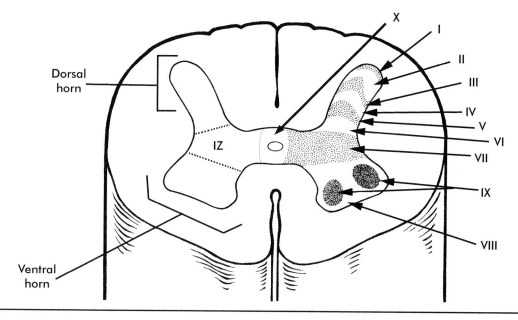

Fig. 2-7. Spinal cord gray matter contains cells, and the white matter contains the ascending and descending tract systems. Specific cell types are located in specific gray matter areas (Laminae I-X). Sensory neurons are mainly located in the dorsal horns, motor neurons are in the ventral horn, and interneurons are within the intermediate zone (*IZ*).

The role of the spinal cord in motor control can be reduced to three primary functions:
1. Sensory processing and integration,
2. Motor output (segmental reflexes and circuitry subserving rhythmic activity), and
3. Autonomic output.

Sensory processing begins with the entry of afferent fibers, primarily via the dorsal root, into the dorsal horn (see Fig. 1-3). These afferent fibers convey a multitude of information from peripheral receptors. Spindles and GTOs have been discussed previously, and many other receptors that convey information regarding touch, pressure, heat, cold, and noxious stimuli also send their messages into the dorsal horn. Once entering the dorsal horn, sensory afferents bifurcate and branch so that a single receptor might impact hundreds of neurons. Most of the neurons in the dorsal horn are interneurons. Sensory processing begins with these interneurons because each interneuron might receive sensory input from a multitude of receptors. These interneurons then send projections to other neurons within the spinal cord, and/or their axons form ascending sensory pathways that will synapse in higher brain centers (e.g., spinocerebellar, spinothalamic, and so forth). Other sensory afferent branches, specifically those of Ia afferents, bypass neurons within the dorsal horn and synapse directly on motor neurons within the ventral horn to form monosynaptic reflex arcs (e.g., the stretch reflex; see Fig. 2-1). Spinal cord neurons and sensory afferents within the spinal cord receive direct or indirect input from descending supraspinal centers. This descending input modulates neural receptivity to sensory input or affects neurotransmitter release from sensory terminals. Some sensory afferents also synapse *presynaptically* (see Chapter 3) on other sensory afferents and affect neurotransmitter release. Thus, sensory afferent input, interneuronal activity, and supraspinal input from the brain stem and cerebral cortex modulate sensory processing and ultimately our perception of our environment.

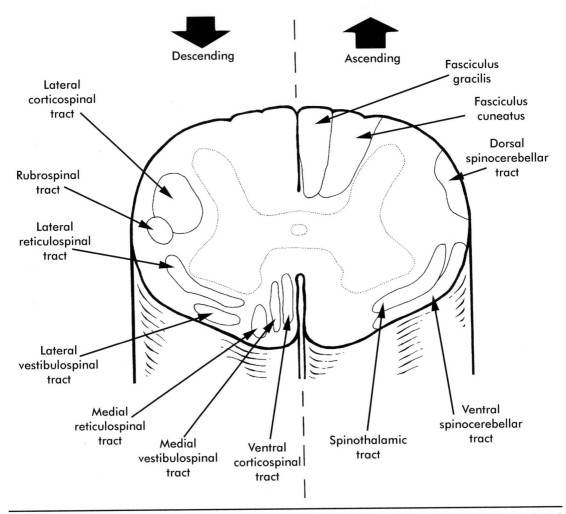

Fig. 2-8. The approximate location of spinal tracts. For illustrative purposes, descending tracts are on the left, and ascending tracts are on the right. In reality, ascending and descending tracts are on both sides of the spinal cord and there is some overlap of tract systems.

Motor output includes segmental reflex reactions, generation of rhythmic activity, and volitional movement. The motor neurons that control muscle contraction are located in the ventral horn of the spinal cord. Alpha motor neurons innervate extrafusal (voluntary) muscle fibers and smaller gamma motor neurons innervate intrafusal fibers (muscle spindle fibers). *Beta motor neurons*, first discovered in amphibians, innervate both extrafusal and intrafusal muscle fibers and are thought to exist in humans also. The axons from motor neurons exit the ventral horn of the spinal cord via the ventral root. From here they form a mixed peripheral nerve (containing motor efferents and sensory afferents) and continue to their target muscle. Motor neurons receive divergent input from sensory afferents, interneurons, and descending pathways. Some of these inputs are inhibitory and others are excitatory. Motor neurons process this input and use it to guide individual muscle contraction and synergistic coordination of muscle groups.

Spinal (segmental) reflexes are one type of motor output. *Reflexes* are defined as a highly automated motor response resulting from a specific sensory input. They can involve monosynaptic (e.g., stretch reflex) or polysynaptic (e.g., flexion withdrawal reflex; see Chapter 3) connections. As the circuitry subserving a given response increases in connective complexity and begins increasingly to involve other pathways, the motor behaviors elicited by activity in these pathways are no longer termed reflexive but rather are referred to as generating rhythmic activity or motor synergies. *Central pattern generator* is a term used to describe neural circuitry within the mammalian spinal cord or brain stem that mediates rhythmic activities such as breathing, chewing, scratching, and locomotion. Supraspinal and afferent inputs influence motor output regardless whether the output involves a simple monosynaptic reflex or complex interactions of several central pattern generators. This modulation of reflex circuitry can involve a number of different mechanisms acting alone or in concert. For instance, the stretch reflex, which involves only an Ia afferent and an alpha motor neuron, can be influenced in several ways.

The Ia afferents can be presynaptically inhibited by descending pathways or by other afferents. *Presynaptic inhibition* results in a decreased amount of neurotransmitter being released by the presynaptic terminal. *Presynaptic excitation*, via a somewhat different mechanism, increases the amount of neurotransmitter released at the presynaptic terminal. Increasing or decreasing presynaptic inhibition or excitation changes the amount of influence the sensory afferent has on the postsynaptic neuron (in this case the alpha motor neuron). The reactiveness of the stretch reflex can also be influenced by the excitability of the alpha motor neuron itself. Other sensory and interneuronal input that has converged on the alpha motor neuron might make it more or less receptive to incoming Ia afferent input. You should become familiar with temporal and spatial summation of inhibitory postsynaptic potentials and excitatory postsynaptic potentials (briefly presented in Chapter 3).

Reflexes, therefore, are not as stereotyped as you might think. A graphic example of the nonstereotyped nature of reflexes was revealed during experiments testing the stretch reflexes of human infants.[41,43] If the infant was content and happy, reflexes tended to be relatively *hypotonic* (i.e., diminished resistance to passive stretching). During breast-feeding this hypotonicity was pronounced. If this same infant became agitated, so did the stretch reflex. Tapping a tendon during this time resulted not only in a very brisk hypertonic response, but the response spread into neighboring muscles as well. The same afferent input resulted in a totally different motor response. Emotional status appears to have an affect on the way sensory information is gated. You have probably experienced a similar phenomenon. An unexpected light touch to your shoulder in a darkened room probably elicits a different response than this same touch in a social situation. In the former instance the light touch would elicit a startle reaction, whereas in the later instance the touch would probably cause you to turn your head in the direction of the stimulus.

Autonomic output is the third primary function associated with spinal cord function. The sympathetic, parasympathetic, and enteric nervous systems that comprise the autonomic system are primarily concerned with body homeostasis. Autonomic output might not typically be thought of by beginning students as having a direct impact on motor control. However, as illustrated in the previous paragraph, background emotional state and changes in systemic biochemistry can have a dramatic effect on motor behavior. Many preganglionic autonomic neurons are located in specific regions in the spinal cord intermediate zone. The clinician needs to be particularly aware of the autonomic nervous system because spinal cord injury can cause autonomic dysfunction that can affect cardiac function, thermoregulation, bladder function, digestion, and sexual function.

Sensory afferents, interneurons, and motor neurons interact within the spinal cord to form simple and complex circuits. Spinal reflexes are involved with more types of movement than you probably realize.

Spinal reflexes will be the subject of Chapter 3. The next major structure to be presented in this chapter is the brain stem.

■ THE BRAIN STEM

Most professors and students alike dread the teaching of the brain stem. The brain stem is the complex rostral extension of the spinal cord. Its complexity is matched only by its mystery. A number of factors combine to make this area difficult to examine. Its location, hidden under the folds of the cerebral cortex, can be likened to a python enveloped by dense jungle foliage. A multitude of diverse nuclei and neurotransmitters are contained within its borders. Furthermore, cranial nerves and their nuclei originate in the brain stem. Finally, contained within the brain stem are neural pathways ascending from the spinal cord and arriving from the cerebral cortex and cerebellum. Further increasing the complexity is the fact that a tremendous amount of species variation exists regarding the structure and function of the brain stem.

Brain stem structures are not only responsible for automatic postural responses, but also their input onto interneurons of spinal reflex pathways dramatically alters spinal cord functioning. Spinal cord reflexes can be conditioned or modified by descending input such that the reflex response to sensory stimulation is modified or even ignored. Brain stem projections may even be able to turn on and off various reflexes, depending on behavioral conditions. Because the cerebral cortex has direct projections to the brain stem, perhaps conscious activity can alter reflex behavior as well.

Nuclei and neural networks within the brain stem are responsible for nothing less than the control of such diverse functions as respiration, cardiovascular function, gastrointestinal function, eye movement, equilibrium responses, postural reactions, and a multitude of reflex reactions. Brain stem structures are intimately involved in locomotion, balance, visual tracking, head and eye orientation to auditory input, and many other movements. An animal with a transection through the rostral part of the brain stem will still walk in a near normal fashion. Unlike animals with spinal cord transections, who exhibit walking movements only when supported and placed on a moving treadmill, animals with a rostral brain stem transection retain equilibrium reactions and can walk overground. To the casual observer, there appears to be no deficit in locomotion—that is, until the animal encounters an obstacle such as a wall. The animal, upon encountering the wall, will butt its head against the wall and continue to walk. In other words, the animal retains all the necessary components to walk but walking has become a completely purposeless act. The brain stem appears to contain the basic motor repertoire for movement, or perhaps it is the driving force that activates central pattern generators within the spinal cord. The brain stem is incapable of attaching meaning to any motor act. Despite this serious limitation, the brain stem is essential to movement and the struggle to gain a handle on its complex nature is worthwhile. To decipher some of the complexity of the brain stem, we must consider some of its structures and nuclei individually. The wide array of the effects on movement by descending systems originating from the brain stem cannot be presented here adequately. For present purposes, only those functions dealing directly with movement will be discussed. Some of the specialized structures and nuclei contained within the brain stem worthy of special attention are the red nucleus of the midbrain, vestibular nuclei, the reticular formation, tectospinal tracts, mesencephalic/pontine locomotor regions, and cranial nerve nuclei.

The major anatomical components of the brain stem are the pons, medulla, and midbrain (see Fig. 1-2). Within each of these structures are nuclei. Some of these nuclei extend beyond a single anatomical component. One such nucleus that extends throughout most of the rostral-caudal extent of the brain stem is a diffusely organized grouping of neurons called the reticular formation.

The reticular formation

There's nothing like starting with one of the most complex and least understood structures of the brain stem. The reticular formation extends throughout the length of the brain stem. It is a mixed bag of interneurons and nerve fibers of diverse function and destination. The reticular formation receives input from widespread areas of the cerebral cortex, including the motor cortex. It also receives input from the spinal cord, collaterals of the spinothalamic tract (involved with pain), hypothalamus (concerned with emotions, motivation, and endocrine functions), limbic system (concerned with emotions and endocrine functions), vestibular nuclei (equilibrium), cerebellum (coordination), basal ganglia (initiation of movement), cutaneous receptors (sense of touch and pressure), and the superior colliculus (involved with eye movements).

The sensory input to the reticular formation is further characterized by a great deal of convergence and divergence. A single cell within the reticular formation may respond to a sensory stimulus applied just about anywhere on the body. Considering this vast convergence of seemingly dissimilar input, no wonder neuroscientists have yet to unravel everything about the reticular formation. Its varied and diffuse afferent input makes determining its specific functions difficult. Its efferent projections are no more enlightening. The reticular formation sends projections to the cerebellum, the spinal cord, the basal ganglia, the thalamus, and the cerebral cortex (most of which are indirect projections via the thalamus). Divergence of the system enables it to influence almost all parts of the nervous system.

Three functions of the reticular system are of particular relevance to movement: wakefulness, modification of sensory input, and motor control.

Wakefulness. The first function of the reticular system deals with keeping us bright and alert. Within the reticular formation is a grouping of cells called the *reticular activating system*. These cells project to the thalamus, which in turn project to widespread areas of the cerebral cortex. It is hypothesized that this pathway is responsible for keeping us awake and regulating sleep-wake cycles. Damage to this area of the brain stem results in coma. The reticular activating system appears to activate the cerebral cortex and enable us to focus our attention.

Fighting off sleep while at work or while driving is an example of the reticular activating system at work. Consider the scenario of driving cross-country. To make the most use of your precious vacation time in Montana, you have decided to drive until you drop. Sleep becomes the enemy. All that matters is your destination. Sleep is a powerful force and even though you are consciously aware of the likely severe consequences of falling asleep on the no-speed-limit Montana autobahns, sleep is a difficult force to overcome. The reticular activating system needs to come to your rescue. Positron emission tomography studies in humans have confirmed that the midbrain reticular formation is involved in arousal and vigilance.[35] You need to fire up the reticular activating system and slap the cortex awake. To mobilize the reticular cavalry, you apparently need stimulation or an attention-demanding task. The reticular activating system thrives on afferent input. So, to fight off sleep, pay attention and stimulate yourself. Change your visual focus periodically, pinch yourself, get some wind in your hair, turn on some music, and invent reaction-time tasks for yourself. Diversity and intensity are the keys. Similar approaches, but more intense in their application, are being applied in some medical centers for the treatment of coma.

Modification of sensory afferent input to spinal cord motor neurons. In addition to the reticular formation's widespread projections to the cerebral cortex, it also projects to the spinal cord. As mentioned earlier, sensory input can trigger or modify a variety of spinal cord reflexes. The reticular formation further complicates matters by modifying sensory input. The reticular system gates sensory input and thereby modifies motor output. Its projections to the spinal cord, similar to vestibular projections, are mainly to interneurons and motor neurons of proximal musculature. This leads to the third function of the reticular system to be discussed.

Motor control. The last function of the reticular system I would like to discuss is its role in directing motor output. This role theoretically has implications for controlling the "big choke," a condition too often experienced by talented athletes during periods of high stress and anxiety. The reticular formation sends projections to motor neurons that control muscles and muscle spindles. This gives the reticular system considerable influence over the muscle tone of the extremities. Remember that the reticular system receives considerable input from the hypothalamus and the limbic system, structures responsible for emotions and their accompanying physiological changes. Ever wonder why it seemed that if you got "fired up" with emotion before a competition you could often exceed your normal level of performance? We have all seen how momentum in a game can affect athletes' performance. The opposite, unfortunately, can also happen. Nervousness and anxiety can destroy coordination and careers.

Perhaps you are the world's greatest basketball free-throw shooter when practicing in the privacy of your backyard court, but come game day, coliseum fright takes over and it is not unusual for you to go 0-for-October. What has likely happened is that your game day nervousness activated the reticular formation, which in turn preset spindles and muscle tone to a different level than those of your practice sessions. All the motor learning that took place in your backyard court occurred under different conditions than what you faced before a crowd. Motor learning involves the proper matching of initial body position and tone, motor output, and resultant afferent feedback. For you to succeed in the performance of a motor task, your practice conditions and muscle tone should replicate as closely as possible those you will face on game day (see Chapter 7 for a discussion of factors affecting motor learning).

The role of emotion in athletic performance and motor skill acquisition is not an imaginary concept. The reticular formation, serving as a link between the limbic system and motor neurons within the spinal cord, provides a very real connection whereby emotion can play a very large role in motor performance. Furthermore, the reticulospinal tract is not the only system by which nervousness can affect motor performance. The interconnectivity of the basal ganglia, cerebellum, thalamus, cerebral cortex, and other brain stem nuclei such as the vestibular system provide ample opportunity for other systems to exert their influences.

Vestibular system

The vestibular system is a complex sensory system of vital importance for balance, head control, and eye-tracking tasks. Vestibular sensory receptors are located in the inner ear. The semicircular canals, utricle, and saccule comprise the peripheral receptors of the vestibular system. This peripheral sensory receptor system is called the *labyrinthine system*. These receptors are huge compared with the other receptors discussed previously. The labyrinthine system detects changes in head position and angular acceleration. Via vestibulo-ocular reflexes, they assist in controlling eye movements, especially during visual tracking of moving objects. They convey their messages via the eighth cranial nerve primarily to the vestibular nuclei located in the medullary portion of the brain stem. Some projections do not go to vestibular nuclei but rather to the cerebellum, the reticular formation, the thalamus, and the cerebral cortex.

The vestibular nuclei receive input from the peripheral labyrinth receptors, the reticular formation, and the cerebellum. The output from vestibular nuclei is primarily to motor neurons within the spinal cord, specifically, to motor neurons innervating proximal muscles and muscle spindles of the neck and back (postural muscles). Vestibular nuclei are responsible for integrating incoming cerebellar information with input from the labyrinths and reticular formation. The cerebellum does not project directly to the spinal cord. Rather, it exerts its influences on spinal cord neural functioning via the vestibular nuclei, the rubrospinal system, and, more indirectly, cerebellocortical circuits.

An example from everyday life might be better for understanding vestibular function than an in-depth discussion of afferent and efferent connectivity. You walk out of a supermarket with grocery bags in both arms. As you direct your attention to crossing the road without becoming windshield chowder, a banana peel escapes your attention—but it does not escape contact with the sole of your shoe. Only your vestibular system can save you now! As your foot slips out from under you, peripheral sensory receptors including labyrinthine receptors and muscle/joint proprioceptors are already in the process of mobilizing the muscular troops to save your butt. The receptors will bypass the brain and first send their alarming message to vestibular nuclei. The first thing the vestibular nuclei will do is fire up the muscles and muscle spindles of proximal antigravity muscles. The spindles will increase muscle tone and increase the body's ability to respond to muscle stretch. The first muscles to be activated are not those of the arms and legs, but rather the back and trunk muscles. Contraction of these postural muscles provides a stable base of support for your flailing arms and legs. All that flailing is an attempt to keep your center of gravity over your feet. Lucky for you that you don't have to think about all of this. If you did, your reactions would be so slow that the humiliation and pain of falling would be an everyday occurrence for you.

Debate continues about whether the vestibular system initiates the body's response to losing its balance, or whether joint proprioceptive receptors or a change in eye position take the lead role and are the first to respond. Which happens first is not exactly something you have time to think or care much about when you are falling, but nonetheless this gives neuroscientists who study equilibrium responses something to argue. For your purposes, it is sufficient to know that the vestibular system is a quickly reacting system that helps you maintain balance primarily by controlling postural muscles.

The vestibular system, together with the superior colliculus and the tectospinal tract, has an equally important role in eye-tracking tasks. Eye movement must be coordinated with head rotations to allow you to maintain visual fixation of an object. This is obviously of vital importance in eye-hand coordination, a topic to be covered in more detail in Chapter 5. Vestibulo-ocular reflexes take care of this task regardless whether your head is stationary and you wish to maintain visual contact with a moving object, or your head is moving and you still need to maintain visual contact.

For instance, let's take the above example of slipping on a banana peel one step further. As you are falling, out of the corner of your eye you happen to see a friend entering a crowded subway station (Fig. 2-9). Not wanting to lose this opportunity to see your friend again, you keep your eyes focused on him so you don't lose him in the crowd. This is a conscious act, but one that is taken care of reflexively by vestibulo-ocular reflexes. In this instance your vestibular nuclei are aiding in maintaining an upright body posture concomitant with the performance of a visual tracking task.

Red nucleus
Within the midbrain of the brain stem is the red nucleus (Fig. 2-10). Unlike the vestibulospinal system, which excites postural muscles (e.g., abdominal, neck, and back muscles), rubrospinal projections tend to excite motor neurons of the arms and legs. I mention this to show how different systems interact to accomplish a desired goal. If you lose your balance, stiffening and stabilizing of the postural muscles is desirable to allow the arms and legs to move, either into flexion or extension, to try to preserve your center of gravity. The vestibular system activates the postural muscles. Other systems, such as the red nucleus via the rubrospinal tract (RST), control the muscles of the extremities. Projections of the RST onto the spinal cord are similar, and overlap those coming from the motor cortex (i.e., the corticospinal tract). Similar to the sensorimotor cortex, neural activation within the red nucleus precedes movement. Neural activity in the red nucleus is related to force, velocity, and direction of movement, especially of distal digit movement. Perhaps future research will show that the RST helps to facilitate corticospinal tract effects.

The corticospinal tract is greatly expanded in humans compared with other species. Concomitant with the expansion of the human corticospinal tract, the relative size and role of the RST have diminished. As the corticospinal tract has expanded, the RST has decreased in size. Perhaps the phylogenetic changes in these projections represent an increased conscious control of motor functions of humans. We still maintain brain stem–spinal projections for automatic responses, but we have evolved an increased capability to direct our actions consciously. Some investigators have suggested that each system is preferentially activated during different movement tasks. The corticospinal tract is most involved during unique,

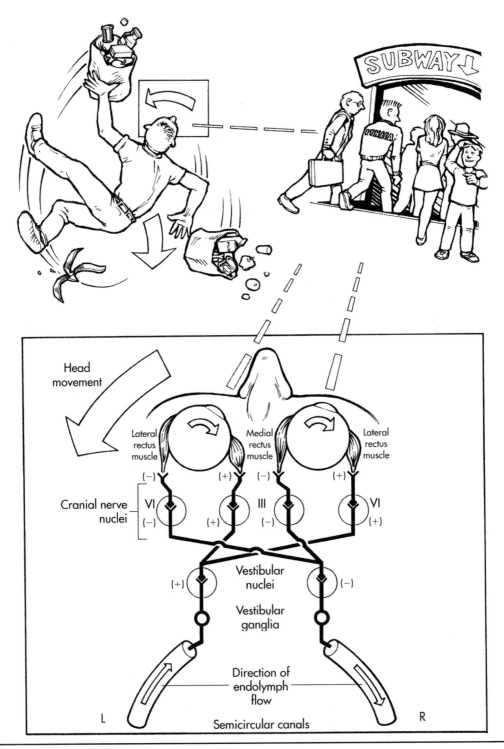

Fig. 2-9. The vestibulo-ocular reflex coordinates eye movements with the vestibular system. It allows you to maintain eye contact with an object even while your head is moving. +, Excitatory synapse; –, inhibitory synapse.

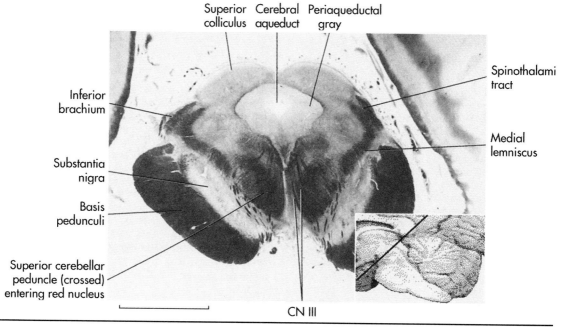

Superior colliculus   Cerebral aqueduct   Periaqueductal gray

Spinothalami tract

Inferior brachium

Medial lemniscus

Substantia nigra

Basis pedunculi

Superior cerebellar peduncle (crossed) entering red nucleus

CN III

Fig. 2-10. Brain stem section at the level of the red nucleus. The basis pedunculi, also shown in this section, contain fibers descending from the cerebral cortex en route to brain stem nuclei and the spinal cord. *Scale mark* = 1 cm. (From Nolte J. The human brain, 3rd ed. St. Louis: Mosby-Year Book, 1993.)

unlearned movements. The RST becomes increasingly involved when a movement sequence becomes learned or when a movement is an automatic reaction. This hypothesis implicates the red nucleus in motor learning. But if the red nucleus is directly involved in motor learning tasks, why is the RST so diminutive in size in humans?

The reduction in the size of the red nucleus and its projections in humans might account for the fact that nonhuman animals tend to recover more fully after cerebral strokes than after similar lesions in humans. Perhaps the RST provides an alternative pathway to compensate for corticospinal tract damage in animals that is not available to humans.

Lesions that involve the sensorimotor cortex or its projections also affect the red nucleus. The sensorimotor cortex normally projects ipsilaterally to the red nucleus. In infant cats, ablation of one sensorimotor cortex results in abnormal bilateral corticorubral projections from the intact sensorimotor cortex.[40] Lesioning the corticospinal tract at spinal levels results in changes in red nucleus neurons.[7] These experiments provide evidence that the functioning of the RST and corticospinal tract are interrelated but in ways that have yet to be identified precisely.

■ THE BASAL GANGLIA

The basal ganglia are mysterious enigmas and have the makings of great science fiction. The basal ganglia consist of a complex group of neural structures that form a foreboding fortress hidden deep inside the protective cavernous covering of the brain (Fig. 2-11). The basal ganglia exert their influences by means not completely understood. At least a dozen science fiction and mystery thrillers have started with not too dissimilar plots. Neuroscientists have begun to unravel their mystery. The mystery has been displaced by marvel and not a small amount of confusion and controversy.

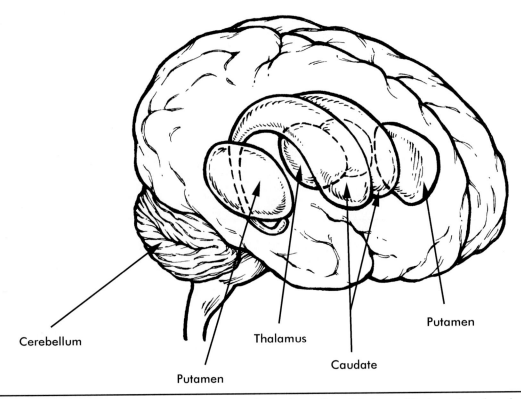

Fig. 2-11. Located deep within the cerebral cortex are the basal ganglia and thalamus. The horseshoe-shaped structure is the caudate. Lateral to it is the putamen and medial to it is the thalamus.

Nomenclature

The caudate nucleus, putamen, globus pallidus, subthalamic nucleus, and substantia nigra are collectively referred to as the basal ganglia (Figs. 2-11 to 2-13). The basal ganglia have been historically thought of as being connected with motor systems. Recent work has shown that this is an oversimplification. It now appears that we should refer to the various components of the basal ganglia not in anatomical terms, but in terms related to their functions. For instance, the amygdala, although physically connected to the caudate and once thought to be one of the basal ganglia, is now referred to separately because it is more closely associated with the limbic and olfactory systems and specifically the emotion of fear. Other structures, such as the caudate, are also being found to be more involved in emotion and cognition than with motor control. The final taxonomy and nomenclature for the basal ganglia remain to be determined. Despite the apparent temporary nature of basal ganglia terminology, you will need some additional vocabulary to understand literature relating to their function.

The putamen and globus pallidus are collectively referred to as the *lenticular nucleus*. The caudate and putamen are called the *striatum*. Corticostriatothalamocortical is the term used to describe the primary anatomical and functional loops within the basal ganglia. Nomenclature confusion is just the beginning. Defining basal ganglia connectivity and function is the real challenge. The confusion will not be easily resolved because the study of the basal ganglia is technically difficult.

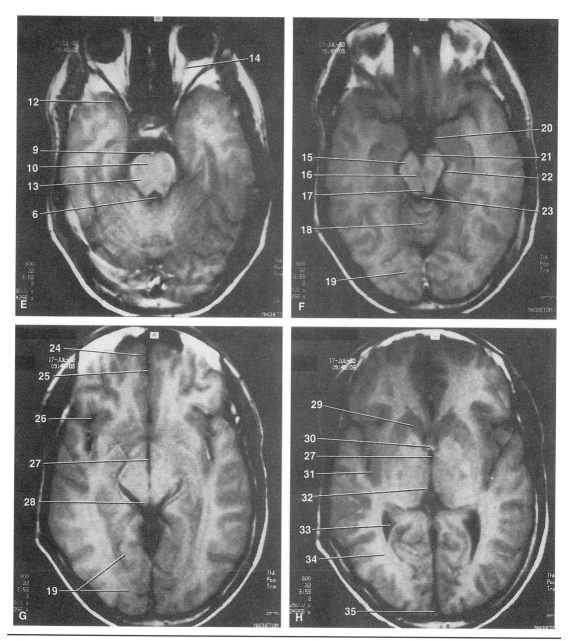

Fig. 2-12. Magnetic resonance image in the horizontal plane shows some internal brain and brain stem structures. *6*, Fourth ventricle; *9*, basilar artery; *10*, basilar pons; *12*, temporal lobe; *13*, tegmentum of pons; *14*, optic nerve; *15*, cerebral peduncle; *16*, red nucleus; *17*, cerebral aqueduct; *18*, vermis of cerebellum; *19*, occipital lobe; *20*, uncus of hippocampus; *21*, interpeduncular cistern; *22*, ambient cistern; *23*, quadrigeminal cistern; *24*, frontal lobe; *25*, interhemispheric fissure; *26*, lateral fissure; *27*, third ventricle; *28*, superior colliculus; *29*, head of caudate nucleus; *30*, fornix; *31*, insula; *32*, habenula; *33*, posterior horn of the lateral ventricle; *34*, visual pathway (geniculocalcarine tract); *35*, superior sagittal sinus. (From Jennes L, Traurig HH, Conn PM. Atlas of the human brain. Philadelphia: JB Lippincott, 1995.)

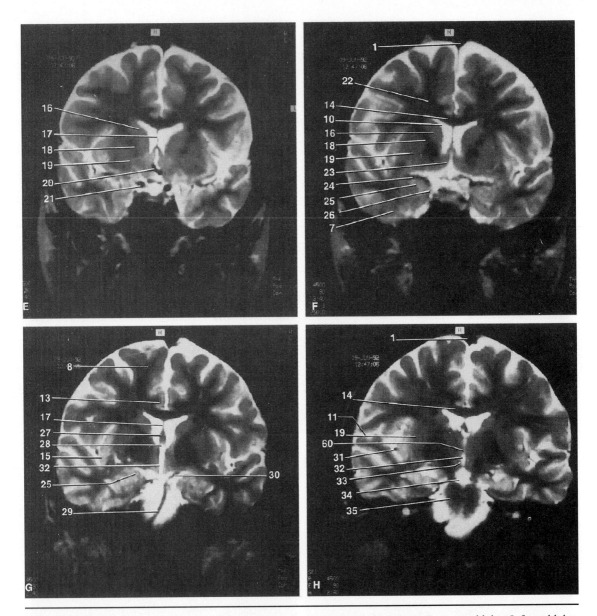

Fig. 2-13. Magnetic resonance image in the coronal plane. *1*, Superior sagittal sinus; *7*, temporal lobe; *8*, frontal lobe; *10*, anterior horn of lateral ventricle; *11*, lateral fissure; *13*, cingulate gyrus; *14*, body of corpus callosum; *15*, insular cortex; *16*, head of caudate nucleus; *17*, septum pellucidum; *18*, anterior limb of internal capsule; *19*, putamen; *20*, anterior cerebral artery; *21*, internal carotid artery; *22*, corona radita; *23*, septum (parolfactory gyrus); *24*, middle cerebral artery; *25*, amygdala; *26*, uncus; *27*, fornix; *28*, interventricular foramen of Monro; *29*, basilar artery; *30*, posterior cerebral artery; *31*, middle cerebral artery, Sylvian branch; *32*, third ventricle; *33*, hypothalamus; *34*, interpeduncular cistern; *35*, basilar pons; *60*, massa intermedia. (From Jennes L, Traurig HH, Conn PM. Atlas of the human brain. Philadelphia: JB Lippincott, 1995.)

Methodologies to examine basal ganglia function

Various methods are used to determine basal ganglia connectivity and function, including neuroanatomical tracing techniques, positron emission transaxial tomography (PET scan), functional magnetic resonance imaging (these latter two techniques combine imaging of the brain to determine structural locations with a measure of the metabolic activity of neurons within specific locations), lesion studies (whereby a certain nucleus or group of cells within the basal ganglia are destroyed to study the effects on behavior), intra- and extracellular recordings of neural activity (techniques that monitor changes in neural activity during various functional tasks or sensory input), and autopsy data (postmortem analysis after diseases known to involve damage to the basal ganglia, such as Parkinson's disease and Huntington's chorea). These methods can also be applied to other areas within the nervous system. Each technique has its drawbacks and limitations. Lesion studies of the basal ganglia are especially difficult to interpret because of the rich and diverse network of basal ganglia interconnectivity. Determining whether an observed behavior after a basal ganglia lesion is due to the loss of function at the lesion site or secondary to the effects of the removal of this input to the thalamus, cortex, or other basal ganglia nuclei is difficult. PET scans investigate the human basal ganglia during different functional tasks. PET scans, however, are limited by the degree of resolution possible. They are not precise enough, as yet, to discriminate between some small adjacent cell groupings within the basal ganglia.[8] To add to the difficulties inherent to discerning the function of the basal ganglia, dramatic species variation appears to exist. Many PET studies in humans do not correlate extremely well with nonhuman animal lesion studies. So much controversy and disparate findings exist that I am somewhat hesitant to attempt an integrative summary of function for fear I will offend someone by failing to include his or her data or hypothesis. So, with that caveat, and my apologies for any unintended omissions, let's press onward through the fog. And remember, as Francis Crick reputedly said, "A theory that accounts for all the facts is bound to be wrong, because some of the facts are bound to be wrong."

The basal ganglia are essential for movement, yet they have no direct projection to the spinal cord and receive no direct sensory information from peripheral receptors. The basal ganglia can influence activity of the corticospinal, rubrospinal, and reticulospinal tracts. Indeed, by the projections to the thalamus, which receives every type of sensory input from all parts of the body, the basal ganglia can potentially influence all sensorimotor activity. Cortical and thalamic inputs provide the afferent input to the basal ganglia and terminate primarily in the striatum. The major basal ganglia efferents are to thalamic nuclei that relay information primarily to sensorimotor cortical areas. In addition, a rich, diverse, and almost totally indescribable interconnectivity exists between the various components of the basal ganglia (Fig. 2-14). Basal ganglia circuitry is so complex that I have yet to meet any neuroscientist who can recite, from memory, its known connections. How could we? New data arrive on an almost weekly basis that add to known connectivity and challenge currently held opinions regarding function. Furthermore, each pathway uses a different neurotransmitter, which further complicates understanding because each transmitter might have a different effect on different structures and pathways. To gain an elementary understanding of basal ganglia function, we'll begin with an examination of some of their neural projections and targets.

Corticostriatothalamocortical loops

Corticostriatothalamocortical projections form five fairly distinct functional loops (Fig. 2-15):

1. motor pathway (Fig. 2-16),
2. oculomotor pathway,
3. dorsolateral prefrontal pathway,
4. lateral orbitofrontal prefrontal pathway and,
5. limbic pathway.

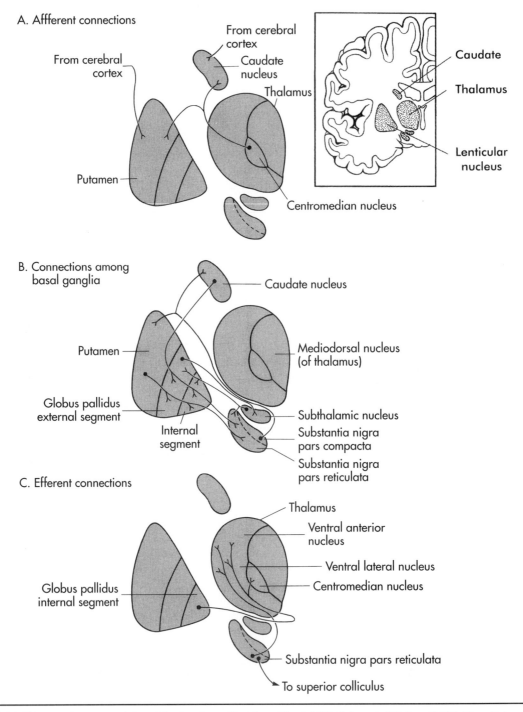

Fig. 2-14. The complex connectivity of the basal ganglia. (From Kandel ER, Schwartz JH, Jessell TM. Essentials of neuroscience and behavior. Norwalk, Conn.: Appleton & Lange, 1995.)

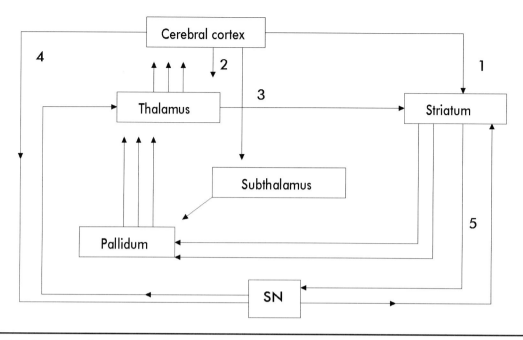

Fig. 2-15. Basal ganglia connectivity forms functional circuits termed corticostriatothalamocortical loops. This diagram illustrates five currently defined loops (see text for details). (Redrawn from Afifi AK. Basal ganglia: functional anatomy and physiology. Part 2. J Child Neurol 1994;9:353.)

Within the motor pathway, the putamen is the primary target of afferent input. The afferent input consists of somatotopically organized inputs from primary motor cortex (Area 4), primary sensory cortex (Areas 3,1,2), association cortex (Area 5), premotor cortex (Area 6), and supplementary cortex (Area 6). Specific target areas within the putamen can also be classified based on behavioral variables. Certain neurons within the putamen respond to target location, others to limb kinematics, and others to muscle activation patterns.[1] The putamen projects to the globus pallidus and the substantia nigra, which in turn project to motor nuclei within the thalamus (i.e., nuclei that project to motor areas of the cerebral cortex) and a brain stem nucleus called the *pedunculopontine nucleus*. This nucleus is associated with cerebellar functioning and forms a connection between the cerebral cortex and the cerebellum. Thalamic projections back to the related sensorimotor cortices complete the corticostriatothalamocortical loop. Considerable convergence exists from multiple sensory systems and between motor and sensory information in the striatum.

Neural activity associated with movement
With some exceptions, most basal ganglia neurons become active after movement initiation and after activation of neurons in the supplementary and primary motor cortex. But here is where it starts to get interesting. Neurons within the basal ganglia function differently during different functional tasks.[14,47,48] And during any specific functional task, some basal ganglia neurons will only respond to sensory input that is directly relevant to the movement taking place.[14] Others respond only if the sensory stimulus is attached to a motor memory. Repetitive exposures to certain sensory input change the functional characteristics of

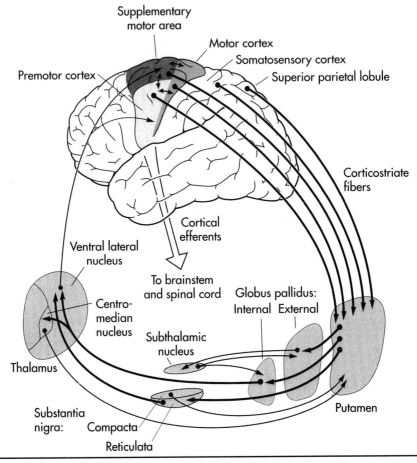

Fig. 2-16. The anatomical structures and the connectivity of the basal ganglia motor loop. (From Kandel ER, Schwartz JH, Jessell TM. Essentials of neuroscience and behavior. Norwalk, Conn.: Appleton & Lange, 1995.)

neurons within the basal ganglia. Striatal interneurons acquire response properties on the basis of experienced reward.[23] Some neurons within the basal ganglia are not tonically active and become active only during movement. Other neurons, such as those in the subthalamus, are tonically active and increase their output during movement. Neurons within the caudate are neither tonically active nor do they change activity levels with movement. Other basal ganglia cells activate before the performance of a learned skill.[22]

Perhaps now you can understand why a concise description of the basal ganglia has eluded neuroscientists. The basal ganglia are composed of a diverse group of neurons, all with an apparently different function. To complicate matters further, their function changes depending on the task, emotional attachment to the task, and whether or not the task involves memory.

Theoretical perspectives on function

Armed with data, we can make some conjectures regarding function. For instance, the fact that caudate neurons are not tonically active and do not change levels of activation during motor activity suggests that the caudate is not involved in the motor pathway and serves some other function. On the other hand, by the nature of its projections to the globus pallidus (the major source of basal ganglia efferents to the thalamus) and its pattern of neural activity, the subthalamus appears to be in a position to regulate the output of the basal ganglia.[2] The next obvious questions are, what does this output from the basal ganglia do, and what is it doing with the tremendous amount of input it receives from the cerebral cortex? At this point, the answers depend on who you talk to and what research techniques were used to assess function. Although differences of opinion exist, a general theme regarding the global functioning of the basal ganglia is beginning to emerge.

The basal ganglia appear to be involved in the cognitive and motivational aspects of movement. Its circuitry reinforces desired motor behaviors and suppresses unwanted behavior. Basal ganglia function is intimately related to cortical, brain stem, extrapyramidal, and cerebellar functioning. There is little doubt that basal ganglia can regulate muscle tone[33] and that they participate in the generation, switching, and termination of movement as dictated by situational demands and emotional or attentive states.[6] Some reports indicate that the basal ganglia are preferentially activated during memorized motor tasks[22] and therefore contribute to the automatic execution of a learned motor plan.[1,34] Novel tasks do not activate the basal ganglia to the same degree as a learned task. Interestingly, the basal ganglia are equally active during an imaginative performance of a task (mental imagery) as during an actual performance.[8] Perhaps, therefore, movement preparation and alteration of muscle tone to changing task demands are important functions that can be attributed to the basal ganglia. Some have suggested that the basal ganglia reformat cortical inputs into distributed and distinct modules of movement and temporally organize the sequencing of these modules to optimize motor performance.[23] Human PET scan data present some contradictory evidence to these hypotheses, but also lend some support.

Some human PET scan studies involving the learning of complex finger movements have led researchers to conclude that the basal ganglia are not involved in motor skill acquisition or the facilitation of sequential movements.[59] Cellular recordings from monkey basal ganglia neurons and human PET scans indicate that basal ganglia neuron activation is independent of movement force, frequency of movement, load, velocity, decisions about movement direction,[8,47] or whether motor skills were being acquired or reproduced from memory.[8,47] The sensorimotor cortex and the cerebellum were important in determining these movement parameters, but the basal ganglia were not.[49]

A proposed theory that does appear compatible with existing data states that higher centers, such as the cerebral cortex and cerebellum, initiate movement and movement sequences. Once this process has been initiated, the basal ganglia optimize patterns of muscle activation so that the desired goal is achieved in the most efficient way. The basal ganglia suppress unwanted movement and continually monitor descending commands, with the resultant afferent feedback.[13] One way to test this global theory of basal ganglia function is to assess whether it is consistent with clinical signs and symptoms that result from lesions of the basal ganglia.

Lessons from patients with damage to the basal ganglia
People with damage to the basal ganglia often cannot control their movements. The hands, arms, and face may exhibit tremors and constant involuntary movement even when the person is resting quietly. Paradoxically, another common symptom is the inability to move voluntarily. When affected by a basal ganglia disorder, a person's hand may be in constant motion, but when the individual attempts to move the hand to reach a glass of water, nothing happens. Then, in a cruel twist, if the individual does manage to initiate movement, often he cannot stop himself appropriately. For example, a person may wish to walk from one end of the room to another. Perhaps a gentle nudge begins him on his way. But instead of stopping at the end of the room, he may continue walking into the next room unless physically restrained.

TABLE 2-2 **Disorders of the basal ganglia with clinical and pathological correlations**

Disorder	Clinical Impairments	Pathophysiology
Parkinson's disease	Resting tremor, rigidity, akinesia, bradykinesia	Degeneration of pathway connecting substantia nigra and striatum; reduction in specific neurotransmitters (dopamine, serotonin, norepinephrine)
Huntington's disease	Chorea, decreased muscle tone, dementia (later stages)	Degeneration of specific neurons within the caudate and putamen
Ballism	Spontaneous, uncoordinated, jerky, involuntary movements of the limbs	Damage to subthalamic nucleus
Tourette's syndrome	Multiple tics, involuntary movement and vocalizations, hyperactivity	Involvement of pathway connecting striatum with globus pallidus. Alteration in dopamine uptake

Data from Adams RD, Victor M. Principles of neurology, 5th ed. New York: McGraw-Hill, 1993; and Kandel ER, Schwartz JH, Jessell TM, eds. Principles of neural science, 3rd ed. Norwalk: Appleton & Lange, 1991.

Some individuals experience a flaccid paralysis after a stroke. Damage to the lenticular nucleus appears to be responsible for this severe impairment.[52] Several other disorders can be attributed to specific lesions or neurotransmitters within the basal ganglia (Table 2-2).

In Parkinson's disease, dopaminergic input to the striatum is lost. Without going into the detailed circuitry or biochemistry involved, the net result is inhibition (or more precisely, decreased disinhibition) of basal ganglia and thalamic neurons. This results in slowness and poverty of movement. Muhammad Ali and Katherine Hepburn are two examples of individuals who exhibit slightly different effects of Parkinson-like symptoms (my understanding is that neither individual has been diagnosed with Parkinson's disease but they manifest impairments attributed to basal ganglia damage).

Muhammad Ali is, in my opinion, one of the greatest athletes and animated personalities of all time. I can still remember staying up late as a kid to listen to the radio broadcast of his first title fight with Sonny Liston. Just listening to his performance was exhilarating. I couldn't wait for my father's next issue of *Sports Illustrated* to arrive because I knew the pages would contain the photographic images my imagination had assigned to the radio commentator's words. I wasn't disappointed. Even with still photographs, the man's physical grace was apparent. One of the greatest sport photographs of all time captured Ali's raw power and emotion as he stood astride the fallen Liston. Contrast this image to the man we now see fleetingly. The float of the butterfly has been reduced to a shackled, shuffling gait. The face that once was alive with emotion and playfulness, is now leaden and belies the spirit of the man.

The lack of emotional expression is a hallmark of Parkinson's disease. This is attributed to the basal ganglia's connections to emotional centers of the brain and its influence over facial muscles. Contrast Ali's lack of facial expression, however, to Katherine Hepburn, who also demonstrates some Parkinson-like symptoms. Katherine Hepburn has resting tremors and a tremulous voice, but her face and eyes continue to light up with emotion during the interviews I've seen. Perhaps this can be attributed to her training as an actress or perhaps to lack of involvement of specific pathways mediating facial emotional expression. Conjecture like this opens up a neurological Pandora's box and is a question not easily answered.

Huntington's chorea is caused by a loss of striatal neurons that results in reduced neural inhibition. This loss manifests clinically as random, flailing, involuntary movement, balance difficulties, and facial grimacing. Woody Guthrie, the famous songster/hipster, is the person who comes to mind when talking about Huntington's chorea. During the early stages of his disease, he was thought to suffer from substance abuse. Slurred speech, movement tics, and balance difficulties are early symptoms of Huntington's chorea. Over time, however, these symptoms worsen and constant, uncontrollable body movements increasingly contribute to a disabling condition.

Treatment of basal ganglia disorders

Treatments initiated in the 1970s and 1980s for basal ganglia disorders focused on drugs that would mimic the neurotransmitters normally secreted by the basal ganglia. For instance, in Parkinson's disease the substantia nigra fails to produce dopamine. Therefore, various drugs are given to try to increase dopamine synthesis. These drugs were, and remain, very beneficial, but in progressive disorders such as Parkinson's disease and Huntington's chorea, the cells of the basal ganglia continue to die and, therefore, the disease progresses. Pharmacological interventions continue to be refined and new protocols are continually being developed that target very specific neurotransmitters and receptors. Neurosurgical approaches, such as a pallidotomy (the surgical production of lesions in the globus pallidus) are also used to treat basal ganglia disorders. These approaches are designed to activate or deactivate specific pathways.

A promising technique currently being developed by neuroscientists involves placing healthy fetal basal ganglia cells into the diseased area. The fetal cells grow, divide, and secrete the neurotransmitters that the diseased neurons were no longer capable of producing. The procedures being developed have the potential to halt the progress of the disease and thereby restore normal movement. This technique is not limited to the basal ganglia but is also being examined to lessen the effects of spinal cord injury. Scientists must determine whether CNS fetal transplants act solely as agents for nonspecific transmitter release or contribute to the establishment of functional connections.

Unfortunately, the use of fetal and embryonic tissue is an ethically and politically sensitive issue, and federal funding for this pioneering work is vulnerable to congressional cutbacks or outright bans. Treatments for basal ganglia disorders will continue to develop and evolve just as the basal ganglia have evolved over phylogenetic time.

Evolutionary development of the basal ganglia and cerebellum

Two subcortical structures enlarged during primate evolution: the basal ganglia and the cerebellum.[4,38] Both are indirectly connected with each other and both are intimately involved in motor control. The basal ganglia are involved in optimization of, and attaching emotional significance to, motor skills. Both of these activities help to define dexterous, thinking animals, so not surprisingly, the basal ganglia have expanded during primate evolution. The basal ganglia, however, do not appear to have changed substantially during subsequent hominid evolution. In contrast, the cerebellum has continued to expand during human evolution.[38] What is it about movements of the human animal that require a cerebellum of a size and complexity that has never before been possessed by any creature that has inhabited this planet? And, what is it about cerebellar functioning that is so essential to human behavior?

■ THE CEREBELLUM: THE COACH WITHIN
An introduction to the mystery

The cerebellum has been studied extensively. Its connections are well known and its neurons have been morphologically and neurophysiologically identified. We know much detail about its component parts and its afferent and efferent projections. The mystery of the cerebellum lies in the fact that we have a fairly good idea about what it does—we just don't know how it manages to it. Mathematicians and computer experts have been called on to study the problem and have yet to come close to devising a theoretical model that approaches the elegance of control that the cerebellum exerts over muscular coordination. The following paragraphs will begin with brief descriptions of cerebellar connections that impact motor control and progress to a discussion of cerebellar function that is uniquely human.

The cerebellum has no direct connections with motor neurons in the spinal cord, yet its control over their activity is considerable. Lesions to the cerebellum have a devastating effect on movement. Damage to the cerebellum results in clumsy, uncoordinated movement. The timing and force production of muscle contraction becomes abnormal. Involuntary movement and tremors appear whenever voluntary movement is attempted.

The cerebellum projects to nuclei within the brain stem (primarily the vestibular nuclei) and the thalamus. It receives input from vestibular nuclei, spinal cord receptors (muscle spindles, cutaneous afferents, joint receptors, etc.), the reticular formation, and the cerebral cortex (primarily the motor and somatosensory cortex). The spinocerebellar pathways relay information to the cerebellum regarding the strength of muscular contraction, the amount of tension generated, the positions and rates of movement of each body segment, and information regarding any external forces acting on the body. It does all this at speeds greater than 100 m/sec, the fastest conduction time of any pathway within the central nervous system.

"Comparator" or "coach" are the best synonyms to describe cerebellar function. Although a hypothetical premise, conventional teaching holds that the cerebellum processes sensory information from the periphery and compares this information to the motor commands emanating from the motor cortex. In this way it compares the actual movement being performed to the movement desired by the brain and somehow contributes to the correction of any mistakes. The cerebellum is not only a feedback system, but also a feed-forward system. It appears to participate in the programming of voluntary movement, particularly learned, skillful movement that becomes more rapid and precise with time and practice. The cerebellum can regulate reflex gain during a movement and produce long-term movement alterations based on experience. The cerebellum prepares the body for a particular motor act before any movement occurs. Thus it participates in motor programming and motor learning. Knowledge of cerebellar connectivity sheds some light on how this might be accomplished.

Anatomical and functional divisions

The anatomical and functional divisions of the cerebellum can be confusing because its various parts can be conceptually organized in many different ways. The surface of the cerebellum is covered with transverse convolutions called *folia*. These folia increase the surface area of the cerebellar cortex, the portion of the cerebellum that contains neural cell bodies. Cerebellar surface area had to expand in humans because the cerebellum has more neurons than the cerebral cortex and the remainder of the central nervous system combined![45] Transverse fissures are enlarged, deep folia that divide the cerebellum into three lobes: anterior, posterior, and flocculonodular. The flocculonodular lobe is evolutionarily the oldest portion of the cerebellum. Two longitudinal fissures divide the cerebellum into a midline vermis, which separates the cerebellum into two symmetrical hemispheres (Fig. 2-17). The areas closest to the vermis are referred to as the intermediate hemispheres. The areas lateral to the intermediate hemispheres are the lateral cerebellar hemispheres, the most recently evolved area of the cerebellum. These longitudinal anatomical distinctions form functional components with fairly distinct and separate afferent input and efferent output.

The vermis receives input from vestibular nuclei and other brain stem descending pathways such as the red nucleus. It projects back to these brain stem nuclei to assist in the control of proximal, postural muscles.

The intermediate hemispheres connect with cortical and brain stem nuclei to participate in the control of distal movements (Fig. 2-18).

The lateral hemispheres receive input from motor, premotor, and prefrontal cortices and project back to these cortical areas via the thalamus (Fig. 2-18). These pathways are probably important in the plan-

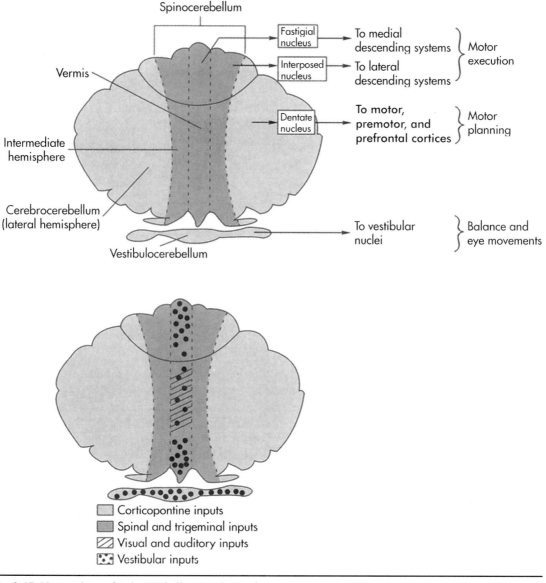

Fig. 2-17. Nomenclature for the cerebellum can be confusing because its component parts can be described anatomically or functionally. Anatomical divisions include the vermis, intermediate hemispheres, and lateral hemispheres. Functional subunits include the vestibulocerebellar, spinocerebellar, and cerebrocerebellar pathways. This diagram illustrates the relationships between anatomical and functional nomenclature. *Top,* Outputs; *bottom,* inputs. (From Kandel ER, Schwartz JH, Jessel TM. Essentials of neuroscience and behavior. Norwalk, Conn.: Appleton & Lange, 1995.)

ning of voluntary movement and are vital for increasing speed of movement associated with motor learning and the acquisition of a motor skill.

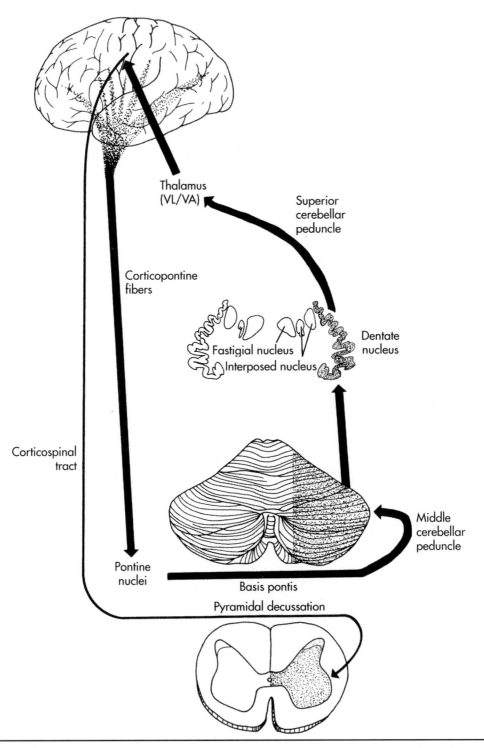

Fig. 2-18. The major cerebellar projections. Different parts of the cerebellar cortex project to different deep cerebellar nuclei. The nuclei comprise the major efferent pathways of the cerebellum. **A**, Major projections of the intermediate zone. *(continued)*

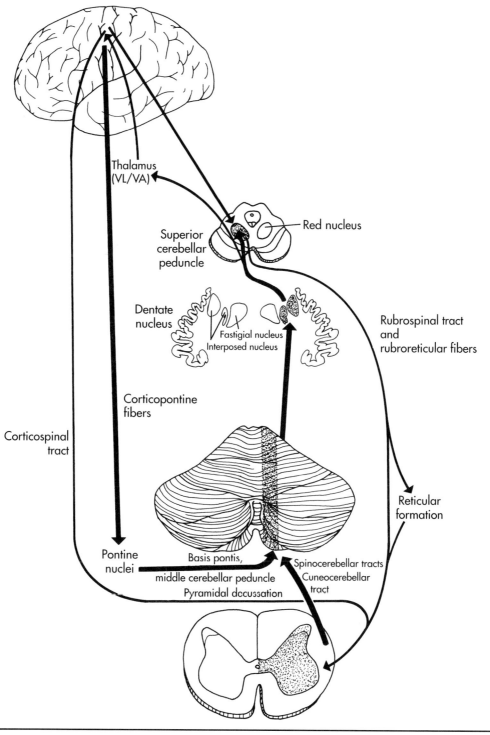

Fig. 2-18, B. Major projections from cerebellar hemispheres. (See text for details.) (From Nolte J. The human brain, 1st ed. St. Louis: Mosby-Year Book, 1981.)

Another way to organize different functional components of the cerebellum is by its afferent input. The primary inputs to the cerebellum are from vestibular nuclei, peripheral receptors via the spinocerebellar tracts, and the cerebral cortex. These inputs are topographically organized within the cerebellum and form three functional subunits. These subunits are somewhat analogous to the anatomical divisions of the cerebellum (vermis, intermediate and lateral hemispheres). However, some inputs and functions are shared by the various anatomical areas. The three functional subunits include the vestibulocerebellar, spinocerebellar, and cerebrocerebellar pathways.

The vestibulocerebellar system receives input from vestibular nuclei and projects directly back to them. The vermis and flocculonodular lobes are the areas of the cerebellum involved in these pathways. It is the only system in which neurons from the cerebellar cortex project directly to a target area (vestibular nuclei). As you will soon read, all other projections from the cerebellar cortex go to deep cerebellar nuclei and do not project out of the cerebellum. The vestibulocerebellar system is the only exception to this organizational rule. The vestibulocerebellar system controls eye movement and balance reactions.

The spinocerebellar system involves projections from the spinocerebellar tracts to the vermis and intermediate hemispheres. The vermis and hemispheres project to deep cerebellar nuclei and ultimately contribute to the control of limb movement.

The cerebrocerebellar system, the most recently evolved and the one about which we know the least, includes direct and indirect inputs from the cerebral cortex, pontine nuclei, and the inferior olivary nucleus to the lateral hemispheres. The lateral hemispheres project back to the premotor, motor, and prefrontal cortices indirectly via a deep cerebellar nucleus that first projects to the thalamus. For now, to keep it simple and nonconfrontational, suffice it to say that the cerebrocerebellar pathway appears to be involved in movement selection and planning.

Taken together, these functional pathways process multisensorial input for purposeful movement. Before an attempt can be made to understand the exact functions of the cerebellum, however, a little more explanation is needed regarding the organization of afferent input and efferent output. For instance, afferent input is received by neurons in the cerebellar cortex, but cerebellar output is not via the cerebellar cortex but rather via structures called *deep cerebellar nuclei*. The second important concept that will assist in an understanding of cerebellar functioning is the separation of afferent input into classifications called *mossy fiber input* or *climbing fiber input*.

Deep cerebellar nuclei

Three deep cerebellar nuclei exist: the *fastigial, interposed,* and *dentate* (Fig. 2-19). These nuclei collectively form almost the entire output of the cerebellum. The fastigial nucleus receives input from the flocculonodular lobe and vermis and projects to vestibular and reticular nuclei. The interposed and dentate nuclei receive input from the intermediate and lateral hemispheres and project to the reticular formation, red nucleus, inferior olivary nucleus, and the thalamus. Interposed fibers preferentially terminate in the red nucleus and most dentate projections are to the thalamus.

One more note about the cerebellar nuclei that is sure to stimulate your curiosity: they receive input from only one type of neuron in the cerebellar cortex. This is the *Purkinje cell*, and its input to the cerebellar nuclei is tonic (always active) and always inhibitory. The extent of Purkinje cell inhibition to the deep cerebellar nuclei is determined by the afferent input to the Purkinje cells (the mossy and climbing fibers).

Mossy fibers, by far, constitute the majority of sensory inputs to the cerebellar cortex. Various brain stem and spinal cord projections comprise mossy fiber input. Mossy fibers do not synapse directly on Purkinje cells, but on other neurons, such as granule cells, contained within different layers of the cerebellar cortex (refer to a neuroanatomy text for details). Granule cells receive dense input from many mossy fibers. Granule cells, which can be inhibitory or excitatory, then synapse on Purkinje cells. Each Purkinje cell might receive as many as 200,000 inputs from granule cells!

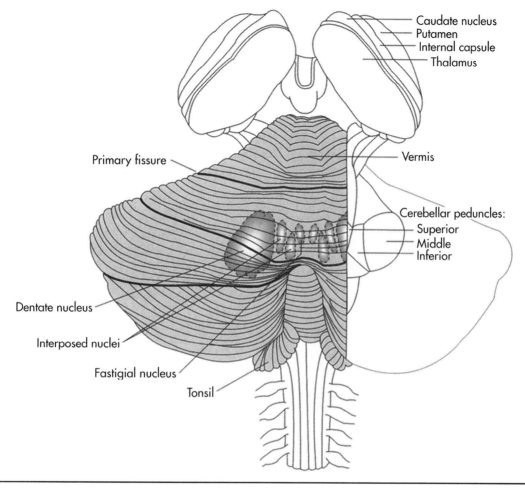

Fig. 2-19. Cerebellar nuclei are imbedded within the cerebellum. This diagram shows their location within the cerebellum and also the anatomical relationship between the cerebellum, thalamus, and portions of the basal ganglia. (From Kandel ER, Schwartz JH, Jessell TM. Essentials of neuroscience and behavior. Norwalk, Conn.: Appleton & Lange, 1995.)

In contrast to the 200,000 synapses from granule cells/mossy fibers, each Purkinje cell receives only one input from a climbing fiber! Yet, the synaptic connection between a climbing fiber and the Purkinje cell is one of the most powerful in the entire nervous system.[19] Each climbing fiber innervates from 1 to 10 Purkinje cells. Climbing fiber input modulates mossy fiber input in dramatic fashion. Together they provide input about what movements are planned and what afferent feedback has resulted from any particular movement or environmental challenge. Climbing fibers originate from the inferior olivary nucleus located in the medulla. The inferior olivary nucleus receives rich input from the cerebral cortex, red nucleus, and the spinal cord. I am tempted to launch into a more detailed description of olivary nucleus anatomy and physiology because its functioning is vitally linked to the cerebellum. I will, however, save you this perhaps overbearing minutia and refer those with inquiring minds to the references listed at the end of this chapter—or, better yet, I advise you to do a MEDLINE computer search, since by the time this book comes out almost certainly more will be known. Current hypotheses regarding function include such diverse thoughts as assigning the olivary nucleus a role in the organization of cerebellar output during well-learned movements[45] or as the initiator of preferential activation of the red nucleus or cerebral cortex depending on movement context.[31] (Remember, red nucleus projections terminate in approximately the same area of the spinal cord as corticospinal tract projections).

Functions of the cerebellum
Despite the many questions that remain regarding cerebellar functioning and its connectivity to structures such as the olivary nucleus, some functions of the cerebellum are widely accepted. The cerebellum aids in visual tracking and helps in predicting movement occurring outside the body. For instance, it helps predict how long a fastball will take to cross home plate. The cerebellum predicts the velocity and course of trajectory, and helps to program the necessary movements for a batter to make contact with the ball. This feed-forward control depends on prior experience and practice (i.e., learning).

Not all learning involves conscious awareness. The cerebellum appears capable of learning. Cerebellar learning evades our conscious perceptions. If a person picks up an object of unknown weight and is asked to move it from point A to point B, initially she will not be able to make an accurate movement. With time and practice, the movement is made quickly and without error. If the cerebellum has been damaged, however, no improvement occurs with practice.

The cerebellum also permits smooth progression from one movement to the next. This is obviously of utmost importance during activities that require muscular coordination. Research has indicated that neural activity within certain nuclei of the cerebellum reflect the direction of the next intended movement rather than the pattern of muscular contraction occurring at the moment. A gymnast, boxer, dancer, or musician all execute one movement after another in rapid succession. Once a particular movement has been initiated, the cerebellum is already preparing the body for its next move. The previous movement appears to trigger the cerebellum to begin the next. Unlike the cortex, which primarily fires at the beginning of a movement and does not appear to be driven by the consequences of the movement, the cerebellum constantly fires and modifies its output during a movement or during a sequence of movements. It gives us the ability to adapt to a changing environment quickly and efficiently.

Insights regarding cerebellar functioning and its connectivity with other CNS structures are constantly evolving from increasingly powerful tools such as functional magnetic resonance imaging, PET, and newly developed scanning techniques. These techniques, combined and correlated with neuroanatomical mapping, single-cell recordings, and behavior, are exploding traditionally held concepts about cerebellar function. One traditionally held concept that recent findings are dispelling is that the cerebellum is only concerned with motor function. Imaging techniques have indicated that the human cerebellum is active during some cognitive and language functions.[3,38] It has also been discovered that the dentate nucleus of the cerebellum and the prefrontal cortex share projections.[46] The prefrontal cortex, among other tasks, is engaged in the business of motor planning. These findings have led to increased research activity into the relationships between the cerebellum, information processing, learning (verbal and nonverbal), and language production.

Different regions of the cerebellum are preferentially activated during motor activities and during cognitive tasks.[32] An example of a cognitive task that involves the cerebellum is solving a pegboard puzzle. This cognitive task causes bilateral activation of the dentate nuclei.[32] The cerebellum is also active when subjects are asked to match verbs to visually presented nouns.[38] The parts of the cerebellum that are metabolically active during this task change as the task becomes more routine. Amazingly, PET scans have confirmed that changes in activation patterns within the cerebellum during the learning of a task take place in as little as 15 minutes.[55]

TABLE 2-3 Cerebellum and cognitive processing tasks

Task	Cerebellar location of activation
Tactile learning	Lateral cortex
Verbal learning (generating verbs to match nouns)	Lateral cortex
Spatial problem solving	Dentate nucleus
Auditory-verbal memory	Lateral and midline cortex
Visual memory tasks	Lateral cortex
Mental imagery	Lateral cortex

Data from Leiner HC, Leiner AL, Dow RS. The underestimated cerebellum. Hum Brain Map 1995;2:244-54.

Broca's area, located in the frontal lobe, receives a projection from the cerebellum. Broca's area is a specialized cortical region that is responsible for coordinating musculature that controls sound and language production. The cerebellum has long been hypothesized to be important for the speed of movement and for the process of performing tasks automatically. Speed and quick changes between muscle groups are essential to the acquisition of language skills. Thus, connections between the cerebellum and Broca's area make intuitive sense. The projections from the cerebellum to prefrontal cortex and Broca's area, via the thalamus, appear to be uniquely human. Perhaps the connection is a prerequisite for language. It would be interesting to know whether "talking" chimps who have been taught sign or a symbolic language possess similar connectivity between the cerebellum and language centers of the brain. Table 2-3 summarizes some of the cognitive/cerebellar interactions that have thus far been determined.

An interesting hypothesis has been introduced that attempts to account for the dentate nucleus' projections to motor and prefrontal cortices and the role of the cerebellum during motor learning. Researchers have proposed that whether the dentate nucleus sends its projections to the prefrontal or motor areas of the brain depends on the task.[38] If the task is a novel one and decisions about movement must be made, the dentate nucleus sends the relevant information to the prefrontal cortex. During well- learned tasks, the prefrontal cortex is not needed and the information from the dentate nucleus is sent directly to the motor cortex. The cerebellum appears to learn combinations of muscle actions and links them to behavioral contexts. Actions are triggered automatically in the presence of previously experienced contexts. Watching Michael Jordan on the basketball court is a perfect example of this concept at work. The man's bodily control and quick reactions are out of this planet.

To be sure, Michael Jordan is a gifted athlete. But he did not achieve his current level of performance without practice. It was practice that enabled his cerebellum to react so quickly to changing conditions on the basketball court. It is Michael's reactions in mid-air that set him apart from his peers. Although practice requires conscious effort, the resultant enhanced cerebellar functioning that leads to superior reactions does not. Michael's cerebellum appears to put him on automatic pilot, bypassing slower cortical decision making processes and thus putting him milliseconds ahead of his competition. My guess is that elite musicians are in the same league.

Cerebellar damage

The cerebellum appears to be involved in the timing of voluntary movement. During rapid movement, the cerebellum likely assesses the rate of movement and calculates the amount of time necessary for the body or limb to reach the intended position. Once the target is reached, the cerebellum then activates the motor cortex to inhibit the agonist muscles and activate the antagonist muscles, thus braking the movement. The more rapid the movement, the earlier the antagonists are activated. The processes of carrying out a movement and simultaneously correcting for errors probably occur too rapidly for the motor cortex to control. In individuals with cerebellar lesions, this braking control is lacking and these individuals experience "past pointing." A patient with a cerebellar lesion will, when reaching for a glass, not stop the arm in time and probably knock the glass over. He may be able to sit quietly, but as soon as movement is initiated, tremors become apparent. This is one way that cerebellar lesions are differentiated from basal ganglia lesions. A person with a cerebellar lesion has no resting tremors; the tremors only appear with movement. With basal ganglia disorders, tremor activity occurs even at rest. The individual with a cerebellar lesion loses the ability of ongoing correction of movement. He may eventually hit the target but only by trial and error. The cerebral cortex can consciously control past pointing after cerebellar lesions, but the control is slow and clumsy and requires much concentration.

Lesions to different areas of the cerebellum result in different impairments. Lesions to the flocculonodular or anterior lobes result in postural deficits.[15] The anterior lobe, however, does not appear to be as involved as the flocculonodular lobe in the routine maintenance of balance. Rather, the anterior lobe adjusts postural responses based on prior experience.[26] In other words, it scales postural responses to be appropriate to environmental context. Without an anterior lobe, you would have a difficult time learning to adjust to the pitch and sway on board a ship. Lesions to cerebellar lateral hemispheres do not result in observable postural or gait deficits. The timing and coordination of arm and hand movements are most obviously affected.[27]

Lesions to the vermis or the anterior and flocculonodular lobes result in loss of proximal stability. Distal extremity movements are likely to become ataxic secondary to this loss of proximal stability. One easy way clinicians can differentiate between cerebellar lesions that involve midline structures versus lateral hemisphere involvement is to provide proximal stability during a movement. Providing proximal stability to someone with lateral hemisphere involvement will not improve the movements, whereas considerable improvement will likely be seen for individuals with midline cerebellar problems.

The cerebellum controls the temporal coordination of multijoint synergists[26,60] and controls segmental central pattern generators for maximal coordination.[5,28] Activity in the cerebellum constantly changes depending on the activity of these generators.[5] Information from central pattern generators is conveyed via spinocerebellar tracts. Therefore, any damage to these tracts can result in a loss of cerebellar control of gait, reaching, mastication, or other activities that rely on these generators.

Because of the role of the cerebellum in cognitive tasks, cerebellar damage can also impact these functions. Practice-related learning (error detection), planning sequenced movements, shifting response to changes in sensory input, visuospatial tasks, tracking, spatial memory, and judging trajectory velocity are examples of cognitive tasks that are likely to be affected after certain types of cerebellar damage.[32,38,46]

The cerebellum is a complex feedback and feed-forward system that still eludes understanding. It has captured neuroscientists' imagination, much the same way Itzhak Perlman, Van Cliburn, Michael Hedges, Muhammad Ali, and Michael Jordan have captured their fans' imagination and wonder. And to think that the cerebellum accomplishes its plethora of motor and cognitive responsibilities without direct projections to the spinal cord or cerebral cortex. The majority of its connections first go to the thalamus. It is through the thalamus that the cerebellum exerts its tremendous influence on our world. The cerebellum is by no means alone in its dependency on the thalamus. Every single sensory and motor system in the human body sends projections to the thalamus.

■ THE THALAMUS

The thalamus is a beautiful structure. It allows us to perceive our world and thus attach meaning to it. Without the thalamus there would be no beauty, nor would there be any emotional connection to a soft,

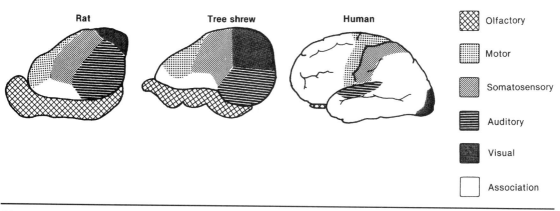

Fig. 2-20. Associational cortical areas have greatly expanded in man. Brains from a rat, shrew, and a person are drawn the same size to show the relative increase in associational areas of man. (From Nolte J. The human brain, 3rd ed. St. Louis: Mosby-Year Book, 1993.)

caressing touch. The thalamus receives input from every sensory system within the body. It receives this sensory information, processes it, begins to interpret the information, and can form and alter our perceptions of it. It integrates cognitive processes such as memory and emotion with sensory input. Some would argue that the thalamus is where we are first consciously aware of incoming sensations.

Evolutionary development
The thalamus has evolved along with the cerebral cortex. The areas within the thalamus and the cerebral cortex that have expanded most dramatically in humans have been the "association" areas. Association areas perform a task identical to their name: they associate various stimuli, make interpretations, and send their cumulative information to primary areas of the brain so that their interpretations can be acted upon (Fig. 2-20).

A rat has very little area within the cerebral cortex or thalamus devoted to associative functions. Rats basically respond to sensory stimuli in rather predictable ways. In contrast, the human cerebral cortex and thalamus are dominated by association areas. These areas allow us to interpret sensory input in a multitude of ways and thus respond in an equally complex manner. No wonder we tend to confuse each other.

Structure and function
The thalamus is actually just one component of a group of structures referred to as the *diencephalon*. The diencephalon consists of the thalamus (dorsal thalamus), epithalamus, hypothalamus, and subthalamus. Only the thalamus will be discussed in this section.

The thalamus is a bilaterally symmetrical structure that straddles the third ventricle (Fig. 2-21). One half of the thalamus resides hidden within the left hemisphere and its identical half resides in the right hemisphere. Each half is no bigger than your thumb. Contained within the thalamus are a multitude of nuclei. Each nucleus receives afferent input and projects to a specific cortical region (Fig. 2-22). Table 2-4 summarizes these projections.

Somatosensory information is carried to the thalamus primarily via two tract systems: the *posterior column/medial lemniscus pathway* and the *spinothalamic tract*. The posterior column/medial lemniscus pathway conveys information from joint, cutaneous, and muscle receptors. Touch, pressure, and joint

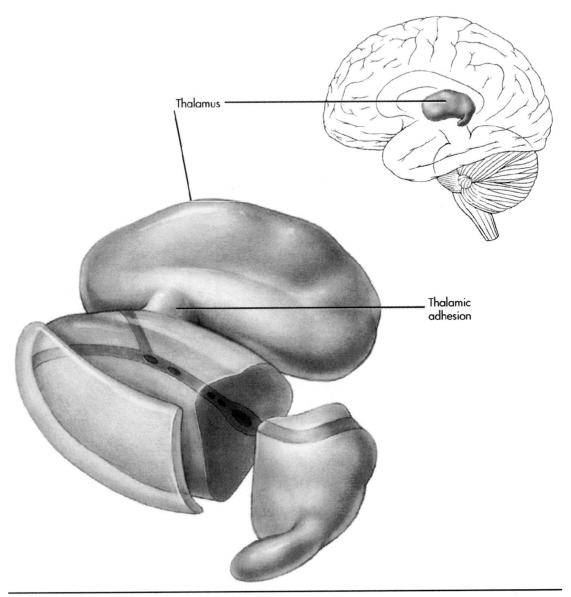

Thalamus

Thalamic
adhesion

Fig. 2-21. The thalamus is a bilateral structure deeply imbedded within the cerebral cortex. The two halves of the thalamus are separated by the third ventricle. This illustration provides a 3-D representation of the thalamus and its location within the cerebral cortex. (From Martin JH. Neuroanatomy: text and atlas. Norwalk, Conn.: Appleton & Lange,
1989.)

position are among the principle sensations represented in this pathway. The spinothalamic tract conveys
nociceptive and temperature sensations from the body. The *trigeminothalamic tract* serves the same functions for the face. Two sensations that receive less attention than pain and temperature that are also conveyed in the spinothalamic and trigeminothalmic tracts are the itch and tickle.[51]

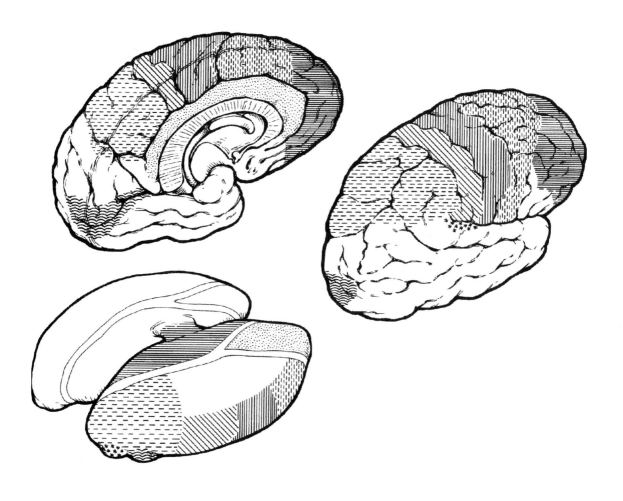

Thalamic nucleus	Cortex area		Thalamic nucleus	Cortex area
Medial	Frontal		Ventral anterior	Premotor
Anterior	Cingulate		Ventral posterolateral	Sensory
Ventral lateral	Motor		Lateral geniculate	Visual
Pulvinar	Posterior parietal		Medial geniculate	Auditory

Fig. 2-22. The thalamus contains numerous nuclei that receive specific afferent input and project to specific areas within the cerebral cortex. The differently shaded regions correspond to thalamic nuclei and their primary projections to the cerebral cortex.

TABLE 2-4 Thalamic nuclei input and output			
Name of nucleus	**Subcortical input**	**Major output**	**Function**
Lateral geniculate	Optic tract	Visual cortex	Vision
Medical geniculate	Inferior colliculus	Auditory cortex	Hearing
Ventral posterolateral	Somatosensory pathways: posterior columns/medial lemniscus, spinothalamic tract	Somatosensory cortex	Sensation (body)
Ventral posteromedial	Trigeminothalamic tracts	Somatosensory cortex	Sensation (face)
Ventral lateral and ventral anterior	Cerebellum, basal ganglia, red nucleus	Motor/premotor cortex	Motor
Anterior	Mammillothalamic tract	Cingulate gyrus	Limbic
Pulvinar	Retina, superior colliculus	Parietal association cortex	Sensory
Lateral posterior	Superior colliculus	Parietal association cortex	Sensory
Lateral dorsal	Cingulate gyrus	Cingulate gyrus	Emotion
Medial dorsal	Amygdala, olfactory cortex	Prefrontal	Limbic
Intralaminar	Other thalamic nuclei, reticular formation, cerebellum, somatosensory pathways	Widespread throughout cortex	?
Reticular	Thalamus	Thalamus	Modulates thalamus

Adapted from Nolte J. The human brain, 3rd ed. St. Louis: Mosby-Year Book, 1993; and Kandel ER, Schwartz JH, Jessell TM, eds. Principles of neural science, 3rd ed. Norwalk: Appleton & Lange, 1991.

The thalamus and cerebral cortex share reciprocal connections. For instance, projections originating in the sensorimotor cortex will terminate within the ventrolateral nucleus of the thalamus. This nucleus will, in turn, send a projection back to the sensorimotor cortex. Each area of the cerebral cortex has a representative counterpart in the thalamus. The purposes of these corticothalamic/thalamocortical reciprocal pathways is not entirely clear, but they appear to be a way that the cerebral cortex can actually control its own afferent input. Perhaps they allow the brain to acquire more information about a certain incoming sensation that might be of primary importance during a certain task and to ignore superfluous information. The thalamic reticular nuclei (not to be confused with the brain stem reticular formation) appear to be optimally positioned for these tasks and their function does appear to be the gating of information between the cortex and thalamus.[56]

The primary functions assigned to the thalamus are the integration of sensory input and cortical attentiveness to these various stimuli. Thalamic nuclei, by nature of their projections to every area of the cerebral cortex, appear capable of directing the attentiveness of specific cortical areas and of contributing to consciousness.[50] The thalamus also appears to contribute to the emotional and affective aspects of pain.[39]

Our responses to pain are conditioned by previous experience. Try this experiment with a friend (a very *good* friend!): Hold your friend's hand down on top of a table as you reach for an ice pick. My guess is that a mass reflex action resulting in the forceful withdrawal of your friend's hand will occur. Mass reflex actions are the hallmark of spinothalamic action in response to a painful stimulus. In this experimental paradigm, no actual pain has been inflicted. The mere sight of the ice pick and knowledge of the consequences of its forceful entry into the back of one's hand is enough to elicit the response—which is a response conditioned by cognition and previous experience.

To assign specific functions to the thalamus is difficult. Lesion studies yield limited data because thalamic lesions involve multiple pathways and not just an isolated thalamic nucleus. Each thalamic nucleus of course also has specific functions in addition to functions shared with other nuclei. Human damage to the thalamus is typically of vascular origin and almost always involves structures apart from thalamic nuclei. In the future, increased resolution capabilities of various scanning techniques should provide an enhanced understanding of individual thalamic nuclei function. Clinicians, however, can expect certain sensory and motor problems if the thalamus is damaged.

Thalamic damage

Damage to the thalamus typically results in sensory disturbances. These disturbances may include an inability to distinguish between various types of stimuli or their intensity. Identifying the location of the stimulus may be problematic. Thalamic damage might also result in *thalamic pain syndrome*. In this unfortunate sensory disorder, any type of sensory stimulus evokes a sensation of pain. Neuropsychological problems and hemianopsias are also frequent sequelae to thalamic damage.[36]

Damage to the thalamus can also result in motor disturbances. Dystonias, chorea, sensory ataxia, tremors, and dyskinesia are not uncommon. Some of these disturbances can be attributed to the sensory losses associated with thalamic damage. Others can be attributed to damage to adjacent areas that subserve motor functions, such as the internal capsule and basal ganglia. *Thalamic syndrome* is a clinical term used to describe thalamic damage that results in a combination of thalamic impairments that include pain, hemianesthesia, and sensory ataxia.

The thalamus is incredibly well connected with the rest of the nervous system and its integrative and perceptual functions are nothing less than wondrous. Envision all of these functions occurring in an area the size of your thumb. Now, envision functions occurring in an organ whose evolutionary size expansion so dominates the human cranium that it has exceeded cranial capacity and has been forced to fold and refold upon itself. I am, of course, talking about the cerebral cortex. With regard to CNS integration, complexity, and mystery, the thalamus pales in comparison to the cerebral cortex.

■ THE CEREBRAL CORTEX
Evolution and Aristotle's mistake

The cerebral cortex is the newest evolutionary expansion of the nervous system. Depending on your point of view, it is either the emperor who lords over the kingdom or merely a slave to its constituents' wishes. Regardless, it is 2,500 cm^2 of wondrous mystery.

Thus far, I have discussed the primary players involved in motor control. In review you will find that some mention has been made of each structure's relationship with the cerebral cortex, the part of the nervous system commonly referred to as the brain (Fig. 2-23). To think of any body part or physiological function that does not involve the cerebral cortex is impossible. Cerebral cortical involvement in human movement is considerable and perhaps moreso than in any other species.

Neuroscientists have long known that stimulation of the motor cortex (a portion of the cerebral cortex which comprises about 5% of its total area) elicits movements on the opposite side of the body. We also know that neurons in this area become active before movement. This is also true, however, of the cerebellum and the basal ganglia. Organisms from single-celled creatures all the way up the phylogenetic tree to amphibians, reptiles, and birds are capable of motility and movement without the benefit of a cerebral cortex. Only mammals have evolved a substantial cerebral cortex. If we choose (as I would urge) to discount Aristotles's view that the mammalian and human brain evolved solely to dissipate heat,[24] we are left to determine the exact function of the cerebral cortex with regard to movement.

Association areas of the brain are the most recent and largest expansion of the human brain. More than just associational language, cognitive, or visual areas have expanded tremendously in humans. The num-

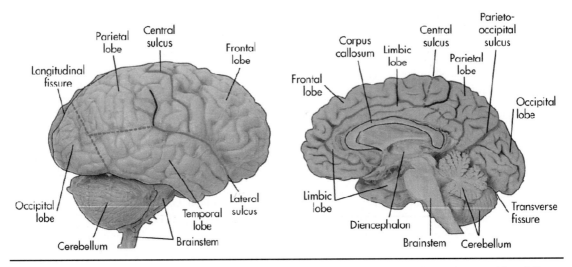

Fig. 2-23. The cerebral cortex is divided into lobes, each of which receives different afferent input and has different functions. A shows the lateral surface and B shows the medial surface of a brain in which the contralateral hemisphere has been removed. (From Nolte J, Angevine J. The human brain in photographs and diagrams. St. Louis: Mosby-Year Book, 1995.)

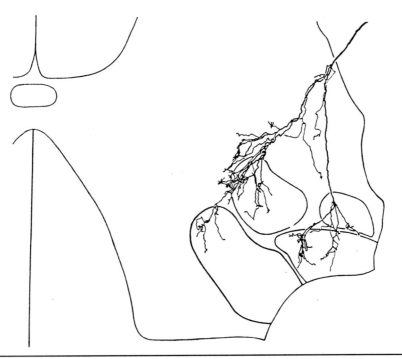

Fig. 2-24. Diagram of the axonal branching within the cervical spinal cord from a single neuron located in the hand area of a monkey's motor cortex. Outlined areas indicate four distinct groups of spinal motor neurons. Primates, including humans, have more direct projections from the cortex to spinal motor neurons (corticospinal tract neurons) than other species. (From Shinoda Y, Yokota JI, Futami T. Neurosci Lett 1981;23:7-12.)

ber of corticospinal tract projections has increased progressively from prosimians to monkeys, apes, and humans. Early in phylogenetic development the corticospinal tract terminated primarily on sensory neurons in the dorsal horn of the spinal cord and modulated sensory information to spinal neurons. Over evolutionary time, the corticospinal tract projections have not only increased but now, in more highly evolved primates including humans, it forms direct projections on motor neurons that control medial and distal limb musculature (Fig. 2-24). Is plantigrade bipedalism somehow related to motor cortical expansion? The chicken or the egg conundrum has considerable relevance in discussions of human brain evolution. Did motor areas of the brain expand to meet the increasing demands of cognitive abilities, or did cognitive abilities expand as our movement repertoire, and thus our ability to explore and perceive our environment, increased?

The study of the nervous system is an intellectual frontier and that of the cerebral cortex the deepest, darkest jungle within that frontier. The cerebral cortex receives information from every nervous system structure thus far discussed and in turn projects to these structures. Because of its importance and because it is here, in the cerebral cortex, that we humans have the most potential to affect and gain control over all other systems involved with motor control, an entire chapter (Chapter 4) is devoted to its exploration. Before jumping ahead to Chapter 4, however, you are encouraged to absorb the next chapter, which discusses some of the subcortical circuitry directly involved in motor control. The chapter begins with local monosynaptic spinal cord reflex arcs and progresses to connectivity involving the cerebral cortex.

SUGGESTED READINGS

Adams RD, Victor M. Principles of neurology, 5th ed. New York: McGraw-Hill, 1993.

al Falahe NA, Nagaoka M, Vallbo AB. Dual response from human muscle spindles in fast voluntary movements. Acta Physiol Scand 1991;141:363-71.

Albright TD. My most true mind thus makes mine eye untrue. Trends Neurosci 1995;18:331-3.

Anastasijevic R, Vuco J. Activity pattern of muscle stretch receptors at the beginning of muscular reflex contraction and its relation to the silent period. Exp Neurol 1982;76:528-37.

Appenteng K, Prochazka A. Tendon organ firing during active muscle lengthening in awake, normally behaving cats. J Physiol (Lond) 1984;353:81-92.

Baldissera F, Hultborn H, Illert M. Integration in spinal neuronal systems. In: Brooks VB, ed. Handbook of physiology: the nervous system II. Baltimore: Williams & Wilkins, 1981:509-95.

Bastian JJ, Thach WT. Cerebellar outflow lesions: a comparison of movement deficits resulting from lesions at the levels of the cerebellum and thalamus. Ann Neurol 1995;38:881-92.

Becker WJ, Morrice BL, Clark AW, Lee RG. Multi-joint reaching movements and eye-hand tracking in cerebellar incoordination: investigation of a patient with com-

plete loss of Purkinje cells. Can J Neurol Sci 1991;18:476-87.

Bloedel JR, Bracha V, Larson PS. Real time operations of the cerebellar cortex. Can J Neurol Sci 1993;20:7-18.

Bogen JE. On the neurophysiology of consciousness: part II. Constraining the semantic problem (see comments). Conscious Cogn 1995;4:137-58.

Boyd IA. The isolated mammalian muscle spindle. In: Evarts E, Wise S, Bousfield D, eds. The motor system in neurobiology. Amsterdam: Elsevier, 1985:154-67.

Brooks DJ. Parkinson's disease—a single clinical entity? Q J Med 1995;88:81-91.

Burchiel KJ. Thalamotomy for movement disorders. Neurosurg Clin N Am 1995;6:55-71.

Burgess PR, Wei JY. Signaling of kinesthetic information by peripheral sensory receptors. Ann Rev Neurosci 1982;5:171-87.

Burke D. Critical examination of the case for or against fusimotor involvement in disorders of muscle tone. Adv Neurol 1983;39:133-50.

Burke D. Muscle spindle function during movement. In: Evarts EV, Wise SP, Bousfield D, eds. The motor system in neurobiology. Amsterdam: Elsevier, 1985:168-72.

Burke D, Gandevia SC, McKeon B. The afferent volleys responsible for spinal proprioceptive reflexes in man. J Physiol (Lond) 1983;339:535-52.

Burke D, Gandevia SC, McKeon B. Monosynaptic and oligosynaptic contributions to human ankle jerk and H-reflex. J Neurophysiol 1984;52:435-48.

Burke D, Gracies JM, Mazevet D, Meunier S, Pierrot-Deseilligny E. Convergence of descending and various peripheral inputs onto common propriospinal-like neurones in man. J Physiol (Lond) 1992;449:655-71.

Burke RE. Control systems operating on spinal reflex mechanisms. J Neurosci Res Prog Bull 1971;9:60-85.

Burke RE. On the central nervous system control of fast and slow twitch motor units. New Dev Electromyogr Clin Neurophysiol 1973;3:69-94.

Calabresi P, Pisani A, Mercuri NB, Bernardi G. The corticostriatal projection: from synaptic plasticity to dysfunctions of the basal ganglia. Trends Neurosci 1996;19:19-24.

Carp JS, Wolpaw JR. Motoneuron plasticity underlying operantly conditioned decrease in primate H-reflex. J Neurophysiol 1995;72:431-42.

Contreras Vidal JL, Stelmach GE. A neural model of basal ganglia-thalamocortical relations in normal and Parkinsonian movement. Biol Cybern 1995;73:467-76.

Cote L, Crutcher MD. The basal ganglia. In: Kandel ER, Schwartz JH, Jessell TM, eds. Principles of neural science, 3rd ed. Norwalk: Appleton & Lange, 1991.

Denise P, Darlot C. The cerebellum as a predictor of neural messages—II. Role in motor control and motion sickness. Neuroscience 1993;56:647-55.

Dominey P, Decety J, Broussolle E, Chazot G, Jeannerod M. Motor imagery of a lateralized sequential task is asymmetrically slowed in hemi-Parkinsons's patients. Neuropsychologia 1995;33:727-41.

du Lac S, Lisberger SG. Eye movements and brainstem neuronal responses evoked by cerebellar and vestibular stimulation in chicks. J Comp Physiol 1992;171:629-38.

Edin BB, Vallbo AB. Dynamic response of human muscle spindle afferents to stretch. J Neurophysiol 1990;63:1297-1306.

Ferster D, Spruston N. Cracking the neuronal code. Science 1995;270:756-7.

Fournier E, Katz R, Pierrot-Deseilligny E. Descending control of reflex pathways in the production of voluntary isolated movements in man. Brain Res 1983;288:375-7.

Gandevia SC, Burke D. Does the nervous system depend on kinesthetic information to control natural limb movements? Behav Brain Sci 1992;15:614-32.

Gandevia SC, McCloskey DI, Burke D. Kinaesthetic signals and muscle contraction. Trends Neurosci 1992;15:62-5.

Gao J, Parsons LM, Bower JM, Xiong J, Li J, Fox PT. Cerebellum implicated in sensory acquisition and discrimination rather than motor control. Science 1996;272:545-7.

Ghez C, Shinoda Y. Spinal mechanisms of the functional stretch reflex. Exp Brain Res 1978;32:55-68.

Glickstein M, Voogd J. Lodewijk Bolk and the comparative anatomy of the cerebellum. Trends Neurosci 1995;28:206-10.

Gottlieb GL, Agarwal GC. Modulation of postural reflexes by voluntary movement. J Neurol Neurosurg Psychiatry 1973;36:529-39.

Griffiths RI. Shortening of muscle fibres during stretch of the active cat medial gastrocnemius muscle: the role of tendon compliance. J Physiol (Lond) 1991;436:219-36.

Heimer L, Switzer RD, van Hoesen GW. Ventral striatum and ventral pallidum. In: Evarts EV, Wise SP, Bousfield D, eds. Amsterdam: Elsevier, 1985:259-69.

Horak FB, Nashner LM. Central programming of postural movements: adaptation to altered support-surface configurations. J Neurophysiol 1986;55:1369-81.

Houk JC. Regulation of stiffness by skeletomotor reflexes. Ann Rev Physiol 1979;41:99-114.

Houk JC, Henneman E. Responses of Golgi tendon organs to active contraction of the soleus muscle of the cat. J Neurophysiol 1967;30:466-81.

Iacono RP, Lonser RR, Oh A, Yamada S. New pathophysiology of Parkinson's disease revealed by posteroventral pallidotomy. Neurol Res 1995;17:178-80.

Inglis JT, Frank JS, Inglis B. The effect of muscle vibration on human position sense during movements controlled by lengthening muscle contraction. Exp Brain Res 1991;84:631-4.

Jahnke MT, Struppler A. Responses of human muscle spindle afferents during isotonic position holding and active movements. Brain Res 1990;515:181-6.

Jami L. Golgi tendon organs in mammalian skeletal muscle: functional properties and central actions. Physiol Rev 1992;72:623-66.

Jankowska E. Interneuronal relay in spinal pathways from proprioceptors. Prog Neurobiol 1992;38:335-78.

Jankowska E, Edgley S. Interactions between pathways controlling posture and gait at the level of spinal interneurones in the cat. Prog Brain Res 1993;971:161-71.

Lackner JR. Some proprioceptive influences on the perceptual representation of body shape and orientation. Brain 1988;111:281-97.

Lee MS, Marsden CD. Movement disorders following lesions of the thalamus or subthalamic region. Mov Disord 1994;9:493-507.

Leigh RJ, Brandt T. A reevaluation of the vestibulo-ocular reflex: new ideas of its purpose, properties, neural substrate, and disorders. Neurology 1993;43:1288-95.

Loeb GE, Duysens J. Activity patterns in individual hindlimb primary and secondary muscle spindle afferents during normal movements in unrestrained cats. J Neurophysiol 1979;42:420-40.

Loeb GE, He J, Levine WS. Spinal cord circuits: are they mirrors of musculoskeletal mechanics? J Motor Behav 1989;21:473-91.

Lundberg A. Control of spinal mechanics from the brain. In: Tower DB, ed. The nervous system. New York: Raven Press, 1975:253-65.

Lundberg A, Malmgren K, Schomburg ED. Reflex pathways from group II muscle afferents. Exp Brain Res 1987;65:294-306.

Macefield G, Hagbarth KE, Gorman R, Gandevia SC, Burke D. Decline in spindle support to alpha motoneurons during sustained voluntary contractions. J Physiol (Lond) 1991;440:497-512.

Maln'ar Z, Blakemore C. How do thalamic axons find their way to the cortex? Trends Neurosci 1995;18:389-97.

Marsden CD. The mysterious motor function of the basal ganglia. Neurology 1982;32:514-39.

Marsden CD. The enigma of the basal ganglia and movement. In: Evarts EV, Wise SP, Bousfield D, eds. The motor system in neurobiology. Amsterdam: Elsevier, 1985:277-84.

Marsden CD, Obeso JA. The functions of the basal ganglia and the paradox of stereotaxic surgery in Parkinson's disease. Brain 1994;118:822.

Masino T. Brainstem control of orienting movements: intrinsic coordinate systems and underlying circuitry. Brain Behav Evol 1992;40:98-111.

Matthews PBC. Evidence from the use of vibration that the human long-latency stretch reflex depends upon spindle secondary afferents. J Physiol (Lond) 1984;348:383-415.

McCrea DA. Spinal cord circuitry and motor reflexes. In: Pandolf KB, ed. Exercise and sport science reviews, vol 14. New York: Macmillan, 1986:105-41.

McCrea DA. Can sense be made of spinal interneuron circuits? Behav Brain Sci 1992;15:633-43.

Messaros A. Age-induced adaptations to the motor unit. Neurol Rep 1994;18:22-5.

Moore JC. The Golgi tendon organ: a review and update. Am J Occup Ther 1984;38:227-36.

Murphy PR, Martin HA. Fusimotor discharge patterns during rhythmic movements. Trends Neurosci 1993;16:273-8.

Ojakangas CL, Ebner TJ. Purkinje cell complex spike activity during voluntary motor learning: relationship to kinematics. J Neurophysiol 1994;72:2617-30.

Paskavitz JF, Lippa CF, Hamos JE, Pulaski Salo D, Drachman DA. Role of the dorsomedial nucleus of the thalamus in Alzheimer's disease. J Geriatr Psychiatry Neurol 1995;8:32-7.

Pastor AM, Delacruz RR, Baker R. Eye position and eye velocity integrators reside in separate brainstem nuclei. Proc Natl Acad Sci USA 1994;91:807-11.

Pearson KG, Collins DF. Reversal of the influence of group Ib afferents from plantaris on activity in medial gastrocnemius muscle during locomotor activity. J Neurophysiol 1993;70:1009-17.

Pearson KG, Ramirez JM, Jiang W. Entrainment of the locomotor rhythm by group Ib afferents from ankle extensor muscles in spinal cats. Exp Brain Res 1992;90:557-66.

Proske U. The Golgi tendon organ. Trends Neurosci 1979;2:7-8.

Reinkling RM, Stephens JA, Stuart DG. The tendon organs of cat medial gastrocnemius: significance of motor unit type and size for activation of Ib afferents. J Physiol (Lond) 1975;250:491-512.

Rispal-Padel L, Harnois C, Troiani D. Converging cerebellofugal inputs to the thalamus. Exp Brain Res 1987;68:47-58.

Rolls ET. Neurophysiology and cognitive functions of the striatum. Rev Neurol Paris 1994;150:648-60.

Rossignol S, Lund JP, Drew, T. The role of sensory inputs in regulating patterns of rhythmical movements in higher vertebrates. A comparison between locomotion, respiration and mastication. In: Cohen AH, Rossignol S, Grillner S, eds. Neural control of rhythmic movements in vertebrates. New York: John Wiley & Sons, 1988:201-84.

Rothwell JC, Gandevia SC, Burke D. Activation of fusimotor neurones by motor cortical stimulation in human subjects. J Physiol (Lond) 1990;431:743-56.

Ryding E, Decety J, Sjoholm H, Stenberg G, Ingvar DH. Motor imagery activates the cerebellum regionally. A SPECT rCBF study with 99mTc-HMPAO. Brain Res 1993;1:94-9.

Saint Cyr JA, Taylor AE, Nicholson K. Behavior and the basal ganglia. Adv Neurol 1995;65:1-28.

Sanes JN, Dimitrov B, Hallett M. Motor learning in patients with cerebellar dysfunction. Brain 1990;113:103-20.

Schafer SS. Regularity in the generation of discharge patterns by primary and secondary muscle spindle afferents, as recorded under a ramp-and-hold stretch. Exp Brain Res 1994;102:198-209.

Scholz JP, Campbell SK. Muscle spindles and the regulation of movement. Phys Ther 1980;60:1416-23.

Schwindt PC. Control of motoneuron output by pathways descending from the brain stem. In: Towe AL, Luschei ES, eds. Handbook of behavioral neuobiology: motor coordination. New York: Plenum Press, 1981:139-230.

Scott SH, Loeb GE. The computation of position sense from spindles in mono- and multiarticular muscles. J Neurosci 1994;14:7529-40.

Shumway-Cook A, Woollacott MH. Motor control: theory and applications. Baltimore: Williams & Wilkins, 1995.

Simard CP, Spector SA, Edgerton VR. Contractile properties of rat hindlimb muscles immobilized at different lengths. Exp Neurol 1982;77:467-82.

Solodkin M, Jiminez I, Rudomin P. Identification of common interneurons mediating pre- and postsynaptic inhibition in the cat spinal cord. Science 1984;224:1453-6.

Stelmach GE, Phillips JG. Movement disorders—limb movement and the basal ganglia. Phys Ther 1991;71:60-7.

Turker KS, Brodin P, Miles TS. Reflex responses of motor units in human masseter muscle to mechanical stimulation of a tooth. Exp Brain Res 1992;100:307-15.

Vallbo AB, al Falahe NA. Human muscle spindle response in a motor learning task. J Physiol (Lond) 1990;421:553-68.

Welsh JP, Lang EJ, Suglhara I, Rodolfo L. Dynamic organization of motor control within the olivocerebellar system. Nature 1995;374:453-7.

Westmoreland BF, Benarroch EE, Daube JR, Reagan TJ, Sandok BA. Medical neurosciences. Boston: Little Brown & Co, 1994.

Wolpaw JR, Maniccia DM, Elia T. Operant conditioning of primate H-reflex: phases of development. Neurosci Lett 1994;170:203-7.

REFERENCES

1. Afifi AK. Basal ganglia: functional anatomy and physiology. Part 2. J Child Neurol 1994;9:352-61.

2. Albin RL, Young AB, Penney JB. The functional anatomy of disorders of the basal ganglia. Trends Neurosci 1995;18:63-4.

3. Allen G, Buxton RB, Wong EC, Courchesne E. Attentional activation of the cerebellum independent of motor involvement. Science 1997;275:1940-3.

4. Armstrong E. A comparative review of the primate motor system. J Motor Behav 1989;21:493-517.

5. Arshavsky YI, Gelfand I, Orlovsky GN. The cerebellum and the control of rhythmical movements. In: Evarts EV, Wise SP, Bousfield D, eds. The motor system in neurobiology. Amsterdam: Elsevier, 1985:87-97.

6. Barinaga M. Social status sculpts activity of crayfish neurons. Science 1996;271:290-1.

7. Bregman BS, Goldberger ME. Infant lesion effect. III. anatomical correlates of sparing and recovery of function after spinal cord damage in newborn and adult cats. Dev Brain Res 1983;9:137-54.

8. Brooks DJ. The role of the basal ganglia in motor control: contributions from PET. J Neurol Sci 1995;128:1-13.

9. Burke D, Hagbarth K, Lofstedt L. Muscle spindle activity in man during shortening and lengthening contractions. J Physiol (Lond) 1978;277:131-42.

10. Carew TJ. Descending control of spinal circuits. In: Kandel ER, Schwartz JH, eds. Principles of neural science. New York: Elsevier, 1981:312-22.

11. Carp JS, Wolpaw JR. Motoneuron properties after operantly conditioned increase in primate H-reflex. J Neurophysiol 1995;73:1365-73.

12. Chen XY, Wolpaw JR. Operant conditioning of H-reflex in freely moving rats [abstract]. J Neurophysiol 1995;73:411-5.

13. Connolly CI, Burns JB. A new striatal model and its relationship to basal ganglia diseases. Neurosci Res 1993;16:271-4.

14. Connor NP, Abbs JH. Sensorimotor contributions of the basal ganglia: recent advances. Phys Ther 1990;70:864-72.

15. Dichgans J, Diener HC. Different forms of postural ataxia in patients with cerebellar diseases. In: Igarashi M, Black FO, eds. Disorders of posture and gait. Amsterdam: Elsevier, 1986:207-13.

16. Evatt ML, Wolf SL, Segal RL. Modification of human spinal stretch reflexes: preliminary studies. Neurosci Lett 1989;105:350-5.

17. Forssberg H, Eliasson AC, Kinoshita H, Westling G, Johansson RS. Development of human precision grip. IV. Tactile adaptation of isometric finger forces to the frictional condition. Exp Brain Res 1995;104:323-30.

18. Garland SJ, McComas AJ. Reflex inhibition of human soleus muscle during fatigue. J Physiol (Lond) 1990;429:17-27.

19. Ghez C, Gordon JG. An introduction to movement. In: Kandel ER, Schwartz JH, Jessell TM. Essentials of neural science and behavior. Norwalk: Appleton & Lange, 1995:485-500.

20. Gordon AM, Forssberg H, Iwasaki N. Formation and lateralization of internal representations underlying motor commands during precision grip. Neuropsychologia 1994;32:555-67.

21. Gray H, Bannister LH, Berry MM. Gray's anatomy: the anatomical basis of medicine and surgery (British ed), 38th ed. Edinburg: Churchill Livingstone, 1996.

22. Graybiel AM. The basal ganglia. Trends Neurosci 1995;18:60-2.

23. Graybiel AM, Aosaki T, Flaherty AW, Kimura M. The basal ganglia and adaptive motor control. Science 1994;265:1826-32.

24. Gross CG. Aristotle on the brain. Neuroscience 1995;1:245-50.

25. Holmqvist B, Lundberg A. Differential supraspinal control of synaptic actions evoked by volleys in the flexion reflex afferents in alpha motoneurones. Acta Physiol Scand 1961;54:5-51.

26. Horak FB, Diener HC. Cerebellar control of postural scaling and central set in stance. J Neurophysiol 1994;72:479-93.

27. Hore J, Wild B, Diener HC. Cerebellar dysmetria at the elbow, wrist and fingers. J Neurophysiol 1991;65:563-71.

28. Houk JC. Cooperative control of limb movements by the motor cortex, brain stem and cerebellum. In: Cotterill RMJ, ed. Models of brain function. London: Cambridge University Press, 1989:309-25.

29. Hulliger M. Fusimotor control of proprioceptive feedback during locomotion and balancing: can simple lessons be learned for artificial control of gait. Prog Brain Res 1993;97:173-80.

30. Hulliger M, Sjolander P, Windhorst UR, Otten E. Force coding by populations of cat Golgi tendon organ afferents: the role of muscle length and motor unit pool activation strategies. In: Taylor A, Gladden MH, Durrbaba R, eds. Alpha and gamma motor systems. New York: Plenum Press, 1995:302-8.

31. Kennedy PR. Corticospinal, rubrospinal and rubro-olivary projections: a unifying hypothesis. Trends Neurosci 1990;13:474-9.

32. Kim SG, Ugurbil K, Strick PL. Activation of a cerebellar output nucleus during cognitive processing. Science 1994;2265:949-51.

33. Kimura M. Physiological bases of involuntary movement. Rinsho-Shinkeigaku Clin Neurol 1994;34:1241-2.

34. Kimura M. Role of basal ganglia in behavioral learning. Neurosci Res 1995;22:353-8.

35. Kinomura S, Larsson J, Gulyas B, Roland PE. Activation by attention of the human reticular formation and thalamic intralaminar nuclei. Science 1996;271:512-4.

36. Kumral E, Kocaer T, Ertubey NO, Kumral K. Thalamic hemorrhage. A prospective study of 100 patients. Stroke 1995;226:964-70.

37. Lance JW, McLeod JG. A physiological approach to clinical neurology. London: Butterworths, 1975.

38. Leiner HC, Leiner AL, Dow RS. The underestimated cerebellum. Human Brain Mapping 1995;2:244-54.

39. Lenz FA, Gracely RH, Romanoski A, Hope EJ, Rowland LH, Dougherty PM. Stimulation in the human somatosensory thalamus can reproduce both the affective and sensory dimensions of previously experienced pain. Nature Med 1995;1:885-7.

40. Leonard CT, Goldberger ME. Consequences of damage to the sensorimotor cortex in neonatal and adult cats. II. Maintenance of exuberant projections. Dev Brain Res 1987;32:15-30.

41. Leonard CT, Hirschfeld H, Moritani T, Forssberg H. Myotatic reflex development in normal children and children with cerebral palsy. Exp Neurol 1991;111:379-82.

42. Leonard CT, Kane J, Perdaems J, Frank C, Graetzer DG, Moritani T. Neural modulation of muscle contractile properties during fatigue: afferent feedback dependence. Electroencephalogr Clin Neurophysiol 1994;93:209-17.

43. Leonard CT, Matsumoto T, Diedrich P. Human myotatic reflex development of the lower extremities. Early Hum Dev 1995;43:75-93.

44. Lundberg A, Voorhoeve P. Effects from the pyramidal tract on spinal reflex arcs. Acta Physiol Scand 1962;56:201-19.

45. McCormick DA. The cerebellar symphony. Nature 1995;374:412-3.

46. Middleton FA, Strick PL. Anatomical evidence for cerebellar and basal ganglia involvement in higher cognitive function. Science 1994;266:458-61.

47. Mink JW, Thach WT. Basal ganglia motor control. I. Nonexclusive relation of pallidal discharge to five movement modes. J Neurophysiol 1991;65:273-300.

48. Mink JW, Thach WT. Basal ganglia motor control. II. Late pallidal timing relative to movement onset and inconsistent pallidal coding of movement parameters. J Neurophysiol 1991;65:301-29.

49. Mink JW, Thach WT. Basal ganglia motor control. III. Pallidal ablation: normal reaction time, muscle cocontraction, and slow movement. J Neurophysiol 1991;65:330-51.

50. Newman J. Thalamic contributions to attention and consciousness [comment]. Conscious Cogn 1995;4:172-93.

51. Nolte J. The human brain. St. Louis: Mosby-Year Book, 1988.

52. Pantano P, Formisano R, Ricci M, et al. Prolonged muscular flaccidity after stroke. Morphological and functional brain alterations. Brain 1995;118:1329-38.

53. Prochazka A, Hulliger M. Muscle afferent function and its significance for motor control mechanisms during voluntary movements in cat, monkey, and man. In: Desmedt JE, ed. Motor control mechanisms in health and disease. New York: Raven Press, 1983:93-132.

54. Prochazka A, Hulliger M, Zangger P, Appenteng K. "Fusimotor set": new evidence of alpha-independent control of gamma-motoneurones during movement in the awake cat. Brain Res 1985;339:136-40.

55. Raichle ME, Fiez JA, Videen TO, et al. Practice-related changes in human brain functional anatomy during nonmotor learning. Cereb Cortex 1994;4:8-26.

56. Raos VC, Savaki HE. Functional anatomy of the thalamic reticular nucleus as revealed with the [14C]deoxyglucose method following electrical stimulation and electrolytic lesion. Neuroscience 1995;68:287-97.

57. Schomburg ED. Spinal sensorimotor systems and their supraspinal control. Neurosci Res 1990;7:265-340.

58. Segal RL, Wolf SL. Operant conditioning of spinal stretch reflexes in patients with spinal cord injuries. Exp Neurol 1994;130:202-13.

59. Shibasaki H, et al. Both primary motor cortex and supplementary motor area play an important role in complex finger movement. Brain 1993;116:1387-98.

60. Thach WT, Goodkin HP, Keating JG. The cerebellum and the adaptive coordination of movement. Ann Rev Neurosci 1992;15:403-42.

61. Wolf SL, Segal RL. Reducing human biceps brachii spinal stretch reflex magnitude. J Neurophysiol 1996;75:1637-46.

62. Wolpaw JR, Herchenroder PA. Operant conditioning of H-reflex in freely moving monkeys. J Neurosci Methods 1990;31:145-52.

63. Wolpaw JR, O'Keefe JA. Adaptive plasticity in the primate spinal stretch reflex: evidence for a two-phase process. J Neurosci 1984;4:2718-24.

Principles of Reflex Action and Motor Control

General Principles of Neural Transmission and Signal Processing
Reflex Circuitry Involved with Agonist Muscle Activation
Reflex Circuitry Involved with Antagonist Muscle Activation
Flexor Reflex Afferents
Central Pattern Generators
Modulation of Reflex Activity
Long-Loop Transcortical Reflexes
Descending Control of Segmental Circuitry
Making Sense and Nonsense of Spinal Cord Connectivity

Rene Descartes was a seventeenth century philosopher most widely remembered for his beliefs that the mind and body were separate entities and that the pineal gland represented the seat of the human soul. Descartes is also widely given credit for being the first to describe reflexes. He presented the idea that sensory stimuli cause events in the nervous system that result in a motor response. He might not have had the mechanisms correct (as you can tell from the legend on the facing page), but, as you will read in this chapter, reflex theory is absolutely correct and forms the basis of much human movement.

The previous chapter focused on the functioning of neural structures that have an impact on human movement. Hopefully you saw that not just the function of the structure is important, but also its connectivity with other structures. In fact, the connectivity between structures actually determines function, because the ionic and chemical processes involved with neural transmission are essentially identical throughout the nervous system. The ionic and chemical processes involved in neural transmission are relatively simple. Behavioral complexity is achieved via diverse divergent and convergent connectivity as well as specific cellular properties.

This chapter will introduce generalized rules regarding neural transmission and nervous system connectivity. The focus will be primarily spinal cord circuitry and descending influences on this circuitry.

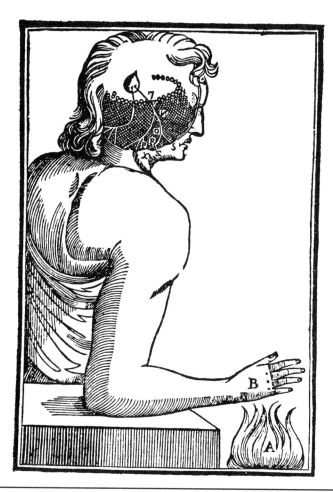

"If fire A burns hand B and causes the spirits entering tube 7 to tend toward O, these spirits find there two pores or principal passages OR and OS. One of them, namely OR, conducts the spirits into all nerves that serve to move the external members in the manner necessary to avoid the force of this action, such as those that withdraw the hand or the arm or the entire body and those that turn the head and the eyes for protection against it. And through the other passage, OS, the spirits enter all those nerves that cause internal emotions like those that pain occasions in us, such as nerves that constrict the heart, agitate the liver, and other such." (From Descartes R: Treatise of man; translation by Hall TS. Cambridge, Mass.: Harvard University Press, 1972.)

Brain stem circuits such as the reticulospinal, rubrospinal, and vestibulospinal tracts were discussed in Chapter 2. The brain stem tectospinal tract will be discussed in Chapter 5 and brain stem locomotor centers will be presented in Chapter 6. The connectivity, of course, differs, but the general principles regarding transmission and input integration are similar for the spinal cord, brain stem, and other central nervous system (CNS) structures.

Processing and interpreting incoming sensory stimuli are two major functions of the human nervous system. These processes begin at the cellular level and increase in refinement and complexity as nerve cells combine to form functional units and connect with neurons subserving different functions. Interpretation of your world, and your place in it, begins far from your conscious awareness; it begins with a peripheral receptor and a cell membrane.

■ GENERAL PRINCIPLES OF NEURAL TRANSMISSION AND SIGNAL PROCESSING

Every neuron has a *resting membrane potential*. This is defined as the difference in the electrical charge between the inside and the outside of the cell. Neurons have a negative resting membrane potential of approximately –65mV. Afferent input to the neuron that moves the resting membrane potential in a negative direction is said to cause *hyperpolarization*. Input that moves the resting membrane potential in a positive direction is termed *depolarization*. Hyperpolarization makes a neuron less likely to reach an *action potential threshold* (*spike threshold*) and is, therefore, referred to as *inhibitory*. Any input that depolarizes the neuron is *excitatory*. The summation of inhibitory and excitatory input onto a neuron determines whether that neuron will achieve an action potential and thus transmit the incoming information to other parts of the nervous system.

Let's consider the sense of touch. You reach out to touch a raindrop that has formed on your window. Several different types of skin receptors will respond to the characteristics of the raindrop and convey the sensations of wet, cold, soft, etc. (or more specifically, signals related to humidity, temperature, and texture) to the sensory neuron located in the dorsal root ganglion. As you lift your hand to look at the tip of your finger, thereby stimulating retinal receptors in the eye (and a quite different receptor physiology story), the droplet gently flows down your finger and forearm, thereby stimulating additional receptors from these parts of your anatomy. Regardless of the sensory neuron involved, receptor stimulation will result in *receptor potentials* (also referred to as generator potentials), which are a change in the sensory neuron's resting potential. The amplitude and duration of receptor potentials vary depending on the intensity of the sensory stimulation. Not all receptor potentials result in an action potential and the propagation of information. Only if the receptor potential exceeds the sensory spike threshold will an action potential result (Fig. 3-1). If the incoming sensory stimulus is intense, it will cause a large receptor potential amplitude. The large receptor potential amplitude will not result in any change in action potential amplitude. An action potential follows the all-or-none principle and does not vary in amplitude. Rather, a large receptor potential will cause an increased rate of action potential firing. The increased action potential rate results in more neurotransmitter being released from the stimulated neuron's presynaptic membrane. The amount of time that a receptor potential exceeds the spike threshold (the *duration* of stimulus) determines the number of action potentials. The greater the number of action potentials, the greater the amount of neurotransmitter release. The greater the amount of a specific transmitter being released, the greater likelihood that it will have an effect on its target (postsynaptic) cell. Thus, sensory neurons convey the intensity of sensory stimulation by changes in the amplitude of its receptor potentials and therefore the rate of action potentials it generates. The duration of the sensory stimulus determines the length of time that action potentials are generated.

Sensory neuron action potentials cause release of neurotransmitters from the presynaptic terminal. The transmitters bind with the postsynaptic membrane of the target neuron if the postsynaptic membrane contains receptors for the transmitter. This will cause a *synaptic potential* in the postsynaptic neuron. If the synaptic potential causes hyperpolarization of the neural membrane, it is termed an *inhibitory postsynaptic potential* (IPSP). If it causes a depolarization, it is termed an *excitatory postsynaptic potential* (EPSP).

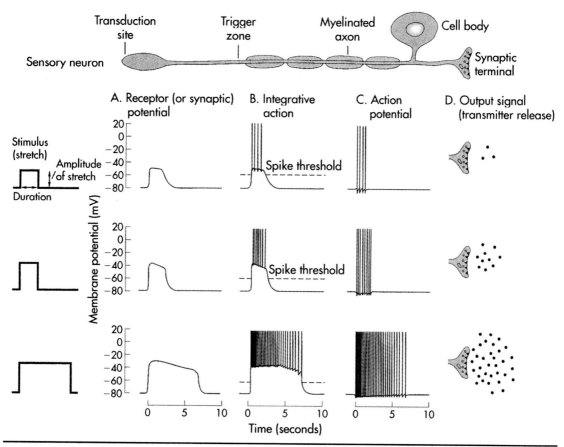

Fig. 3-1. A sensory neuron transforms a physical stimulus into an electrical signal. The receptor potential's amplitude and duration are proportional to the amplitude and duration of the sensory stimulus. Column *A* illustrates three graded receptor potentials. In Column *B* the receptor potentials have exceeded the spike threshold and have generated action potentials. Note that the action potentials have the same amplitude regardless of the receptor potential amplitude. Greater receptor potential amplitudes result in increased action potential rate. In column *C*, we see that the longer the duration of the stimulus, the greater the number of action potentials. Column *D* shows that action potentials cause release of neurotransmitter at the synaptic terminal. The amount of transmitter released depends on the number of action potentials arriving at the terminal per unit time. (From Kandel ER, Schwartz JH, Jessell TM. Essentials of neuroscience and behavior. Norwalk, Conn: Appleton & Lange, 1995.)

The type of receptor on the postsynaptic membrane determines whether the neurotransmitter causes an IPSP or an EPSP.

A single EPSP is not likely to cause an action potential in the postsynaptic neuron. Neurons receive multiple and diverse input. An alpha motor neuron in the spinal cord might receive 10,000 inputs, a Purkinje cell in the cerebellum about 200,000. The neuron's postsynaptic membrane sums incoming IPSPs and EPSPs. If EPSPs summate sufficiently (i.e., to the spike threshold), an action potential results.

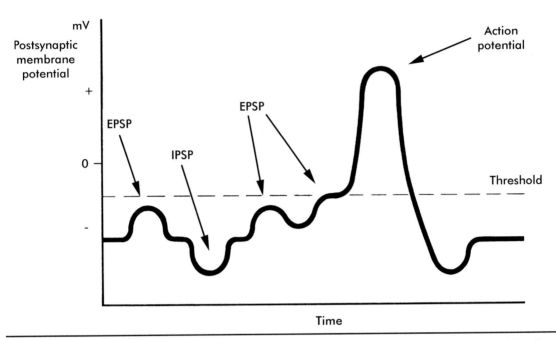

Fig. 3-2. The summation of EPSPs and IPSPs at the postsynaptic terminal. EPSPs move the curve in a positive direction and thus toward an action potential threshold, whereas an IPSP moves the curve in a negative direction and away from threshold. (Adapted from Fredericks CM, Saladin LK. Pathophysiology of the motor systems. Philadelphia: FA Davis, 1996.)

In this way every nerve cell can integrate input from multiple sources. Cell membranes, far from your conscious thoughts, begin the process of interpreting your world.

EPSPs and IPSPs can summate either via temporal summation or spatial summation. The number of inputs per unit time determines whether temporal summation occurs. The more inputs coming in during a short period from a specific source(s) that produce similar effects on the postsynaptic membrane, the more likely these inputs will summate and have an effect on the postsynaptic membrane (Fig. 3-2). In other words, *temporal summation* occurs when inter-event intervals are shorter than the duration of the postsynaptic potential.

Spatial summation refers to EPSPs or IPSPs being caused by multiple neural inputs. EPSPs cause depolarization and IPSPs cause hyperpolarization. The more sources sending either EPSPs or IPSPs increase the likelihood that the neuron will be moved toward depolarization or hyperpolarization, respectively. If EPSP input is sufficient, spike threshold will be obtained and an action potential will result. Similar to temporal summation, spatial summation occurs when inputs arrive during the duration of the postsynaptic potential.

In addition to membrane mechanisms, a single neuron has other means of organizing input. Convergence and divergence are two methods by which this is accomplished (Fig. 3-3). *Convergence* refers to the arrival of diverse input from multiple locations to a single neuron or location. Neural *divergence* refers to a neuron's ability to exert an influence on multiple target sites. This is accomplished by axonal branching and the formation of multiple synapses with more than one neural target. The spinothal-

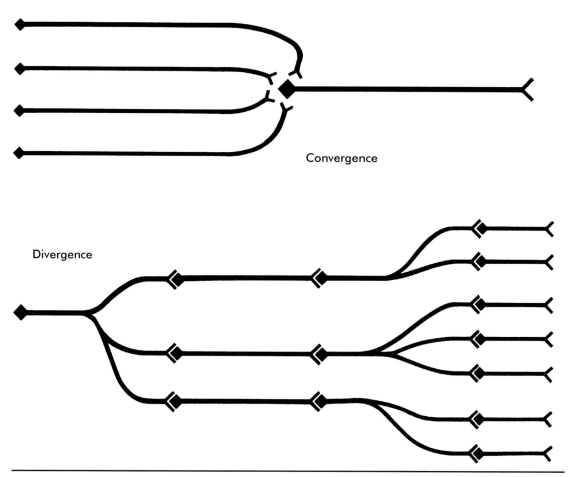

Convergence

Divergence

Fig. 3-3. Convergence refers to neural input from a multitude of sources to a single neuron or location. Divergence refers to the spread of neural output via axonal branching from a single source to multiple locations.

amic tract and postganglionic nerves of the autonomic nervous system are classic examples of divergence and the wide distribution of effects a single neuron can have within the nervous system.

In addition to mechanisms that allow afferent stimuli to spread to different regions of the nervous system, other mechanisms serve to isolate afferent input. *Lateral (surround) inhibition* is a mechanism that assists in the localization and discrimination of incoming sensory information (Fig. 3-4). This effect is achieved by inhibitory interneurons. An incoming sensory stimulus activates sensory receptors that relay this information to sensory neurons. These neurons then convey the sensory message to other parts of the nervous system. In addition, they will also synapse on inhibitory interneurons that will inhibit adjacent sensory neurons. This action creates an isolated point of excitation surrounded by inhibition, which aids in the identification, localization, and interpretation of intensity of the sensory input. Other terms such as feed-forward, feedback, and distal inhibition refer to specific inhibitory mechanisms that contribute to lateral inhibition. These mechanisms interact to filter input so that we can discriminate between multiple inputs and focus attention on those that are most important for a given situation. Increasing the focus of

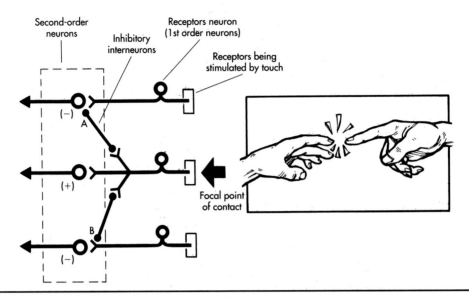

Fig. 3-4. Lateral (surround) inhibition: The receptors in the fingertip that are located at the focus of the touch will have receptor potentials that are greater in amplitude and duration than those receptors located more peripheral to the stimulus. In addition, the receptors at the focal point of contact will synapse on inhibitory interneurons that can inhibit adjacent neurons postsynaptically (*A*) or presynaptically (*B*). These mechanisms allow isolation of a sensory stimulus and a determination of its location.

attention to particular inputs and combining input into meaningful arrays are accomplished by several additional mechanisms.

In some situations within the CNS, filtering out information is not desirable; rather, increasing the information-carrying capacity of a certain pathway or a system of pathways is beneficial. One such information processing mechanism thought to be used throughout the nervous system is parallel processing.

Parallel processing refers to similar information being conveyed by multiple sources. The sources can be as varied as different pathways or be parallel axons within a pathway. The fact that different pathways convey similar information does not necessarily mean they will result in the same outcomes. Perhaps the pathways convey information to different regions within the CNS. Perhaps the pathways synapse on different neurons within the same nucleus. Parallel processing increases information-carrying abilities and appears to be a general feature throughout the human CNS. It results is some redundancy within the CNS, which proves beneficial if one area or pathway becomes dysfunctional through injury or disease.

And don't think that parallel processing is just an esoteric neuroscientific concept. The 1996 world chess champion, Russian Garry Kasparov, has earned the dubious distinction of being the first world champion to lose to a computer that used parallel processing. Deep Blue, the computer, had numerous parallel processors that allowed it to evaluate millions of possible chess piece movements in seconds. Computer modelers have increasingly taken interest in human physiology, especially brain physiology, to create artificial intelligence and thinking machines. But, they still haven't designed a machine that can do standup comedy or scratch an itch.

We will now progress from speaking in generalities about neural membranes and organizational principles, to brief discussions of segmental circuitry that underlie specific functions.

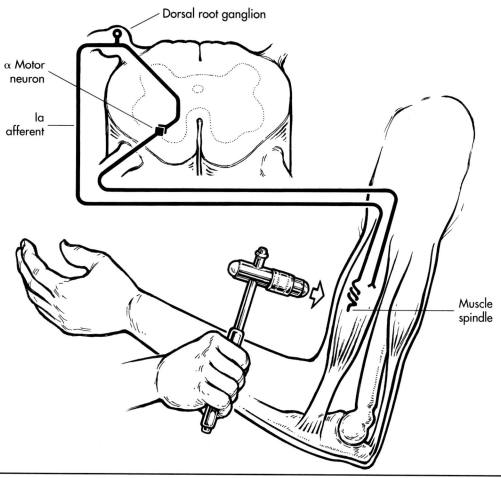

Fig. 3-5. The monosynaptic component of the stretch reflex. Brisk stretching of a muscle causes a stretch receptor (muscle spindle) to respond. These receptor potentials are conveyed via Ia sensory afferents directly to alpha motor neurons. If the stretch is strong enough, the alpha motor neurons cause an action potential that results in the contraction of the stretched muscle.

■ REFLEX CIRCUITRY INVOLVED WITH AGONIST MUSCLE ACTIVATION

We move in response to sensory stimulation. We might be moved to respond verbally to kind words from a friend or we might withdraw a limb from a painful stimulus. Both of these motor acts were initiated by differing sensory inputs. The wiring of humans is consistent with chemical and physical laws: For every action there is a reaction, for every stimulus, a response. Humans have a movement repertoire that is the envy of the planet. Yet, a primary building block of our movements—the monosynaptic reflex—is present even in lowly invertebrates. One of the classic monosynaptic reflexes is the stretch reflex. The stretch reflex is a good place to begin to gain an understanding of how nervous system connectivity dictates movement patterns. It is also a good example of the relationship between sensory input and motor output.

Stretching a muscle activates muscle spindles and causes the stretched muscle to contract. Testing a stretch reflex is one of the first neurological tests taught to clinicians. Tapping a tendon stretches the muscle and elicits a contraction. The circuitry involved is fairly straightforward (Fig. 3-5). Stretch receptors

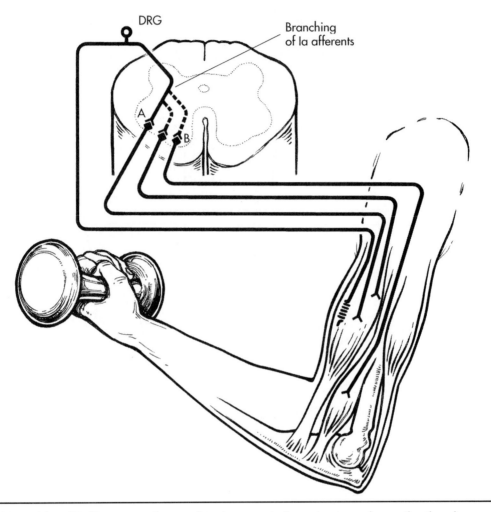

Fig. 3-6. Branching of Ia fibers to muscle synergists: **A** represents the motor neuron innervating the primary mover. It receives a direct projection from the Ia or other sensory fibers. **B** represents synergist motor neurons. They also receive input from the sensory fibers innervating the primary mover. This is one mechanism whereby multiple muscles can be recruited for a particular task.

(i.e., muscle spindles) within the muscle convey their excitatory message via Ia afferent fibers directly to the motor neurons innervating the stretched muscle. Only two neurons, a sensory neuron in the dorsal root ganglion and a motor neuron in the ventral horn of the spinal cord, are involved. It is called a *monosynaptic reflex* because only one synapse is involved. The Ia afferent that is conveying the sensory information from the stretched muscle, however, tends to branch and convey its message elsewhere as well. Some branches will ascend to higher brain centers to inform them of changes in peripheral conditions; others will synapse on various interneurons, and still others will synapse on motor neurons of synergist muscles.

Synergist muscles share a similar mode of action as the primary agonist muscle (the prime mover). For instance, as a load increases, more muscles will be required to lift or counteract the load. Branching of Ia and other sensory fibers to synergist muscles assists with this task (Fig. 3-6). Most tasks require multiple

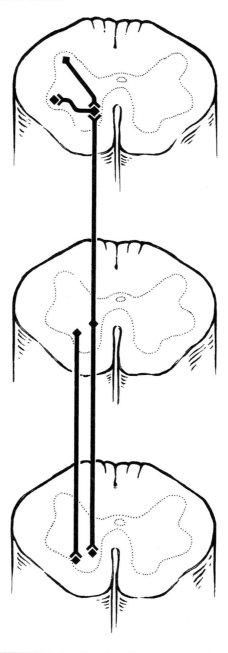

Fig. 3-7. Propriospinal interneurons never exit the spinal cord but ascend and descend the cord to synapse on interneurons and motor neurons up to several segments away. These connections contribute to coordination of postural adjustments with voluntary movement, and coordination between limbs.

muscles from various body segments to act in concert. This effect requires activation of muscles in addition to agonists and synergists. Much of the coordination and activation of diverse muscle groups across several joints is accomplished by propriospinal neurons.

Propriospinal neurons are located in the spinal cord and receive rich convergent input. Propriospinal neurons are interneurons whose axons span multiple spinal cord segments and hence have a range of action that is greater than that of strictly segmental interneurons. Propriospinal neurons send projections to interneurons and motor neurons located several spinal segments away from their cell bodies (Fig. 3-7). The connections made by these propriospinal neurons allow multiple muscles to coordinate their activity for postural adjustments and voluntary movement. Any type of arm or leg movement depends first on the stability of proximal, postural muscles and the coordination of these postural muscles with distal movements. Coordinated activations of my fingers as I type on the keyboard require interactions among wrist, elbow, shoulder, and back muscles in addition to finger musculature. These activities use propriospinal neurons to provide the necessary linkage.

◼ REFLEX CIRCUITRY INVOLVED WITH ANTAGONIST MUSCLE INHIBITION

The circuitry discussed in the previous section dealt with the activation of muscles. It is important to realize that smooth movement relies not only on muscle activation, but on muscle deactivation as well. For you to reach out and touch someone would be impossible if muscles that opposed that movement were contracting. The best way to explain antagonist muscle inhibition during movement is to go back to the stretch reflex.

Disynaptic Ia inhibitory interneuron–mediated inhibition

As discussed in the previous section, the Ia afferents that convey stretch receptor information branch when they enter the spinal cord. Some of these branches synapse on interneurons. One type of interneuron that is contacted is the Ia inhibitory interneuron. This interneuron, when stimulated, secretes a neurotransmitter that will have an inhibitory effect on motor neurons innervating muscles that are antagonists to the stretched muscle (Fig. 3-8). This process is also referred to as *disynaptic inhibition* because two synapses are involved in the inhibitory pathway. The Ia inhibitory interneuron, similar to most interneurons, receives rich convergent input from many other sources in addition to Ia afferents (Fig. 3-9). The Ia interneuron processes this divergent input so that the appropriate amount of antagonist muscle inhibition is achieved. Different tasks require varying degrees of antagonist muscle inhibition and synergist muscle activation.

Disynaptic Ia inhibitory interneuron–mediated inhibition is not the only means by which the nervous system can cause inhibition.

Inhibition of antagonists and other muscle groups can also be accomplished by Renshaw cell–mediated inhibition, Ib-mediated inhibition, and presynaptic inhibitory mechanisms. These mechanisms, together with descending influences, can grade muscle contractions based on situational demands.

Renshaw cell–mediated recurrent inhibition

Renshaw cells are interneurons that directly synapse on alpha motor neurons and Ia inhibitory interneurons (Fig. 3-10). Similar to Ia inhibitory interneurons, they also receive convergent input from multiple descending and segmental inputs, but their primary input is from alpha motor neurons. Any given Renshaw cell projects to an alpha motor neuron and this very same alpha motor neuron, in addition to projections to extrafusal muscle fibers, projects directly back to the Renshaw cell! The collateral from the alpha motor neuron to the Renshaw cell is termed a recurrent collateral and thus the name, *recurrent inhibition*. The alpha motor neuron that initiates a contraction within its target muscle will also activate its Renshaw cell. The Renshaw cell, in turn, will synapse back upon the alpha motor neuron and inhibit it and, via collaterals, its synergists. Thus, any activation of the Renshaw cell, whether from its alpha motor neuron or from descending sources, will decrease motor neuron output. What possible function could having an activated alpha motor neuron inhibit its own output serve? To be quite honest, no one really knows,

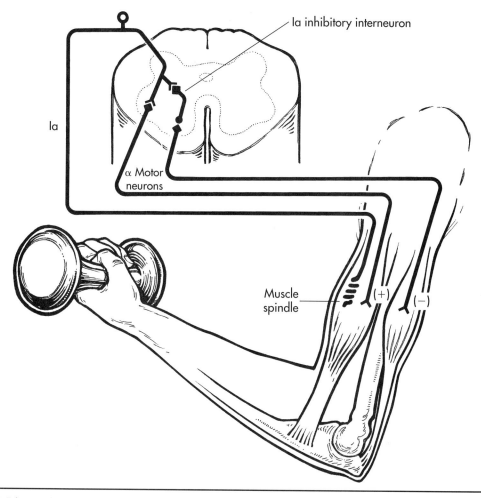

Fig. 3-8. Disynaptic Ia interneuron reciprocal inhibition: The Ia inhibitory interneuron mediates disynaptic inhibition of a muscle that is an antagonist to the contracting muscle. The Ia afferent of the contracting muscle synapses on its own alpha motor neuron and also collateralizes to synapse on a Ia inhibitory interneuron that will inhibit the antagonist motor neuron.

but quite a bit of speculation has been put forward. To begin to answer this question, you must know more about the connectivity of the Renshaw cell, motor control, and muscle origins and insertions.

The Renshaw cell inhibits the alpha motor neuron that caused its activation, and it also inhibits alpha motor neurons that innervate synergist muscles about the joint. Renshaw cells also inhibit the gamma motor neurons of these same muscles. In addition, they inhibit antagonist muscle Ia inhibitory interneurons. At this point you should reexamine Fig. 3-10; this is one of those cases where a diagram is worth a thousand words. Refer to the diagram as you read the following paragraphs.

One possible way to think about Renshaw cells is as variable gain regulators.[11,55] Renshaw cells inhibit agonist muscles and disinhibit, by nature of their antagonist Ia inhibitory interneuron connections, antagonist muscles. *Disinhibition* reduces inhibition. Renshaw cells, therefore, bring opposing muscles

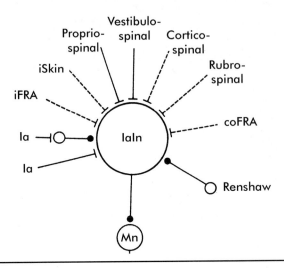

Fig. 3-9. Examples of the wide array of convergence onto interneurons. *i*, Ipsilateral; *co*, contralateral; *FRA*, flexor reflex afferents; *Mn*, motor neurons; *dotted lines*, polysynaptic pathwys; *filled circles*, inhibition; *lines*, excitation. (Modified from Brookhart JM, Mountcastle VB, Brooks VB, Geiger SR, eds. Handbook of physiology: the nervous system II. Bethesda, Md.: American Physiological Society, 1981.)

into closer approximation with regard to contraction levels. Thus, in some ways they function as the opposites of Ia inhibitory interneurons.

Some activities require muscle cocontraction, and Renshaw cells appear to contribute to situationally appropriate muscle cocontraction. Guided arm movements to a target appear to involve Renshaw cells. Preparing for a forearm tennis volley requires that you use the triceps to extend the arm. But to hit your target, the tennis ball, you need to control this elbow extension and also prepare for rapid elbow flexion as you make contact with the ball. The preparatory phase of this movement requires a degree of cocontraction between antagonist muscles but not so much to limit freedom of movement. Activation of the triceps and the cocontraction between the triceps and the biceps are then replaced as you swing toward the ball by stronger activations of the biceps and inhibition of the triceps. The Renshaw cell may help you coordinate these tasks and attain the proper amount of muscle balance. It will do so without any conscious intervention on your part. One can speculate, however, that by nature of the descending connections with the Renshaw cell, some degree of control can be exerted when needed.

Renshaw cells are under central control from descending brain stem and cortical pathways. Their relative output is modulated by these descending systems and thus the Renshaw cells, with or without your conscious efforts, can probably modify the relative excitation and inhibition of multiple heteronymous muscles during any given movement. *Heteronymous muscles* are muscles that are involved in a movement task but are not the primary movers. All activities require muscle activation from muscles other than the prime mover. The functioning of these muscles is essential to muscle balance. Gain modulation mediated by Renshaw cells is not limited to disinhibition of antagonist muscles. They also contribute to heteronymous muscle control.

During a movement, synergists (heteronymous muscles) receive collateralized Ia afferent input from the primary mover. The postsynaptic excitatory effects of this Ia afferent input will be counterbalanced by recurrent inhibition from Renshaw cells of the primary mover. Heteronymous muscles receive weaker Ia

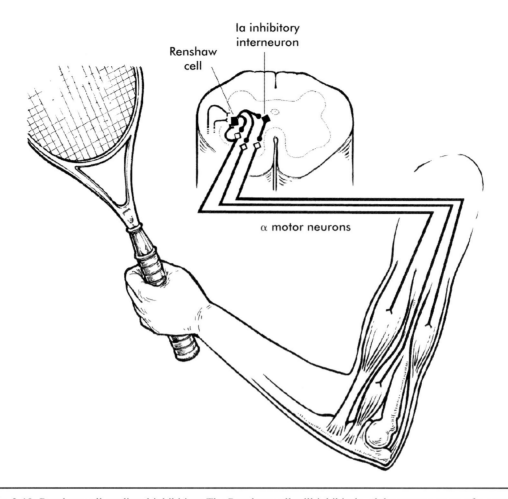

Fig. 3-10. Renshaw cell mediated inhibition: The Renshaw cell will inhibit the alpha motor neuron of a contracting muscle and its synergists. In addition, it will inhibit the antagonist muscle's Ia inhibitory interneuron (disinhibition). This aids in grading muscle contractions and assisting task-appropriate agonist/antagonist cocontraction. As indicated by the *arrows*, the Renshaw cell receives other input in addition to input from an alpha motor neuron.

input than the primary mover and are thus more affected by Renshaw cell inhibition. In this way, muscle contraction can be focused and gradations of muscle contraction, depending on the position of the limb and the task, can be accomplished smoothly. This is also a convenient way for the body to conserve energy. Why use multiple muscles to perform a task when one or two will do? You don't need a sledge hammer to drive a thumbtack.

Individuals with upper motor neuron damage (i.e., damage to descending motor pathways) appear to have accentuated levels of Renshaw cell activity.[61,97,105] Spasticity, excessive muscle cocontraction, an inability to fractionate movement, and an inability to grade muscle forces are common impairments that accompany upper motor neuron damage. At this point it should make some sense to you as to why and how abnormally heightened Renshaw cell activity might contribute to these impairments.

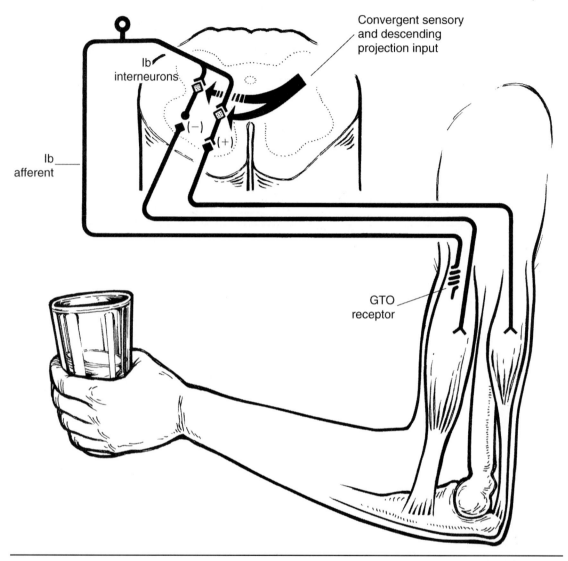

Fig. 3-11. Ib fiber mediated inhibition: GTOs monitor changes in muscle force. Ib afferent fibers convey this information to Ib interneurons, which inhibit the contracting muscle and excite its antagonists. This type of inhibition assists with the matching of muscle forces to the requirements of a task.

Ib fiber–mediated nonreciprocal inhibition (autogenic inhibition)

Golgi tendon organs (GTOs) detect changes in muscle force (see Chapter 2). Their messages are conveyed via Ib afferents that synapse on Ib interneurons. Similar to Renshaw cells, increased activity in the Ib interneuron results in inhibition of the motor neurons that innervate the muscles that generated the initial muscle force (Fig. 3-11). The more force being generated by a muscle, the more active the Ib inhibition back to its motor neuron pool. The Ib interneuron receives rich convergent input from sources other than the GTO. It receives substantial input from Ia afferents as well as joint and cutaneous afferents. The Ib interneuron is also under central control via projections from the corticospinal tract, rubrospinal tract, and the lateral reticulospinal tract. As discussed previously, GTOs are very sensitive to even small changes in muscle force. The Ib interneuron appears to be very involved in movements that require the processing of tactile, stretch, and force receptors. Via this processing, we can grade muscle forces to match the requirements of the task, such as picking up a dime from a smooth table. Matching grip force to object size, weight, and texture appears to be a learned activity.[29,40] Young children need repetitive exposures to objects before they begin to exhibit appropriate grip forces. Whether Ib interneuron firing changes during the learning of these tasks would be interesting to know.

Choreographing inhibitory mechanisms

Other forms of segmental inhibition exist in addition to the ones listed above. My guess is that as more becomes known about interneurons, we will find that they meld afferent and descending neural inputs in ways not yet defined or imagined. For instance, one type of inhibition is referred to as Group Ia nonreciprocal inhibition.[51] Different muscle groups appear to use this pathway, which involves a different type of interneuron other than the Ia inhibitory pathway.[91] I am sure that before this book is published, other interneuronal functions and interactions will be discovered. Interneurons remain a relatively unexplored mine field of information.

You will probably need to think about each previously discussed pathway individually to grasp the significance of its function. But don't envision the operation of each pathway existing in isolation. The pathways interact in intricately choreographed synaptic dances. The temporal sequencing and muscle balance that must be achieved even in the operation of daily mundane tasks is nothing short of phenomenal.

What is simpler and more commonplace to daily human existence than feeding yourself? Imagine yourself at your favorite drinking establishment with a mug of your favorite drink and a pile of peanuts sitting in front of you. The muscles and biomechanics involved in lifting the mug are slightly different than those involved in cupping a handful of peanuts into your mouth. Drinking from the mug requires flexing and pronating the forearm, whereas eating peanuts out of the palm of your hand requires elbow flexion and supination. The biceps and brachioradialis are involved in both tasks. Both contribute to lifting the mug. During the peanut eating task, however, the brachioradialis (being an elbow pronator) is an antagonist to the biceps (which supinates the elbow and will need to be inhibited somewhat). And of course the mug is heavier than the handful of peanuts, so this must be taken into account by peripheral receptors, interneuronal pathways, and synergist muscles. Try to map out what pathways would be involved with these multiple tasks. Once you have it figured out, imagine someone interrupting the arc of your arm movement. What receptors and pathways are involved now? Aren't you glad you don't have to think about these things on a regular basis to satisfy your thirsts and hungers? Imagine what it would be like if you had consciously to control multiple pathways and multiple circuits within a pathway. Reflex pathways that involve more than one neural circuit are the topic of the next section.

■ FLEXOR REFLEX AFFERENTS
Definition and description

Some reflex pathways involve multiple circuits. *Flexor reflex afferents* (FRAs) are a good example of this. Recall that stepping on a sharp shell (or any other object that causes pain) results in a flexion withdrawal of the ipsilateral leg and concomitant extension of the contralateral leg. We referred to this response as the crossed extension reflex. This very same response can also be elicited by stimulating a multitude of receptors that don't involve the pain pathways. Stimulation of Groups II, III, and IV joint afferents and cutaneous afferents evokes polysynaptic actions that result in ipsilateral flexion and contralateral crossed extension reflex responses. FRAs describe a common reflex activation of flexor motor neurons from multiple sensory sources.[6] In addition, these polysynaptic pathways share similar interneurons and are under the control of descending projections from the brain and brain stem.[6,21,22,54,96]

FRAs involve different short (monosynaptic) and long (polysynaptic) latency reflex pathways that include both facilitatory and inhibitory interneurons. A characteristic of FRAs is the extensive multisensorial convergence onto interneurons involved in the pathways. Despite the diverse nature of the afferent input, stimulation of FRAs results in a typified motor output. This output, however, is not invariable. Motor output, as a result of FRA stimulation, can be modified by the limb's position at the time of stimulation,[27] descending commands,[41,54,75] and afferent input.[87,93] An awareness of FRAs is important not only as a general organizational principle within the CNS, but also because it has implications for clinical neurology and the generation of rhythmical motor acts such as locomotion.

Involvement of FRAs in spasticity

Clinicians who treat patients with neurological problems become very familiar with spasticity and its devastating affects on movement. *Spasticity* is an impairment that results from various forms of neural damage or disease. Damage that involves corticofugal pathways (pathways originating from cerebral cortex and descending to brain stem and spinal cord) often result in spasticity. Spasticity and the spastic condition results in a multitude of signs and symptoms including hypertonia (resistance to passive stretch), accentuated tendon reflexes, abnormal patterns of muscular coordination, paresis, and muscle cocontraction during voluntary movement.[39,68] FRAs possibly contribute to the typical patterns of spasticity observed after damage to supraspinal centers. Supraspinal control of FRAs appears to gate afferent input so that not all movements elicit a reflexive response. This is the means by which activity within FRA pathways matches descending commands.[96] Disruption of descending control of FRA interneurons alters this control, such that the integration of descending commands and FRA afferents is no longer possible. This disruption of interneuronal functioning contributes to the spastic condition and associated movement disorders. One of the disorders, common to damage to supraspinal centers, is the disruption of limb coordination so necessary for behaviors such as locomotion. FRA pathways also appear to contribute to these sequential, rhythmic motor behaviors.

Involvement of FRAs in locomotion

In the early 1900s, Graham Brown attempted to outline the neural basis of mammalian locomotion. Inherent to his explanation was the half center theory.[57] This theory states that rhythmic stepping depends on the inhibition of ipsilateral limb antagonists coupled with the coordination of contralateral limb flexors and extensors. This coordination requires circuitry that not only inhibits ipsilateral antagonists, but also inhibits circuitry controlling the contralateral limb. This action involves, at the very least, two groups of interneurons connected by reciprocal inhibitory connections. This connectivity is capable of generating alternating activity. The theory was without direct scientific evidence of its existence until the description of FRAs. FRAs transform peripheral inputs to activate flexors and extensors alternately. Interneurons activated by FRAs, therefore, might represent the circuitry underlying the rhythmic bilateral activation of flexors and extensors proposed by Brown's half center theory. Further evidence for the involvement of FRAs in the generation of locomotor-like behavior was provided by experiments that involved electrical stimulation of a brain stem nucleus (mesencephalic locomotor region). Stimulation of this area results in stepping movements.[82] Electrical stimulation of the mesencephalic locomotor region at intensities subthreshold for locomotion, evoked FRA-like responses that ultimately yielded to locomotor activity as electrical stimulation intensity increased.[98] Locomotion, therefore, must use at least some of the same circuitry as involved with FRA responses.

Locomotion, however, is a more complex motor act than reflexive removal of a limb from an afferent stimulus. Other afferents, notably Ias and Ibs, contribute to transitions during the gait cycle. Equilibrium, propulsion, upper and lower body coordination, fast sequencing of muscles, and the control of multiple body parts and degrees of freedom become increasingly involved. FRAs alone do not appear capable of this type of integration. Additional neural mechanisms are likely involved in the generation and mainte-

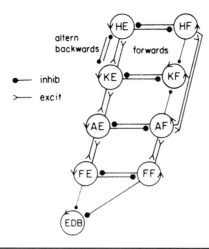

Fig. 3-12. Diagrammatic representation of a central pattern generator (*CPG*) controlling cat quadrupedal locomotion. *E*, Extensor; *F*, flexor; *H*, hip; *K*, knee; *A*, ankle; *F*, foot; *EDB*, extensor digitorum brevis. (From Grillner S. In: Brooks VB, ed. Motor control. Handbook of physiology vol 2. Bethesda, Md.: American Physiological Society, 1981.)

nance of human locomotion. A natural sequelae to a discussion of FRAs and circuitry subserving rhythmical motor activities is the concept of central pattern generators.

■ CENTRAL PATTERN GENERATORS
Definition and description
Central pattern generators (CPGs) refer to a grouping of neurons or neural circuits that can generate coordinated, rhythmic movements autonomously.[26,42,44,48] CPGs exist in the brain stem and spinal cord and contribute to various vertebrate motor acts including mastication, respiration, scratching, and locomotion. CPGs for locomotion have been identified in the spinal cord of several vertebrate species[44,59,74] (Fig. 3-12).

For instance, cats with a total transection of the spinal cord are capable of overground and treadmill locomotion. The animals must be supported because they lack equilibrium control. Nonetheless, appropriate reciprocal muscle activations and a weight-bearing gait are apparent.[30,32,43,90,92] Locomotion, therefore, is possible without input from higher brain centers. The locomotion exhibited by animals that have had their spinal cords transected, however, is not purposeful locomotion. Rather, it resembles automatic behavior.

CPGs can generate coordinated locomotor movements in the absence of movement-related afferent feedback.[46,48] Although CPGs form an innate neural network that independently can activate coordinated stepping, this does not imply that the network, or its output, is invariant. CPGs can change output depending on speed requirements[30,100] and in response to obstacle avoidance.[2,32] Although CPGs can operate without afferent input, CPG activity is constantly modified by available sensory input.[44]

At any given moment, or stage, of a step cycle, the importance and consequences of various afferent inputs change. For instance, during the transition from stance to swing, hip flexor stretch receptors may be the primary sensory input that initiates change in CPG output.[47] During other stages and conditions, other sensory input may be of primary importance. These differences have yielded the concept of command neurons. Command neurons are defined as those neurons that respond to sensory or descending inputs and initiate CPG activity. Regardless of the input, different movements or different conditions

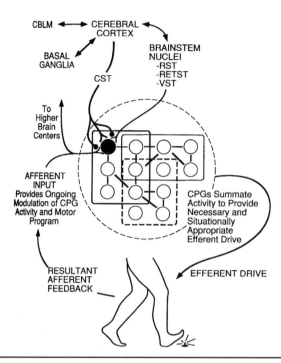

Fig. 3-13. Factors contributing to CPG functioning during human locomotion. *Circles* within each domino represent neural populations innervating a specific muscle group. Projections as drawn do not necessarily represent a monosynaptic connection (see text for details). *Solid circle*, Command neuron that triggers CPG pattern of activation; *CST*, corticospinal tract; *VST*, vestibulospinal tract; *RST*, rubrospinal tract; *RETST*, reticulospinal tract. (From Leonard CT. In: Craik RL, Oatis CA, eds. Gait analysis: theory and application. St. Louis: Mosby-Year Book, 1995.)

might activate different command neurons. Command neurons, in turn, activate specific neural discharge sequencing within the CPG. Thus, different movements are possible depending on which command neurons within the CPG are activated. Thus far, command neurons have only been identified in invertebrate neural networks. Direct experimental evidence of their existence or importance in vertebrates such as humans remains to be determined.

Activity within the CPG, and the patterns of movement that result from CPG activation, appear to be influenced primarily by three factors:

1. Supraspinal center input,
2. The type and degree of afferent feedback, and
3. The influences of limb and body position on afferent feedback (Fig. 3-13).

CPGs and human locomotion

The spinal CPG concept, with regard to human locomotion, is not without controversy. Debates continue about whether the coordination of human locomotion is solely a function of spinal CPG, or whether higher brain centers are essential for the maturation of the human gait pattern.

The innate stepping movements of human fetuses[18] and the bipedal ambulation exhibited from birth by human infants (both infants who are developing normally[28] and those with anencephaly[104]) support the existence of spinal cord locomotor-generating circuits in humans, at least early in ontogeny. A study examining adults after spinal cord damage suggested that locomotor CPGs are present in humans.[12] However, verifying the completeness of the spinal cord lesion in this and other studies is impossible. The reason for this is that in experiments other than those in humans, the spinal cord can be transected surgically and the completeness of the transection can be verified by a number of procedures. In humans, spinal cord injury typically results from trauma and compression. Only indirect methods of assessing spinal cord and descending pathway function can be used. None of these methods can rule out the sparing of small fractions of descending input.

Although autonomous spinal cord–mediated locomotion has been demonstrated in many mammals and in simian infants, it has not been demonstrated convincingly by fully mature simians or humans.[23] It is highly unlikely, however, that CPGs do not exist in some form in humans. Entire neural pathways are rarely lost during evolutionary development.[84,95] Not surprisingly, however, the role of the CPG in generating locomotion has potentially changed with phylogenetic development and with the transition from quadrupedal to bipedal locomotion.

The limited research that is available in humans suggests that spinal cord CPGs might not have the same primacy of control as in other species. Perhaps the autonomy of the CPG is lessened in humans. The role of higher brain centers, such as the cerebral cortex, may be considerably different in humans than it is in other species. Data from humans, in fact, suggest that learning and development of the cerebral cortex play critical roles in the attainment of an adultlike, bipedal, plantigrade gait pattern.[71,79,81]

Of all mammals, humans have the densest corticospinal projections to the ventral horn of the spinal cord, and thus stronger direct control of motor neurons.[4,66] Mammalian cortical projections are not fully developed at birth.[65,70,102] Perhaps the apparent differences in CPG functioning between human infants and adults can be attributed to integration of descending projections with existing CPG circuitry during maturation. Initially, infant walking might be modulated by spinal cord circuitry (CPGs), but with maturity proper CPG functioning becomes dependent on integration with higher centers. Strong evidence suggests that certain motor behaviors in other mammals is first mediated by segmental pathways but then becomes dependent on the sensorimotor cortex during maturation.[69,70,89] It has been hypothesized that human temporal sequencing of muscle activation involves spinal CPGs and integration of these neural circuits with input from higher brain centers.[17,45,72]

The role of descending input and spinocortical afferent pathways on reflex actions will comprise the focus of the last two sections of this chapter. Before we enter this nebulous netherworld bridging reflexive and willed movements, it is necessary to introduce you to mechanisms that can modulate the activity of any neural pathway.

▪ MODULATION OF REFLEX ACTIVITY

The flow of information within a neural pathway can be modulated, modified, or altered by numerous mechanisms. For instance, inputs onto the presynaptic neuron can influence its transmitter release, and certain substances (proteins, enzymes, transmitters) can change the affinity of a postsynaptic receptor for a particular neurotransmitter. The following paragraphs will discuss presynaptic inhibition, presynaptic facilitation, neural modulators, and long-term potentiation. Each of these mechanisms can potentially affect each neural circuit discussed previously. Although they will, no doubt, add some confusion for you, they contribute to clarity within the nervous system. As you will read, these mechanisms can influence functions such as sensory perception, motor learning, and cognitive abilities.

Presynaptic inhibition

Axons make synaptic contact with another neuron's dendrites, cell body, or axon. These synapses are referred to as axodendritic, axosomatic, and axoaxonic, respectively. Previous discussions have focused on the transfer of information from one neuron to another via the interactions between the pre- and post-

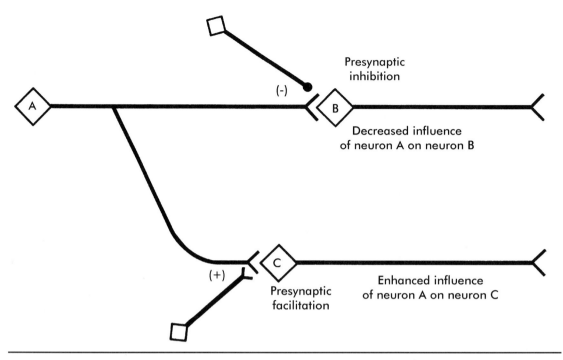

Fig. 3-14. Presynaptic inhibition and facilitation: Via axoaxonic synapses, presynaptic events can alter the amount of neurotransmitter released by a single axon without affecting the functioning of other axons of the same neuron.

synaptic neurons. These synapses involve axodendritic or axosomatic connections. One intriguing synapse, the axoaxonic synapse, functions a bit differently than these others and represents a mechanism by which neural signals of a single axonal branch can be modulated. The two types of modulation that can occur via axoaxonic synapses are termed presynaptic inhibition and presynaptic facilitation (Fig. 3-14).

   Presynaptic inhibition causes inhibition along a neural pathway by decreasing the amount of neurotransmitter released by the presynaptic terminal. This decreases its effect on the postsynaptic neuron. Presynaptic inhibitory mechanisms are not the same as those involved with postsynaptic inhibition. *Postsynaptic inhibition* is the result of neurotransmitter binding, influx of charged ions through the postsynaptic membrane, and a resultant hyperpolarization and IPSP. Presynaptic inhibition works by limiting the amount of transmitter released by the presynaptic axon terminal. Several mechanisms have been identified and the different presynaptic pathways probably involve different mechanisms. The mechanisms thus far identified involve interference with calcium (Ca^{++}) influx or binding. Calcium is essential to neurotransmitter release. Another mechanism involves short-circuiting the action potential in the presynaptic terminal by increasing chloride (Cl^-) conductance. Again, refer to a neurophysiology text for more detailed descriptions of these mechanisms. The main points to be made at this time are that axoaxonic synapses can selectively inhibit transmission along certain axonal pathways and that the mechanisms involved in presynaptic inhibition differ from those involved with postsynaptic inhibition.

The differences in mechanisms between pre- and postsynaptic inhibition are of potential importance for clinicians involved with neurological rehabilitation. Deficits in presynaptic inhibition have been identified for certain patient groups (e.g., those with spinal cord injury, Parkinson's disease, cerebral palsy, or stroke).[56,86,103] Pharmacological enhancement of the pathways might assist in ameliorating some of the motor control and motor learning problems attributed to loss of presynaptic inhibition. Furthermore, because presynaptic mechanisms (such as Ca^{++} transport) are also involved in cognitive learning processes, the relevance of studying these mechanisms is not limited to movement impairments.

Presynaptic facilitation

Presynaptic facilitation is the antithesis of presynaptic inhibition. Presynaptic facilitation increases the amount of transmitter released by the presynaptic neuron. This increase enhances the amplitude of the postsynaptic potential (Fig. 3-14). The mechanisms by which this is accomplished involves increased Ca^{++} influx and a prolongation of the action potential of the presynaptic neuron.

Because presynaptic inhibition and presynaptic facilitation involve axoaxonic synapses, the impact of individual axonal branches can be altered without altering neurotransmitter release from other branches of the neuron. Hypothetically, therefore, the divergent outflow to various neural targets from the presynaptic neuron is not necessarily identical to all targets. This principle remains hypothetical at this point because it has not been directly tested in humans.

Neuromodulators and neural modulation

The function of neurotransmitters is to induce a short-term synaptic current that changes membrane ion conductance and thus either hyperpolarizes or depolarizes the cell. Certain criteria have been established to define whether a certain substance is indeed a neurotransmitter. These criteria include:

1. The chemical must be localized in presynaptic neurons,
2. A specific transport system for the substance must be present in the neuron,
3. Specific postsynaptic binding sites or receptors for the substance must be present,
4. Stimulation of afferents should cause release of the substance,
5. Direct application of the substance to the synapse should produce effects identical to those produced by physiological stimulation,
6. Interaction of the substance with a receptor should cause IPSPs or EPSPs, and
7. Inactivating mechanisms (e.g., diffusion, metabolizing enzymes, reuptake system) should exist to terminate substance effects on the receptor.

Some substances have an affect on the conductance properties of various neurons, but they do not fit all of the above criteria. Some of these substances are referred to as neuromodulators. *Neuromodulators* can alter the input-output properties of neurons, decrease the resting potential of different neurons, and increase the degree of afterhyperpolarization (after an action potential, the neuron experiences a brief hyperpolarization and is thus less responsive to incoming EPSPs).[8,64]

Without going into detailed membrane physiology, neuromodulators tend to work by binding in close proximity to the actual ion channel. A chemical cascade follows this binding that results in altered functioning of the ion channel. The effects of neuromodulators tend to last much longer than the typical effects of a neurotransmitter. Binding of a neuromodulator can alter synapse functioning for seconds, hours, and potentially even longer. In fact, habitual activity of this circuit might lead to long-term changes in the membrane. Neuromodulators do what their name implies: they modulate the behavior of the neuron. In fact, neuromodulators have been implicated in habitual responses to stress.[7,110] Perhaps this helps explain why childhood experiences can have such a long-lasting effect on personality development. Neuromodulators might tonically increase the excitability of the neuron, thereby rendering it more sensitive to afferent input. Our responses to stress become habitual because certain neural pathways might have been "primed" by neuromodulation. Neuromodulators also appear to be involved in long-term potentiation and learning.

Long-term synaptic potentiation and long-term facilitation

In 1890, psychologist William James proposed his "Law of Neural Habit" as an explanation for the physiological basis of memory.[57] This concept was expanded upon in the 1940s by another psychologist, Donald Hebb. "Hebb's Postulate for Learning" states that[52]:

> "When an axon of cell A is near enough to excite a cell B and repeatedly or persistently takes
> part in firing it, some growth process or metabolic change takes place in one or both cells such
> that A's efficiency, as one of the cells firing B, is increased."

It wasn't until the 1970s, when Timothy Bliss and colleagues, working with the rabbit hippocampus (an area in the brain associated with memory), first presented physiological evidence of James' and Hebb's ideas.[9,10] Bliss' group showed that intense afferent stimulation could produce long-term enhancement of synaptic functioning. Synaptic enhancement is defined as an increase in the amplitude of an EPSP above what would normally be expected from a given afferent input. They called this synaptic enhancement *long-term potentiation*. These experiments were the first to show that synaptic efficacy (i.e., synaptic ability to conduct a synaptic potential) might depend on activity. Experiments conducted since then have confirmed that repeated activity within a neural pathway eases transmission along this pathway.[1,63,79,101,106] Jonathan Wolpaw and colleagues have linked changes in spinal cord motor neuron physiology with the learning of specific motor tasks.[13,14] In addition, they have shown that these conditioned changes persist for weeks and even after removal of supraspinal influences.[108] Therefore, motor learning might involve actual physiological changes in the membranes of neurons within the spinal cord. Long-term potentiation appears to aid learning and retention of new information. Agents that block long-term potentiation inhibit learning and retention.[5]

Long-term potentiation involves changes in the postsynaptic neuron in response to intense or repeated afferent input. *Long-term facilitation*, which also enhances synaptic transmission and might also be a mechanism involved in learning, operates somewhat differently. Repetitive (not necessarily intense) afferent input to a neuron results in accentuation of synaptic potential amplitudes and enhancement of transmission that lasts for hours after afferent input is terminated.[5] Long-term facilitation is typically a presynaptic event (as opposed to long-term potentiation, which involves postsynaptic mechanisms). It also involves some fairly complex membrane physiology. The bottom line is that long-term facilitation increases the amount of neurotransmitter released by the presynaptic neuron. This increases its effectiveness on the postsynaptic neuron. As mentioned previously, Ca^{++} is essential for transmitter release from the presynaptic vesicle. Long-term facilitation results in the accumulation of Ca^{++} in the presynaptic terminal. Therefore, when an action potential arrives at the terminal, more Ca^{++} is available and, therefore, more transmitter is released from the terminal than normal. Over time, long-term facilitation increases the strength of synaptic connections and appears to contribute to the formation of new synapses.[60] The formation of new synapses equates to the storage of new memories, whether they are related to cognitive, emotional, or motor functions.

Long-term facilitation alone is not sufficient to produce new synapses. Formation of new synapses also depends on the synthesis of new proteins.[60] This relates back to the function of the neural cell body. A neuron's cell body can synthesize new proteins depending on the needs of the cell. What triggers the neuron to switch to synthesizing the proteins that are necessary for synapse formation remains an attractive mystery.

The take-home message for both long-term potentiation and facilitation is that memory formation and skill acquisition probably depend on enhancement of synaptic functioning. Enhancement of synaptic functioning is activity dependent. The more you use a pathway, the easier the transmission along that pathway becomes. This is something to think about when that last half hour of practice arrives and you don't think you can possibly repeat a drill one more time. This is also a concept that clinicians should impart to patients. Repetition can be boring, and many musicians, athletes, and patients will quit before a sufficient number of trials has occurred to move a novel task into the physiological realm of a memory or acquired skill.

Forcing yourself to do something involves conscious intervention and obvious involvement of the cerebral cortex. Voluntary movements, therefore, involve more than reflex circuitry. The involvement of the cerebral cortex during a movement, however, does not necessarily always involve a conscious thought. The cerebral cortex has reflex loops of its own.

■ LONG-LOOP TRANSCORTICAL REFLEXES

Long-loop reflexes (LLR) refer to pathways that involve *transcortical loops*. These pathways appear well positioned to integrate peripheral information with one's intention and the needs of a task. LLRs modulate segmental reflexes according to intentions and needs.[16] Some have suggested that LLRs be referred to as long-loop responses rather than long-loop reflexes,[11] not because they don't have a short enough latency to be regarded as a reflex or because the LLR responses involve the cerebral cortex. The suggestion was made because LLRs represent an ill-defined no-man's-land between reflex and willed movement.

By definition, LLRs involve intention, usually thought of as involving a conscious act. In the 1950s, Dr. Hammond and colleagues were the first to show that segmental reflexes could be modified by prior instructions to their human subjects.[50] Subjects were instructed either to oppose or to relax during a stretch to the biceps muscle. Quick stretch to the biceps muscle typically resulted in a short latency reflex spike in the stretched muscle. This spike, however, generated little torque. When subjects were instructed to oppose the stretch, the initial spike was followed within milliseconds by a stronger contraction that could not be solely attributed to monosynaptic spinal mechanisms. When subjects were instructed to relax when the biceps was stretched, the initial short-latency response decreased after a series of trials. Therefore, the stretch reflex showed modulation dependent on the task and instructions to the subject. These findings were attributed to the influences of descending cortical projections onto the segmental circuitry. Other investigators[24,25,49,85] have expanded these studies and we now know that LLRs involve motor cortical neurons. Studies in humans and animals indicate that LLRs provide input to segmental circuitry to mediate responses to external perturbations during volitional movements. LLRs are reflexive adjustments by the motor cortex to sudden load disturbances. However, to assume that this is the only behavior in which LLRs are involved might be a mistake. The functional significance of LLRs probably extends well beyond responses to load or limb trajectory responses. Pyramidal tract neurons fire most intensely during the smallest movements of the hand[25] and appear to sense errors automatically during precise movements.[85] LLRs might be one way the motor cortex specifies segmental mechanisms needed to match direction and speed of intended movements with an intended trajectory.[11,35-37] Intention is a key word when thinking about LLRs.

LLRs are highly dependent on prior instruction to or the intent of the subject[24]—hence the difficulty in categorizing LLRs as reflexes. We have long known that sensory afferent input constantly modifies segmental reflexes.[2,20,33,87,93,107] Should we regard descending cortical input as just another afferent input onto segmental pathways?

Neurons within the motor cortex of monkeys respond to peripheral afferent input within 20 msec. The output from these neurons reach the spinal cord within an additional 5 msec.[25] Certainly these speeds would enable cortical pathways to influence segmental reflexes. Muscular responses to a muscle stretch can be divided into M1, M2, and M3 phases.[67] In the human wrist, the M1 response occurs at about 25 msec, the M2 at 50 to 80 msec, and the M3 at 85 to 100 msec. Human M2 and M3 responses depend on an intact sensorimotor cortex.[15,83] Again, these data demonstrate the influence of the cerebral cortex on spinal cord circuitry.

Some investigators have suggested that mechanisms other than transcortical pathways might account for LLRs (specifically M2 and M3).[38,76] Their data have suggested that other peripheral afferents, in addition to Ia afferents, might contribute to long-latency responses and that intact cortical pathways were not necessary for their expression. These apparently contradictory results were obtained from studies in cats. Perhaps species variation underlies the apparent differences. Or, perhaps not. Yet another ongoing debate. Regardless, currently available data from humans strongly support that LLRs are cortically dependent and can provide modulatory feedback to segmental circuitry. LLRs are also probably involved in segmental feed-forward regulation in addition to its feedback responsibilities (feed-forward refers to proactive modulations that precede movement, as opposed to feedback, which refers to reactive modulation to movement and afferent signals).

Via feed-forward mechanisms, LLRs preset muscle stiffness and reflex gain depending on the requirements of a specific task and as a consequence of motor learning. Afferent input produces different motor outputs depending on where on the body the input occurs and when it occurs during a particular phase of the gait cycle.[3,33] Studies in animals other than humans have also shown that repetition of a movement will result in an increased or decreased reflex gain. Reflex gain changes depend on the desired movement outcomes.[25,109] If a reflex contributes to a desirable outcome, it appears that it will be enhanced. If it proves to be detrimental to performance, it will likely be dampened. Conscious control of these modulatory changes does not appear to be necessary.

Data from studies in humans are consistent with these animal studies. Certain segmental reflexes are enhanced when they are useful and contribute to a desired motor and functional outcome. These same reflexes are diminished when they are counterproductive to successful completion of a task.[24,34,53,78] The modulations become enhanced when subjects are repetitively exposed to the same stimuli over and over again. Imagine someone standing behind you and unexpectedly pulling a rug out from under your feet. The tug on the rug will displace your body forward and stretch the calf musculature. The reflexive response to this stretch will be a contraction of the calf muscles and a resultant ankle plantarflexion. The plantarflexion will assist you in maintaining an upright balance. Now imagine yourself on your snowboard shredding down a mogul run. As you hit each consecutive mogul, your ankle will be pushed rapidly into a dorsiflexed position, thus eliciting a stretch reflex. In this instance, you want to absorb the impact and not react with ankle plantarflexion. Plantarflexing the ankle in this case is detrimental to staying on your board. Repetitive exposure to a rug being pulled out from underneath you will result in an accentuation of calf muscle stretch reflexes, whereas repetitive exposure to your mogul run will dampen reflex responses. This is exactly what Dr. Nashner and colleagues found in a slightly more controlled environment.[78]

New and novel neural pathways do not have to be imagined to provide an anatomical basis for LLR physiological findings. Monosynaptic corticospinal projections to alpha motor neurons[99] and to inhibitory interneurons[94] are numerous in humans. Alpha motor neurons and inhibitory interneurons appear to be controlled in parallel by descending cortical pathways.[75,94] The cerebral cortex, therefore, has direct projections that can inhibit as well as excite neurons involved in the stretch reflex, FRAs, CPGs, and presumably other segmental reflexes.

LLRs are yet one additional mechanism by which the CNS tunes movement. Of all reflexes discussed within this chapter, LLRs are the first mechanism that provides a direct theoretical link between a person's intention and adaptation within reflex circuits to that intention. Descending projections from the motor cortex, however, are not the only descending pathways involved in the modulation of reflex activity during movement.

■ DESCENDING CONTROL OF SEGMENTAL CIRCUITRY

Direct (monosynaptic) supraspinal influences onto spinal circuitry are not limited to corticospinal tract input. Additional direct supraspinal inputs descend via the reticulospinal, vestibulospinal, and rubrospinal tracts. The cerebellum and basal ganglia, via indirect projections, can also greatly influence segmental responses. Neurons within these pathways are rhythmically active during activities such as locomotion. Groupings of neurons within the brain stem, such as the mesencephalic and pontine locomotor regions, will also elicit rhythmical firing of spinal cord neurons and limb musculature when stimulated.

These supraspinal pathways are discussed in some detail in Chapters 2 and 6. You should review these chapters especially in light of the new information presented previously within this chapter. The integration of your knowledge regarding segmental reflex mechanisms and the various supraspinal pathways by which descending influences regulate these reflexes is not dissimilar to the physiological integration that occurs: Clarity and ease of transmission accompanies repetitive exposure. The following paragraphs will cursorily review some of the influences exerted by various supraspinal descending pathways onto segmental circuitry.

The reticulospinal tract

The reticulospinal tract has direct projections onto alpha and gamma motor neurons. Its primary projections are to extensor motor neurons and it can be facilitatory or inhibitory to these neurons. The reticulospinal tract is a major contributor to muscle tone and helps to preset musculature to appropriate levels of arousal needed for a particular task. You will recall that the limbic system greatly influences this tract. Emotions, therefore, can greatly influence muscle tone. This is an important concept for all of us, but particularly so for athletes and clinicians. Most athletes are familiar with the bell-shaped curve of arousal and know that a certain amount of emotion is beneficial to performance but that overarousal can be detrimental. Patients who are stressed will experience changes in muscle tone, concentration, and motor control. Clinicians working with an agitated or stressed patient will have to deal with these changes and the treatment challenges they present.

The vestibulospinal tract

The vestibulospinal tracts have been subject to extensive studies and numerous textbook reviews. They are major players in the regulation of postural reflexes. Similar to the reticulospinal tract, most of their connections are to extensor motor neurons of the spinal cord. The vestibulospinal tract is tonically active and helps us maintain an upright posture. Output from the cerebellum inhibits the various vestibular nuclei. Any voluntary movement is preceded by changes in postural set.[53] These anticipatory changes are mediated, to a large part, by the cerebellum and vestibular system and the cerebral cortex. The vestibulospinal tract, therefore, must interact with cortically mediated responses in addition to segmental circuitry. Dysfunctions of the vestibular system result in deficits in postural reactions and voluntary movement.

The rubrospinal tract

The rubrospinal tract has diminished in size in humans, yet its terminations within the spinal cord are similar to those of the corticospinal tract, one of the most recently expanded projection systems. Both the corticospinal and the rubrospinal tracts innervate motor neurons controlling distal musculature. The red nucleus also connects directly and indirectly with the cerebellum, olivary nucleus, and the reticular system. Perhaps the red nucleus is more closely aligned with the basal ganglia and the cerebellum than it is to the cerebral cortex.[62] Isolated lesions to the red nucleus result in intention tremors similar to those that result from certain cerebellar lesions. Or, perhaps because it receives projections from both the cerebral cortex and cerebellum, the red nucleus somehow merges their input before relaying its information to the spinal cord and elsewhere.

Regardless of the descending system being considered, the vast majority of the spinal cord synapses are occurring on interneurons and not directly on motor neurons. The same statement applies for peripheral afferent input. This implies that descending information is processed together with peripheral afferent activity. The apparent increase in direct connectivity in humans from supraspinal centers (such as the motor cortex) onto motor neurons suggests, however, that these higher centers can drive motor neurons rather independently of afferent input. Do these direct projections represent the neural substrate underlying human will? If I can control motor activity and ignore sensory input such as pain, cramps, or an overstretched muscle, am I not driving motor neurons and muscle contraction by sheer will and determination? Some people handle pain better than others. Some aerobic athletes handle "the wall" better than others. And, with risk-taking sports, a few athletes are willing to push the limits to further extremes. Are these examples of willpower—literally the power of the cerebral cortex over the neural circuitry? This is an interesting premise, but premises based on neural connectivity alone are open to debate if not outright ridicule.

■ MAKING SENSE AND NONSENSE OF SPINAL CORD CONNECTIVITY

The Appalachian Trail is a hiking path extending the length of the eastern United States. Walking even a short segment of its northern length reveals a floral diversity that challenges and delights the senses. Cherry, oak, walnut, ash, elm, and dogwood trees abound, each with its own arbor, each with its own characteristics, yet when viewed from the forest floor, virtually indistinguishable from one another. Where does the elm arbor end and the oak arbor begin? Count the number of trees and places the swaying walnut branches contact the branches of a grouping of oak and cherry trees growing at its base. This is an exercise in futility that also results in the loss of the aesthetic as you attempt to quantify the experience. Are attempted explanations of neural synaptic contacts and interactions so different? Neurons have arbors and connections that rival those of the most enchanted forest. Can sense really be made of complex CNS circuitry?

No shortage of opinions exist regarding this question. A brief sampling of published comments by some exceptional neuroscientists include such diverse views as: "...trying to explain how any real neural network works on a cell-by-cell, reductionist basis is futile..."[88] "Those whose experiments have forced us to confront the embarrassment of riches in the workings of the spinal cord must ask whether it is useful to continue to collect more inexplicable data."[73] But, to ensure that you do not put this book down in total frustration, some researchers have a considerably more upbeat appraisal. "There is considerable optimism about arriving at an understanding of spinal motor systems."[78]

Several excellent published reviews of spinal cord circuitry[6,58,76,96] reveal the enormous complexity involved in identifying and deciphering the functions of individual neurons and neural circuitry. Making matters worse, or more interesting depending on your perspective, is that neurons and neural circuits can alter their responses based on the task at hand. To regard spinal reflexes as invariant afferent input/efferent output circuits is no longer tenable. A rich convergent input exists onto spinal neurons and especially to interneurons. This convergence includes afferent and descending supraspinal inputs. Descending input does not trigger a certain spinal reflex. Rather, its input is processed with current afferent information. The output of any spinal reflex circuit is the result of the summation of these inputs and the excitability levels of various interneurons. Therefore, a movement reflects the current status of multisensorial input and the intentional wishes of the individual. Mechanisms such as presynaptic inhibition further mold segmental responses, probably by lessening the effects of some inputs depending on the functional demands at any particular moment during a movement. Altering input in this way might result in preferential selection of certain neural circuits over others.[77] Together with other mechanisms, it also contributes to interactions among spinal circuits. Spinal circuits do not operate in isolation or independently of each other. Intrinsic circuitry might be close to meaningless: It is the neuromodulatory environment that dictates synaptic function and behavior. As with biophysics, optimization of function and energy appear to be guiding principles in the nervous system. Whether we will ever really make sense of it all remains an open question.

SUGGESTED READINGS

Boorman G, Windhorst U, Kirmayer D. Waveform parameters of recurrent inhibitory postsynaptic potentials in cat motoneurons during time-varying activation patterns. Neuroscience 1994;63:747-564.

Brooke JD, McIlroy WE. Effect of knee joint angle on a heteronymous Ib reflex in the human lower limb. Can J Neurol Sci 19889;16:58-62.

Brooke JD, McIlroy WE. Vibration insensitivity of a short latency reflex linking the lower leg and the active knee extensor muscles in humans. Electroencephalogr Clin Neurophysiol 1990;75:401-9.

Brown TH, Chapman PF, Kairiss EW, Keenan CL. Long-term synaptic potentiation. In: Kelner KL, Koshland DE, eds. Molecules to models: advances in neuroscience. Washington, DC: American Association for the Advancement of Science, 1989:196-204.

Burke D, Gracies JM, Mazevet D, Meunier S, Pierrot-Deseilligny E. Convergence of descending and various peripheral inputs onto common propriospinal-like neurones in man. J Physiol (Lond) 1992;449:655-71.

Burke D, Gracies JM, Meunier S, Pierrot-Deseilligny E. Changes in presynaptic inhibition of afferents to propriospinal-like neurones in man during voluntary contractions. J Physiol (Lond) 1992;449:673-87.

Capaday C, Lavoie BA, Comeau F. Differential effects of a flexor nerve input on the human soleus H-reflex during standing versus walking. Can J Physiol Pharmacol 1995;73:436-49.

Carew TJ. Descending control of spinal circuits. In: Kandel ER, Schwartz JH, eds. Principles of neural science. Amsterdam: Elsevier, 1981:312-22.

Goldberger ME. Spared-root deafferentation of a cat's hindlimb: hierarchical regulation of pathways mediating recovery of motor behavior. Exp Brain Res 1988;73:329-42.

Goldberger ME. The extrapyramidal systems of the spinal cord: results of combined spinal and cortical lesions in the macaque. J Comp Neurol 1995;124:161-74.

Grillner S. Control of locomotion in bipeds, tetrapods, and fish. In: Brooks VB, ed. Handbook of physiology: the nervous system II. Bethesda: American Physiological Society, 1981:1179-1236.

Hultborn H, Jankowska E, Lindström S. Relative contribution from different nerves to recurrent depression of Ia IPSPs in motoneurones. J Physiol (Lond) 1971;215:637-64.

Jankowska E, Edgley S. Interactions between pathways controlling posture and gait at the level of spinal interneurones in the cat. Prog Brain Res 1993;971:161-71.

Kandel ER, Schwartz JH, Jessell TM. Principles of neural science, 3rd ed. Norwalk: Appleton & Lange, 1991.

Katz R, Pierrot-Deseilligny E. Facilitation of soleus-coupled Renshaw cells during voluntary contraction of pretibial flexor muscles in man. J Physiol (Lond) 1984;355:587-603.

Laouris Y, Windhorst U. Time constraints of facilitation and depression in Renshaw cell responses to random stimulation of motor axons. Exp Brain Res 1988;72:117-28.

Leiner HC, Leiner AL, Dow RS. The underestimated cerebellum. Human Brain Mapping 1995;2:244-54.

Leonard CT. The neurophysiology of human locomotion. In: Craik R, Oates C, eds. Gait analysis: theory and application. St. Louis: Mosby-Year Book, 1993.

Loeb GE, He J, Levine WS. Spinal cord circuits: are they mirrors of musculoskeletal mechanics? J Motor Behav 1989;21:473-91.

Lundberg A, Malmgren K, Schomburg ED. Reflex pathways from group II muscle afferents. Exp Brain Res 1987;65:294-306.

McCurdy ML, Hamm TM. Topography of recurrent inhibitory postsynaptic potentials between individual motoneurons in the cat. J Neurophysiol 1994;72:214-26.

Meunier S, Pierrot-Deseilligny E, Simonettamoreau M. Pattern of heteronymous recurrent inhibition in the human lower limb. Exp Brain Res 1994;102:149-59.

Nielsen J, Crone C, Sinkjaer T, Toft E, Hultborn H. Central control of reciprocal inhibition during fictive dorsiflexion in man. Exp Brain Res 1995;104:99-106.

Pearson KG, Ramirez JM, Jiang W. Entrainment of the locomotor rhythm by group Ib afferents from ankle extensor muscles in spinal cats. Exp Brain Res 1992;90:557-66.

Pierrot-Deseilligny E. Evidence for Ib inhibition in human subjects. Brain Res 1979;166:176-9.

Pompeiano O. The role of Renshaw cells in the dynamic control of posture during vestibulospinal reflexes. Prog Brain Res 1988;76:83-95.

Schieppati M, Gritti I, Romano C. Recurrent and reciprocal inhibition of the human monosynaptic reflex shows opposite changes following intravenous administration of acetylcarnitine. Acta Physiol Scand 1991;143:27-32.

Sinkjaer T, Nielsen J, Toft E. Mechanical and electromyographic analysis of reciprocal inhibition at the human ankle joint. J Neurophysiol 1995;74:849-55.

Windhorst U. Activation of Renshaw cells. Prog Neurobiol 1990;35:135-79.

Windhorst U, Boorman G, Kirmayer D. Renshaw cells and recurrent inhibition: comparison of responses to cyclic inputs. Neuroscience 1995;67:225-33.

Windhorst U, Kokkoroyiannis T, Laouris Y, Meyer-Lohmann J. Higher-order non-linear phenomena in Renshaw cell responses to random motor axon stimulation. Neuroscience 1996;35:687-97.

REFERENCES

1. Alkon DL. Memory storage and neural systems. Sci Am 1989;261:42-50.

2. Andersson O, Forssberg H, Grillner S. Peripheral feedback mechanisms acting on the central pattern generators for locomotion in fish and cat. Can J Physiol Pharmacol 1981;59:713-26.

3. Andersson O, Forssberg H, Grillner S, Lindquist M. Phasic gain control of the transmission in cutaneous reflex pathways to motoneurones during 'fictive' locomotion. Brain Res 1978;149:503-7.

4. Armstrong E. A comparative review of the primate motor system. J Motor Behav 1989;21:493-517.

5. Atwood HL, MacKay WA. Essentials of neurophysiology. Toronto: BC Decker, 1989.

6. Baldissera F, Hultborn H, Illert M. Integration in spinal neuronal systems. In: Brooks VB, ed. Handbook of physiology: the nervous system II. Baltimore: Williams & Wilkins, 1981:509-95.

7. Barinaga M. Social status sculpts activity of crayfish neurons. Science 1996;271:290-1.

8. Binder MD, Brownstone RM, Heckman CJ, Kiehn O, Powers RK. Do neuromodulators and classical neurotransmitters play different roles in shaping motor output? Lecture, Maui, Hawaii, April 1994.

9. Bliss TVP, Gardner-Medwin AR. Long-lasting potentiation of synaptic transmission in the dentate area of the unaesthetized rabbit following stimulation of the perforant path. J Physiol (Lond) 1973;232:357-74.

10. Bliss TVP, Lomo T. Long-lasting potentiation of synaptic transmission in the dentate area of the anesthetized rabbit following stimulation of the perforant path. J Physiol (Lond) 1976;232:331-56.

11. Brooks VB. The neural basis of motor control. New York: Oxford University Press, 1986:1-330.

12. Bussel B, Roby-Brami A, Yakovleff A, Bennis N. Late flexion reflex in paraplegic patients. Evidence for a spinal stepping generator. Brain Res Bull 198922:53-6.

13. Carp JS, Wolpaw JR. Motoneuron plasticity underlying operantly conditioned decrease in primate H-reflex. J Neurophysiol 1995;72:431-42.

14. Carp JS, Wolpaw JR. Motoneuron properties after operantly conditioned increase in primate H-reflex. J Neurophysiol 1995;73:1365-73.

15. Chan CWY, Melvill Jones G, Kearney RE, Watt DGD. The "late" electromyographic response to limb displacement in man. I. Evidence for supraspinal contribution. Electroencephalogr Clin Neurophysiol 1979;46:173-81.

16. Conrad B, Meyer-Lohmann J. The long-loop transcortical load compensating reflex. In: Evarts EV, Wise SP, Bousfield D, eds. The motor system in neurobiology. Amsterdam: Elsevier, 1996:208-14.

17. Crone C, Hultborn H, Jespersen B, Nielsen J. Reciprocal Ia inhibition between ankle flexors and extensors in man. J Physiol (Lond) 1987;389:163-85.

18. de Vries JIP, Visser GHA, Prechtl HFR. Fetal motility in the first half of pregnancy. In: Prechtl HFR, ed. Continuity of neural functions from prenatal to postnatal life. Oxford: Spastics International Medical Publications, 1984:46-64.

19. Descartes R. Treatise of man. Cambridge: Harvard University Press, 1972.

20. Dubuc R, Bongianni F, Ohta Y, Grillner S. Dorsal root and dorsal column mediated synaptic inputs to reticulospinal neurons in lampreys: involvement of glutamatergic, glycinergic, and gabaergic transmissions. J Comp Neurol 1993;327:251-9.

21. Eccles JC, Eccles RM, Lundberg A. The convergence of monosynaptic excitatory afferents onto many different species of alpha motoneurones. J Physiol (Lond) 1957;137:22-50.

22. Eccles RM, Lundberg A. Synaptic actions in motoneurones by afferents which may evoke the flexion reflex. Arch Ital Biol 1959;97:199-221.

23. Eidelberg E, Walden JG, Nguyen LH. Locomotor control in macaque monkeys. Brain 1981;104:647-63.

24. Evarts EV, Granit R. Relations of reflexes and intended movements. Prog Brain Res 1976;39:1-14.

25. Evarts EV, Tanji J. Reflex and intended responses in motor cortex pyramidal tract neurons of monkey. J Neurophysiol 1976;39:1069-80.

26. Feldman JL, Grillner S. Control of vertebrate respiration and locomotion: a brief account. Physiologist 1983;26:310-6.

27. Forssberg H. Stumbling corrective reaction: a phase-dependent compensatory reaction during locomotion. J Neurophysiol 1979;42:936-53.

28. Forssberg H. Ontogeny of human locomotor control I. Infant stepping, supported locomotion and transition to independent locomotion. Exp Brain Res 1985;57:480-93.

29. Forssberg H, Eliasson AC, Kinoshita H, Westling G, Johansson RS. Development of human precision grip. IV. Tactile adaptation of isometric finger forces to the frictional condition. Exp Brain Res 1995;104:323-30.

30. Forssberg H, Grillner S, Halbertsma J. The locomotion of the spinal cat. I. Coordination within a hindlimb. Acta Physiol Scand 1980;108:269-81.

31. Forssberg H, Grillner S, Halbertsma J, Rossignol S. The locomotion of the spinal cat. II. Interlimb coordination. Acta Physiol Scand 1980;108:283-95.

32. Forssberg H, Grillner S, Rossignol S. Phase dependent reflex reversal during walking in chronic spinal cats. Brain Res 1975;85:103-7.

33. Forssberg H, Grillner S, Rossignol S. Phasic gain control of reflexes from the dorsum of the paw during spinal locomotion. Brain Res 1977;132:121-39.

34. Forssberg H, Hirschfeld H. Phasic modulation of postural activation patterns during human walking. Prog Brain Res 1988;76:221-7.

35. Georgopoulos AP, Caminiti R, Kalaska JF, Massey JT. Spatial coding of movement: a hypothesis concerning the coding of movement direction by motor cortical populations. Exp Brain Res 1983;7:327-36.

36. Georgopoulos AP, Kalaska JF, Caminiti R, Massey JT. On the relations between the direction of two-dimensional arm movements and cell discharge in primate motor cortex. J Neurosci 1982;2:1527-37.

37. Georgopoulos AP, Schwartz AB, Kettner RE. Neuronal population coding of movement direction. Science 1986;233:1416-9.

38. Ghez C, Shinoda Y. Spinal mechanisms of the functional stretch reflex. Exp Brain Res 1978;32:55-68.

39. Glenn MB, Whyte J. The practical management of spasticity in children and adults. Philadelphia: Lea & Febiger, 1990.

40. Gordon AM, Forssberg H, Johansson RS, Westling G. Integration of sensory information during the programming of precision grip: comments on the contributions of size cues. Exp Brain Res 1991;85:226-9.

41. Gracies JM, Meunier S, Pierrot-Deseilligny E. Evidence of corticospinal excitation of presumed propriospinal neurones in man. J Physiol Paris 1994;475:509-18.

42. Grillner S. Locomotion in the spinal dogfish. Acta Physiol Scand 1973;87:31A-32A.

43. Grillner S. Locomotion in the spinal cat. In: Stein RB, Pearson KB, Smith RS, Redford JB, eds. Control of posture and locomotion. New York: Plenum Publishing, 1976:515-35.

44. Grillner S. Neurobiological bases of rhythmic motor acts in vertebrates. Science 1985;228:143-9.

45. Grillner S, Dubuc R. Control of locomotion in vertebrates: spinal and supraspinal mechanisms. Adv Neurol 1988;47:425-53.

46. Grillner S, Perret C, Zangger P. Central generation of locomotion in the spinal dogfish. Brain Res 1976;109:255-69.

47. Grillner S, Rossignol S. On the initiation of the swing phase of locomotion in chronic spinal cats. Brain Res 1978;146:269-77.

48. Grillner S, Zangger P. How detailed is the central pattern generation for locomotion? Brain Res 1975;88:367-71.

49. Hagbarth KE. EMG studies of stretch reflexes in man. In: Widen L, ed. Recent advances in clinical neurophysiology, EEG and clinical neurophysiology. Amsterdam: Elsevier, 1967:74-9.

50. Hammond PH. The influence of prior instruction to the subject on an apparently involuntary neuro-muscular response. J Physiol 1956;132:17-8.

51. Harrison PJ, Jankowska E, Jahannisson T. Shared reflex pathways of group I afferents of different cat hind-limb muscles. J Physiol 1983;338:113-27.

52. Hebb DO. The organization of behavior. New York: Wiley, 1949.

53. Hirschfeld H, Forssberg H. Phase-dependent modulations of anticipatory postural activity during human locomotion. J Neurophysiol 1991;66:12-9.

54. Holmqvist B, Lundberg A. Differential supraspinal control of synaptic actions evoked by volleys in the flexion reflex afferents in alpha motoneurones. Acta Physiol Scand 1961;54:5-51.

55. Hultborn H, Lindstrm HS, Wigstrm H. On the function of recurrent inhibition in the spinal cord. Exp Brain Res 1979;37:399-403.

56. Iles JF, Roberts RC. Presynaptic inhibition of monosynaptic reflexes in the lower limbs of subjects with upper motoneuron disease. J Neurol Neurosurg Psychiatry 1986;49:937-44.

57. James W. Psychology: briefer course. Cambridge: Harvard University Press, 1989.

58. Jankowska E. Interneuronal relay in spinal pathways from proprioceptors. Prog Neurobiol 1992;38:335-78.

59. Jankowska E, Jukes MGM, Lund S, Lundberg A. The effect of DOPA on the spinal cord. 5. Reciprocal organization of pathways transmitting excitatory action to

alpha motoneurones of flexor and extensors. Acta Physiol Scand 1967;70:369-88.

60. Kandel ER. Cellular mechanisms of learning and the biological basis of individuality. In: Kandel ER, Schwartz JH, Jessell TM, eds. Principles of neural science, 3rd ed. Norwalk: Appleton & Lange, 1991:1009-31.

61. Katz R, Pierrot-Deseilligny E. Recurrent inhibition of alpha-motoneurons in patients with upper motor neuron lesions. Brain 1982;105:103-24.

62. Kennedy PR. Corticospinal, rubrospinal and rubro-olivary projections: a unifying hypothesis. Trends Neurosci 1990;13:474-9.

63. Kocsis JD. Competition in the synaptic marketplace: activity is important. Neuroscientist 1995;1:185-7.

64. Kravitz EA, Treherne JE. Neurotransmission, neurotransmitters and neuromodulators. Cambridge: Cambridge University Press, 1981.

65. Kuypers HG. Corticospinal connections: postnatal development in the rhesus monkey. Science 1962;138:678-80.

66. Kuypers HGJM. Anatomy of the descending pathways. In: Brooks VB, ed. Handbook of physiology: the nervous system. Baltimore: Williams & Wilkins, 1981:597-666.

67. Lee RG, Tatton WG. Motor responses to sudden limb displacement in primates with specific CNS disorders and in human patients with motor system disorders. Can J Neurol Sci 1975;2:285-93.

68. Leonard CT. Motor behavior and neural changes following perinatal and adult-onset brain damage: implications for therapeutic interventions. Phys Ther 1994;74:753-67.

69. Leonard CT, Goldberger ME. Consequences of damage to the sensorimotor cortex in neonatal and adult cats. I. Sparing and recovery of function. Dev Brain Res 1987;32:1-14.

70. Leonard CT, Goldberger ME. Consequences of damage to the sensorimotor cortex in neonatal and adult cats. II. Maintenance of exuberant projections. Dev Brain Res 1987;32:15-30.

71. Leonard CT, Hirschfeld H, Forssberg H. The development of independent walking in children with cerebral palsy. Dev Med Child Neurol 1991;33:567-77.

72. Leonard CT, Moritani T, Hirschfeld H, Forssberg H. Deficits in reciprocal inhibition in children with cerebral palsy as revealed by H reflex testing. Dev Med Child Neurol 1990;32:974-84.

73. Loeb GE. Hard lessons in motor control from the mammalian spinal cord. Trends Neurosci 1987;10:108-13.

74. Lundberg A. Reflex control of stepping. In: The Nansen Memorial Lecture, October 10, 1968. Oslo: Universitetsforlaget, 1969:1-42.

75. Lundberg A, Voorhoeve P. Effects from the pyramidal tract on spinal reflex arcs. Acta Physiol Scand 1962;56:201-19.

76. McCrea DA. Spinal cord circuitry and motor reflexes. In: Pandolf KB, ed. Exercise and sport science reviews, vol 14. New York: Macmillan, 1986:105-41.

77. McCrea DA. Can sense be made of spinal interneuron circuits? Behav Brain Sci 1992;15:633-43.

78. Nashner LM. Adapting reflexes controlling human posture. Exp Brain Res 1976;26:59-72.

79. Nelson PG, Yu C, Fields RD, Neale EA. Synaptic connections in vitro: modulation of number and efficacy by electrical activity. Science 1989;244:585-7.

80. Okamoto T, Goto Y. Human infant preindependent and independent walking. In: Kondo S, ed. Primate morphophysiology, locomotor analyses and human bipedalism. Tokyo: University of Tokyo Press, 1985:25-45.

81. Okamoto T, Kumamoto M. Electromyographic study of the learning process of walking in infants. Electromyography 1972;12:149-59.

82. Orlovsky GN. Electrical activity in brainstem and descending paths in guided locomotion. Sechenov Physiol J USSR 1969;55:437-44.

83. Palmer E, Ashby P. Evidence that a long latency stretch reflex in humans is transcortical. J Physiol (Lond) 1992;449:429-40.

84. Passingham RE. Changes in the size and organization of the brain in man and his ancestors. Brain Behav Evol 1975;11:73-90.

85. Phillips CG. Motor apparatus of the baboon's hand. Proc R Soc Lond [Biol] 1996;173:141-74.

86. Pierrot-Deseilligny E. Electrophysiological assessment of the spinal mechanisms underlying spasticity. New Trends Adv Tech Clin Neurophysiol 1990;41:264-73.

87. Prochazka A. Proprioceptive feedback and movement regulation. In: Rowell L, Shapard J, Smith J, et al, eds. American handbook of physiology. New York: Oxford University Press, 1995:1-29.

88. Robinson DA. Implications of neural networks for how we think about brain function. In: Cordo P, Harnard S, eds. Movement control. Cambridge: Cambridge University Press, 1994:42-53.

89. Robinson GA, Goldberger ME. The development and recovery of motor function in spinal cats. I. The infant lesion effect. Exp Brain Res 1986;62:373-86.

90. Robinson GA, Goldberger ME. The development and recovery of motor function in spinal cats. II. Pharmacological enhancement of recovery. Exp Brain Res 1986;62:387-400.

91. Rossi A, Decchi B, Zalaffi A, Mazzocchio R. Group Ia non-reciprocal inhibition from wrist extensor to flexor motoneurones in humans. Neurosci Lett 1995;191:205-7.

92. Rossignol S, Barbeau H, Julien C. Locomotion of the adult chronic spinal cat and its modification by monoaminergic agonists and antagonists. In: Goldberger ME, Gorio A, Murray M, eds. Development and plasticity of the mammalian spinal cord. New York: Fidia Research Series, 1984:323-45.

93. Rossignol S, Lund JP, Drew T. The role of sensory inputs in regulating patterns of rhythmical movements in higher vertebrates. A comparison between locomotion, respiration and mastication. In: Cohen AH, Rossignol S, Grillner S, eds. Neural control of rhythmic movements in vertebrates. New York: John Wiley & Sons, 1988:201-84.

94. Rothwell JC, Day BL, Berardelli A, Marsden CD. Effects of motor cortex stimulation on spinal interneurones in intact man. Exp Brain Res 1984;54:382-4.

95. Sarnat HB, Netsky MG. Evolution of the nervous system. London: Oxford University Press, 1974.

96. Schomburg ED. Spinal sensorimotor systems and their supraspinal control. Neurosci Res 1990;7:265-340.

97. Shefner JM, Berman SA, Sarkarati M, Young RR. Recurrent inhibition is increased in patients with spinal cord injury. Neurology 1992;42:2162-8.

98. Shik ML, Severin FV, Orlovsky GN. Control of walking and running by means of electrical stimulation of the mid-brain. Biofizika 1966;11:659-66.

99. Shinoda Y. Divergent projection of individual corticospinal axons to motoneurons of multiple muscles in the monkey. Neurosci Lett 1981;23:7-12.

100. Shurrager PS, Dykman RA. Walking spinal carnivores. J Comp Psychol 1951;44:252-62.

101. Small SA, Kandel ER. Activity-dependent enhancement of presynaptic inhibition in aplysia sensory neurons. Science 1989;243:1603-6.

102. Stanfield BB. The development of the corticospinal projection. Prog Neurobiol 1992;38:169-202.

103. Stein RB. Presynaptic inhibition in humans. Prog Neurobiol 1995;47:533-44.

104. Thomas A, Autgaerden S, eds. Locomotion from pre- to post-natal life. London: Medical Books Ltd, 1966:1-88.

105. Veale JL, Rees S, Mark RF. Renshaw cell activity in normal and spastic man. New Dev Electromyogr Clin Neurophysiol 1973;3:523-37.

106. Walters ET, Alizadeh H, Castro GA. Similar neuronal alterations induced by axonal injury and learning in aplysia. Science 1991;253:797-9.

107. Windhorst U. Shaping static elbow torque-angle relationships by spinal cord circuits: a theoretical study. Neuroscience 1994;59:713-27.

108. Wolpaw JR, Lee CL. Memory traces in primate spinal cord produced by operant conditioning of H-reflex. J Neurophysiol 1989;61:563-72.

109. Wolpaw JR, O'Keefe JA. Adaptive plasticity in the primate spinal stretch reflex: evidence for a two-phase process. J Neurosci 1984;4:2718-24.

110. Yeh SR, Fricke RA, Edwards DH. The effect of social experience on serotonergic modulation of the escape circuit of crayfish. Science 1996;271:366-9.

The Role of the Cerebral Cortex in Movement

T o say that the human brain is full of fascination and wonder is an understatement of unbelievable proportion. For me, or any author, to write about the functioning of the human brain during movement is a presumptuous act. It is presumptuous because although a vast amount of knowledge has been acquired over the years, we still have no idea how the brain functions. Much of what will be presented in this chapter is conjectural. I have attempted to present available data and synthesize this information into generalized statements regarding how the cerebral cortex contributes to movement and motor control. The role of the cerebral cortex in movement spans the spectrum from thought formation and motivation to the actual generation of a muscle contraction. We remain largely in the dark about how this is accomplished. A quick review of a few statistical tidbits should provide some insight into why an understanding of brain function during movement or any other task remains such a daunting assignment.

■ TERMINOLOGY AND BASIC ORGANIZATIONAL PRINCIPLES

Cerebral statistics

The human brain has a surface area of approximately 1,100 cm^2 per hemisphere and weighs about 1,500 gm. Its volume is approximately that of a quart of milk. The composition of the brain is unremarkable, being composed of 78% water, 10% fat, 8% protein, and 4% "other stuff" (the infamous inert ingredients of consumer product labeling). Despite its rather mundane biochemical profile and the fact that it comprises less than 2.5% of our total body weight, the brain receives over 15% of the body's blood supply and uses 25% of all available oxygen. The brain uses glucose, the jet fuel of human energy sources. It is a self-

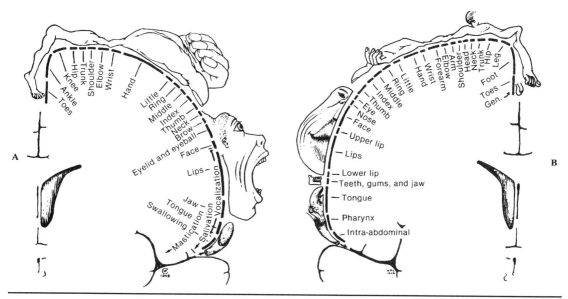

Fig. 4-1. Dr. Penfield's homunculus is an organizational map of the primary motor and somatosensory cortices. Electrical stimulation of the areas depicted in the figure cause movement or sensation of that body part. Notice that more cortical area is devoted to dexterous body parts such as the face and hands. (From Penfield W, Rasmussen T. The cerebral cortex of man. New York: Macmillan Publishing Co., 1950.)

centered metabolic furnace. Deprive it of oxygen or energy for less than a minute and it begins to shut down all bodily processes.

Studies have estimated that the human brain contains 10^{11} (100 billion) neurons that form 10^{14} (100 trillion) synapses and from 10^5 to 10^{15} discrete interconnected cortical circuits.[133] Its convoluted, gyrencephalic surface is more irregular than the surface of the earth. All of this information makes for fascinating trivia but reveals little about the functioning of the human cerebral cortex. Neuroscientists are a clever bunch, however, and behind the closed doors of laboratories around the world, the black box of cerebral functioning is being illuminated a bit more with each passing day. The study of brain circuitry and function is at a stage, however, where scientists aren't even certain what to call various areas of the brain. As more discrete functional areas and circuits are discovered, terminology must change to accommodate these findings.[48] Much of the nomenclature that has been used for the past century to define subdivisions within the cerebral cortex is beginning to lose relevance.

Introduction to brain nomenclature

The homunculus is dead. The significance of this revolutionary, but far from original, opinion is probably lost on new students. To seasoned clinical veterans it might sound like heresy. The homunculus is an organizational map of the primary motor cortex. In the 1930s, Dr. Wilder Penfield, a Canadian neurosurgeon, electrically stimulated the brains of patients with epilepsy during surgery. He found that stimulation of certain cortical areas caused reproducible movements of different body parts. The cortical areas appeared to be organized in such a way that one cortical area controlled one body part. The more agility required of the body part, and the broader the movement repertoire, the larger the cortical area devoted to its control. For instance, the hands and face have a broader representation than the less dexterous legs and trunk. Dr. Penfield characterized his findings with a drawing (Fig. 4-1) of a man draped across the motor strip area of the cerebral cortex. This motor strip corresponds to Brodman's area 4 or the primary motor cortex (MI). Penfield's drawing depicted the cortical representation of each body part and thus the drawn figure, or homunculus, illustrated the relative proportions of the cortex devoted to the control of a body part. Findings of the past decade, however, have displaced the notion of one cortical area controlling one body part. Rather, the current notion is that multiple and diffuse cortical areas interact to control various aspects of a movement or body part.

The demise of the homunculus actually began before its conception. In 1909, Dr. Korbinian Brodman published "Verleichende Lokalisationslehre der Grosshirnrinde in ihren Prinzipien dargestellt auf Grund des Zellenbaues." The book summarized Dr. Brodman's neuroanatomical findings relating to localization of cell types and laminar organization within the cerebral cortex. Based on his *cytoarchitectonic* analysis, Dr. Brodman proposed and described 47 different functional areas within the human brain (Fig. 4-2). Although Dr. Brodman described 47 discrete areas, in his writings he speculated that multiple representations of functional areas could exist and that interconnectivity between cortical areas would impact movement. Thus, he foresaw the limitations of his taxonomy and foreshadowed the demise of the homunculus and his own organizational scheme. One obvious problem with the idea of a homunculus or a 1:1 representation of cortical area to body part is that movement involves multiple body parts and muscles. During any particular movement, some muscles contract to stabilize a joint while others contract synergistically to initiate and perpetuate a movement. Some muscles contract isometrically while others contract eccentrically or concentrically. In the 1950s, experiments by Dr. Clinton Woolsey provided hard data for Dr. Brodman's speculations that motor behaviors would be broadly represented in the cerebral cortex. His experiments showed that multiple areas within the brain could elicit movement. These experiments resulted in the abandonment of the idea of a "motor strip" in favor of somatic "sensorimotor areas." Recent scanning techniques indicate that the diffuse representation of somatic sensorimotor areas is even greater than originally proposed by Woolsey. Brodman's nomenclature has expanded from 47 discrete areas to over 10^3 discrete functioning centers within the brain.[133] Obviously these new findings have not only expanded and clouded our notions about the role of the cerebral cortex in movement, they have also challenged existing nomenclature. As more becomes known about the organizational principles guiding cortical control of movement, the less relevant the organizational taxonomy based solely on cytoarchitectonics appears to be. Techniques that allow the examination of the brain's functional physiology have greatly expanded our knowledge and have challenged neuroscientist's ability to attach organizational order to new findings.

Confounding variables that need to be considered when attempting to name and classify brain regions are: (1) the considerable amount of species variation with regard to functioning areas within the cerebral cortex, (2) the evolutionary expansion of the human brain, and (3) individual differences that result from genetic and epigenetic factors.

Only mammals have developed a *neocortex* (*isocortex*). The differences in the organization and relative sizes of various functional regions within the neocortex (as well as other central nervous system [CNS] structures) of various mammalian species are dramatic (see Figs. 2-18 and 4-3). For instance, each human cerebral hemisphere has a surface area of approximately 1,100 cm^2, whereas that of a rodent is about 3.5 cm^2. The proportional sizes of association cortical areas, cerebellar nuclei and connections, and brain stem nuclei are very different.[19,133] Even within a species, the variability among individuals is considerable. Epigenetic factors profoundly affect some aspects of cortical organization and function. New brain imaging techniques are increasingly revealing the individual uniqueness we all possess.

Brain mapping/brain scanning techniques

Brain imaging techniques permit concomitant analysis of brain structure and function in humans. Imaging is noninvasive and can be used to examine cognitive, emotional, sensory, and motor functions of awake

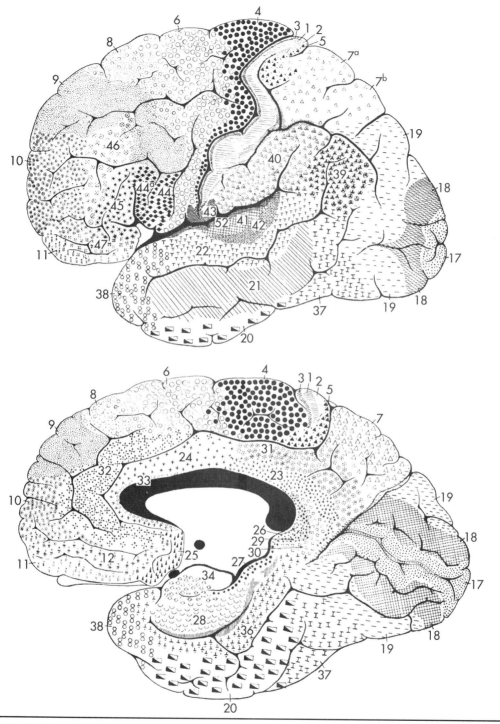

Fig. 4-2. Dr. Brodman, based on cytoarchitectonics, divided the cerebral cortex into 47 different areas, each with a different function. (From Von Economo G, Koskinas GN: Die cytoarchitektonik der Hirnrinde des erwachsenen Menschen. Heidelberg: Julius Springer, 1925.)

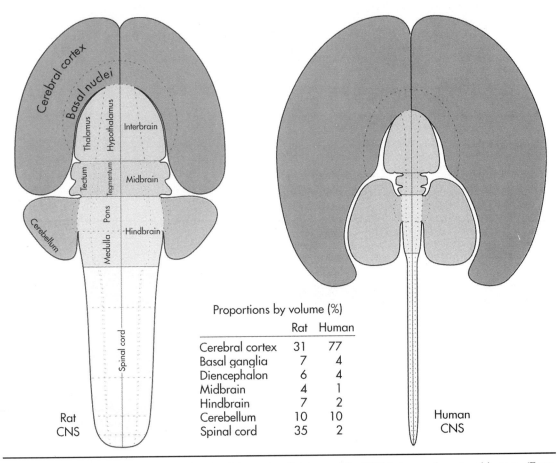

Fig. 4-3. Comparison of the relative volumes of the major divisions of the CNS between the rat and human. (From Swanson L. Trends Neurosci 1995;18:471-4.)

human beings. The capabilities of different imaging techniques range from discerning structures hidden within the folds of the cerebral cortex such as the basal ganglia, to identifying the neurotransmitters used in a certain pathway during a specified function. The following paragraphs describe briefly some of the techniques now being used to assess human brain function.

The pneumoencephalogram. The pneumoencephalogram was once the clinical tool of choice to examine cerebral structures such as the ventricles. Hydrocephalus is a condition in which one or more of the ventricles becomes enlarged, usually secondary to blockage of one of the foramen that drain the cerebrospinal fluid from the ventricles. A pneumoencephalogram involves removing a bit of cerebrospinal fluid from the lumbar cistern and replacing it with air. The air rises through the ventricles and, being less dense than the fluid, can be detected by x-ray studies. The procedure, however, is rather unpleasant for the patient and does not reveal any of the internal structures of the brain. CT scans have now largely displaced the pneumoencephalogram.

Computed tomography. Computed tomography (CT) is perhaps the oldest of the new scanning techniques for imaging the brain. CT uses x-ray radiation and computerized technology to detect variations in the radiodensity of tissues. Its resolution is better than conventional x-rays and one can obtain images of different planes of the brain at various angles and depths of penetration. CT scans can differentiate gray and white matter, blood, and cerebrospinal fluid (Fig. 4-4).

CT scans can not only show the size and symmetry of the ventricles or obstructive masses, it can also image deep cortical structures. They can also show the general size of an infarct after stroke or brain trauma. CT scans show internal structures but reveal nothing about the functioning of the brain. They remain, however, a very useful, noninvasive, and safe clinical tool.

Magnetic resonance imaging. Magnetic resonance imaging (MRI) does not use x-rays but rather magnetic fields to detect both structure and function of the human brain. Exposure to a brief magnetic field causes atomic nuclei to spin in a certain rotation. When the magnetic pulse is turned off, the nuclei return to their original positions and release energy in the form of radio waves. The frequency of these radio waves differs for different tissues. Different aspects of these radio waves can be detected and used to image brain structures or various elements (iron, sodium, phosphorous) within these structures.[94]

MRI scans provide better visual resolution than CT scans (Fig. 4-5). MRI is better able to distinguish gray matter from white matter and is thus able to detect demyelinating disease processes such as multiple sclerosis. Although MRIs can be used to detect metabolic activity within the brain, positron emission tomography (PET) is better suited for these types of analyses.

MRI is being used in conjunction with PET scans to provide the best of two worlds: the high resolution of brain structures by MRI and the ability to detect metabolically active neurons within the brain by PET. This methodology is termed functional magnetic resonance imaging (fMRI).

Positron emission tomography. When the human brain is actively engaged in a mental activity (whether it is a cognitive or motor control task), the metabolic activity of the neurons within certain areas of the brain increases. Metabolic activity is most enhanced in those areas most directly involved in the behavior. During a visual task, the visual cortex will be very active, and during execution of certain motor tasks, the motor cortex will be active. PET scans can detect changes in the metabolic activity of neurons and thus allow investigators to examine the functioning of the brain during various tasks.

Neurons use glucose for their energy source. A radioactive analog of glucose, 2-deoxyglucose, competes with glucose and is taken up by a metabolically active neuron. Unlike glucose, 2-deoxyglucose cannot be broken down and becomes trapped within the cell. This radioactive isotope emits radiation that can be detected by the scanning device. PET scans, therefore, can be used to show what areas of the brain are most active during specific tasks. PET has been used to show differences in cortical structures involved in motor learning and to show differences in the pattern of activity within the brain of people with schizophrenia and those with learning disorders.

Use of PET scans is not limited to detecting metabolic activity within the brain. By binding radioactive isotopes to neurotransmitters, the distribution of various transmitters and their receptors can be determined. By using these techniques, investigators can determine whether a certain transmitter or pathway is used preferentially during a certain activity, whether certain clinical syndromes are associated with changes in transmitter release, and whether pharmacological interventions have an effect on transmitters or their locations during functional activities.

Cortical evoked potentials. Cortical evoked potentials involve applying a stimulus to a peripheral nerve or sense organ and recording the accompanying cortical electrical activity with an electrode placed over the scalp of the appropriate cortical region (i.e., the cortical area that is receptive to that particular sensory input). In this way the integrity of the entire sensory pathway, from receptor to cortex, can be assessed. Recording from several subcortical regions is possible as well.

Visual evoked potentials or pattern-shift visual evoked responses tests the integrity of the visual system. A light stimulus flashed onto the retina results in activity in the occipital lobe of the brain. This test is used to diagnose lesions of the optic nerve and also CNS diseases such as multiple sclerosis.

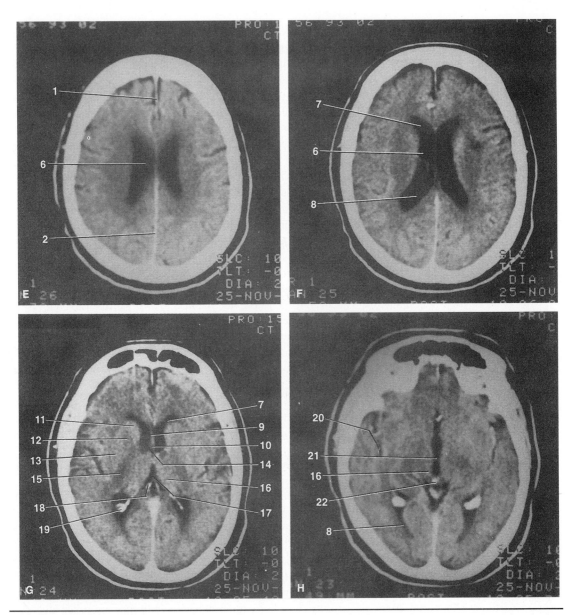

Fig. 4-4. A computed tomography (CT) image shows grey and white matter, ventricles, and some CNS structures within the cerebral cortex. *1.* Anterior falx; *2,* posterior falx; *6,* body of the lateral ventricle; *7,* anterior horn of the lateral ventricle; *8,* posterior horn of the lateral ventricle; *9,* septum pellucidum; *10,* fornix; *11,* head of caudate nucleus; *12,* internal capsule, anterior limb; *13,* lenticular nucleus; *14,* interventricular foramen of Monro; *15,* internal capsule, posterior limb; *16,* thalamus; *17,* cavum velum interpositum; *18,* internal cerebral vein; *19,* choroid plexus in trigone of lateral ventricle; *20,* insula cistern; *21,* third ventricle, *22,* pineal. (From Jennes L, Traurig HH, Conn PM. Atlas of the human brain. Philadelphia: JB Lippincott Co., 1995.)

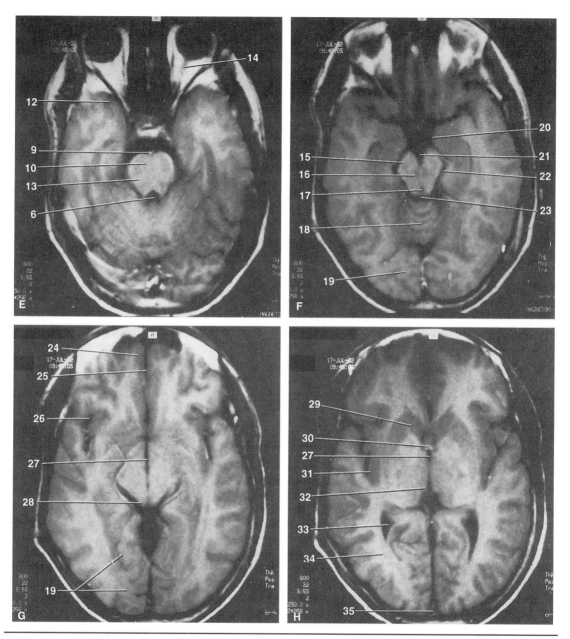

Fig. 4-5. Magnetic resonance image (MRI) shows some of the same structures as the CT scan of Fig. 4-4. *6*, Fourth ventricle; *9*, basilar artery; *10*, basilar pons; *12*, temporal lobe; *13*, tegmentum of pons; *14*, optic nerve; *15*, cerebral peduncle; *16*, red nucleus; *17*, cerebral aqueduct; *18*, vermis of cerebellum; *19*, occipital lobe; *20*, uncus of hippocampus; *21*, interpeduncular cistern; *22*, ambient cistern; *23*, quadrigeminal cistern; *24*, frontal lobe; *25*, interhemispheric fissure; *26*, lateral fissure; *27*, third ventricle; *28*, superior colliculus; *29*, head of caudate nucleus; *30*, fornix; *31*, insula; *32*, habenula; *33*, posterior horn of the lateral ventricle; *34*, visual pathway (geniculocalcarine tract); *35*, superior sagittal sinus. (From Jennes L, Traurig HH, Conn PM. Atlas of the human brain. Philadelphia: JB Lippincott Co., 1995.)

Brain stem auditory evoked potentials are recorded over the auditory portions of the cortex after stimuli presented to one or both ears. A scalp electrode records a series of waves after the sound stimulus. Each distinct wave represents a different portion of the auditory pathway. A lesion that affects a certain part of the pathway will result in changes in the amplitude and latency of one of the waves. Certain CNS diseases and tumors cause changes in brain stem auditory evoked potentials.

Somatosensory evoked potentials or short-latency somatosensory evoked potentials are used to assess sensory pathways to the brain. Electrical stimuli are applied to various peripheral nerves and the resulting potentials are recorded from the sensory cortex of the parietal lobe by scalp electrodes. These procedures can be used to detect peripheral nerve disease, nerve root lesions, and lesions involving the medial lemniscus and thalamoparietal pathway.

Electroencephalography. The electroencephalogram (EEG) records electrical activity generated in the cerebral cortex. It reflects the summation of the excitatory and inhibitory synaptic potentials occurring throughout the brain. Electrodes (usually 8 to 16) are placed on the scalp in a standardized array. The placement of the electrodes permits detection of brain electrical activity and patterns of activity (rhythms) from the various lobes of the brain. Electrical activity within the brain typically occurs at certain frequencies and amplitudes. Depending on the frequency and amplitude of the sinusoidal waves, they are assigned names such as alpha (8 to 12 Hz), beta (>12 Hz), theta (4-7 Hz), and delta (1-3 Hz). Alpha waves are typically recorded over the parietal and occipital lobes and beta activity is generally recorded from the frontal lobes.

The EEG is particularly useful in the diagnosis of seizure disorders. It is also helpful in the diagnosis of sleep disorders. EEGs also used in cases of brain injury, degenerative diseases, and brain tumors.

The EEG has been used for many years as a biofeedback tool for relaxation and stress relief. An evolving, and potentially therapeutic, use of the EEG involves training individuals to alter EEG activity to control computer cursor movement.[147] This application may contribute to a severely disabled individual's ability to control his environment. For instance, an individual who has lost the use of his arms might be able to turn lights on and off, change radio stations, and perform other tasks by moving a computer cursor to a certain icon on the screen, thereby activating the necessary electronics.

The EEG is also being combined with PET scans to show brain activations during thought processes and visual perception tasks. This approach has the advantage of not only showing what areas of the brain are metabolically active, but also of revealing the patterns of activity throughout the brain during a given task. Electroencephalography is associated with less of a time lag than PET is. The use of EEGs with other scanning techniques such as PET is referred to as *multimodal imaging.* Magnetoencephalography is another technique that is being used in conjunction with PET scans.

Magnetoencephalography. Magnetoencephalography is closely related to electroencephalography. It measures magnetic field distributions of the entire cerebral cortex. This imaging technique can detect changes that occur spontaneously and those evoked by external sensory stimuli. It is a painless, noninvasive technique that, unlike EEG recordings, does not rely on time-consuming electrode placements. Magnetoencephalography has been used to study sensory processing and to examine the functional organization of sensorimotor areas of the human brain.[62]

By using magnetoencephalography in conjunction with MRI, one can identify functions of cerebral structures that are involved in sensory activities. It has been used to identify the source of epileptic seizures and to trace parallel pathways involved in the processing of visual information.[62]

Cortical magnetic stimulation. Cortical magnetic stimulation is not a brain mapping technique similar to CT, MRI, or PET. Nor does it detect magnetic field changes like magnetoencephalography. Rather, cortical magnetic stimulation uses electric current and the generation of a magnetic field to stimulate specific cortical areas. It has proven to be particularly useful for the study of motor areas of the brain. Before magnetic stimulation procedures were developed, one could elicit muscle contractions and limb movements by applying an electrical stimulation over the scalp. This is a rather uncomfortable procedure and has now been replaced by painless magnetic stimulation procedures. An insulated coil of wire is placed on the scalp. Passing an electric current through the coil creates a magnetic field perpendicular to the coil. The magnetic field essentially transfers an electrical impulse to cortical tissues, with very little spread to the scalp and no pain to the individual being tested.

Cortical magnetic stimulation activates monosynaptic, corticospinal neurons. The muscular contractions evoked with the stimulation are stronger when subjects are voluntarily contracting a muscle versus when they are at rest. This is because the motor neurons innervating a contracting muscle are in a more excitable state and are more susceptible to activation by descending input.[121] Magnetic stimulation has been used to map the motor cortex and to differentiate areas that preferentially activate hand, finger, and forearm muscles. It has also been used to show the plasticity of motor cortical projections after injury.[15,39]

One experiment showed that a patient with an amputation of the arm below the shoulder had a wider cortical distribution for the activation of the deltoid muscle on the amputated side than on the intact side.[121] This finding provided support for cortical reorganization after injury in humans, similar to that described for nonhuman mammals.[96] Cortical magnetic stimulation has also been used to study the distribution of corticospinal tract neurons,[15,16] patients with neurological disorders,[20,68] cortical contributions to postural reactions,[85] and cerebral plasticity.[39]

I would like to emphasize one cautionary note regarding the use of any of the aforementioned scanning or mapping techniques. As beautiful and as useful as they are, they cannot as yet compete with the level of accuracy of microscopic neuroanatomical and neurophysiological techniques. Gliosis of a cell (a prelude to cell death) can only be detected microscopically. Spared spinal cord projections can only be identified by invasive neuroanatomical or neurophysiological methods and not by any type of clinical scans available today. These are important points. An MRI can grossly identify lesion sites, but it usually cannot indicate whether a small lacunar infarct has compromised a brain stem cranial nerve nucleus. Nor can MRI accurately show whether a lesion, thought to be isolated to the internal capsule, has actually spared the thalamus or basal ganglia. Scans have not replaced a skilled clinical examination or displaced the neuropathologist.

Furthermore, a specific cortical area might be more efficient in a certain task and thus have less relative metabolic activity than another cortical area that is involved but not as efficient in the task. This possibility makes interindividual comparisons very difficult. Knowing what area is active during a task does not tell us how well that particular area is functioning or what the area is doing.[64]

Scanning techniques have greatly contributed, and will continue to contribute, to our understanding of the functional characteristics of the human brain. For the first time in history we can actually visualize the human brain at work. The following section provides a general overview of currently held opinions regarding the functions of various cortical areas that contribute to motor control and the associated nomenclature. Bear in mind that any statement made today regarding principles of brain circuitry organization is likely to need modification in the not-too-distant future.

Organization of cortical fields and functional modules

At the outset I would like to stress that multiple cortical areas and other CNS structures contribute to the control of movement. The individual functioning of any one area of the cerebral cortex does not necessarily indicate how it will interact with other cortical and subcortical pathways and ultimately impact movement. Human PET and fMRI scans have verified data from electrophysiological experiments in monkeys showing that movements of even a single finger are controlled by diffuse networks of neurons.[5] The more complex the movement, the more cortical networks need to be involved. The neocortex consists of a number of functionally and anatomically defined areas that interconnect to form neural networks (Fig. 4-6).

The following paragraphs outline some of the functional characteristics associated with the major sensorimotor cortical areas. The listing is not complete. Virtually all areas of the cortex are directly or indirectly involved in motor control. For instance, the auditory and visual cortices will not be discussed, yet they are intimately connected to sensorimotor areas of the brain. Table 4-1 summarizes the relationship between cortical field nomenclature and Brodman's taxonomy. Note that this is a listing of convenience. The array of organizational schemes from which to choose is bewildering. Almost weekly, new classification systems are developed to accommodate newly discovered unique functional features of cortical areas.

Primary motor area. The primary motor area (MI) was the first cortical area to be directly associated with motor functions. Earlier investigators referred to it as the motor strip. Electrical stimulation to this area of the brain causes movement of various body parts depending on the location of the stimulation. The leg, arm, and head representations within the MI are located in fairly distinct regions. However, within these regions exist multiple representations of the same body part. For instance, the MI arm region contains multiple, overlapping representations of arm muscles and movements.[122] This is rather different than the strict somatotopy proposed by Penfield's homunculus.

The MI is the home of Betz cells, large pyramidal cells that, among other projections, monosynaptically connect with motor neurons in the spinal cord. Forty percent of all pyramidal tract neurons (PTNs) originate in the MI. Of these, the majority terminate in the spinal cord.[112] These *corticospinal* projections have a unique distribution in humans.

In most mammals, the corticospinal tract (CST) terminates in the dorsal horn of the cervical spinal cord.[4,19] If you remember back to previous chapters of this book, this fact should be rich with functional significance. The cervical spinal cord is mainly concerned with the upper extremity and the dorsal horn primarily contains sensory neurons. The fact that the CST of nonprimate mammals synapses in the cervical dorsal horn indicates that the mammalian CST is most likely involved with modulation of sensory information from the upper extremities. In primates, the CST extends throughout the rostral-caudal extent of the spinal cord. It is only in humans, however, that the CST projects to laminae IX, located in the ventral horn of the spinal cord.[4] Laminae IX contain discrete groupings of motor neurons that primarily innervate extremity musculature. It would appear, therefore, that in humans the CST has direct control over the activation of alpha motor neurons and muscle contraction.

PTNs are active during all phases of a movement. Some are active before movement onset and others change activity during the movement.[29,37,38,40] PTNs are activated with voluntary contractions and reflexively during stretch to a muscle. The same neuron that is active during a voluntary contraction will also become activated during stretch of that muscle (e.g., neurons that are active during voluntary elbow flexion will also be active during a stretch to elbow flexors; Fig. 4-7)

All PTNs appear to be excitatory. Any inhibitory effects on motor neurons appear to be mediated by segmental inhibitory interneurons. Via this type of connectivity, PTNs can mediate reciprocal muscle activity. In other words, they will excite agonists and their synergists and, via an interneuron, inhibit muscles antagonist to the movement. Most PTNs synapse on motor pools innervating more than one muscle. One PTN might synapse on multiple synergist motor neuron pools (see Figs. 2-22 and 4-8). A small population of MI cells has been discovered, however, that mediates muscle cocontraction (i.e., innervates both agonist and antagonist muscles).[50,66] Fast frequency movements require stabilization and muscle cocontraction. This appears to be accomplished, at least in part, by a population of PTNs that concomitantly excite agonists and antagonists.

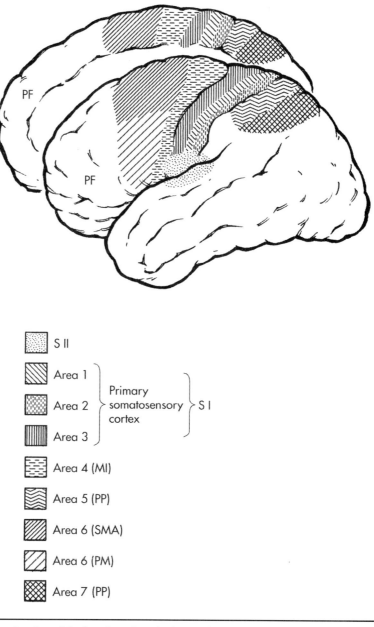

Fig. 4-6. An approximate estimation of the location of cortical areas devoted to motor control.

The MI receives diverse input from other cortical regions and from peripheral sensory afferents and subcortical structures via the thalamus. The MI apparently sums this input and initiates movement in rela-

TABLE 4-1 Brain regions closely associated with motor functions

Cortical field nomenclature	Approximate Brodman location
Primary motor area (MI or MsI)	Area 4
Premotor areas	
Supplementary motor cortex (SMA or MII)	Area 6
Premotor cortex (PM)	
Primary somatosensory (SI or SmI)	Areas 1, 2, 3
Secondary somatosensory (SII or SmII)	Caudal area 2
Posterior parietal	Areas 5,7
Prefrontal	Rostral to area 6

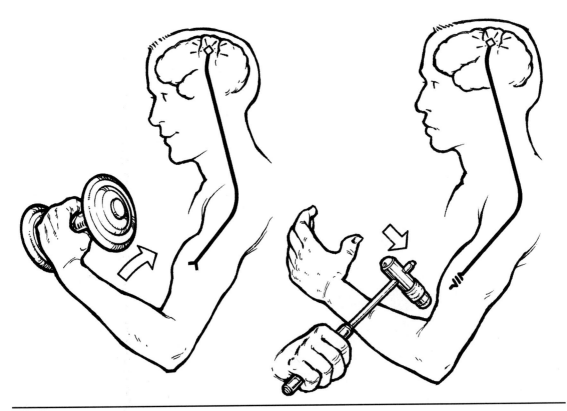

Fig. 4-7. A pyramidal tract neuron located within the primary motor cortex increases its rate of firing during either a voluntary contraction or a stretch to the muscle.

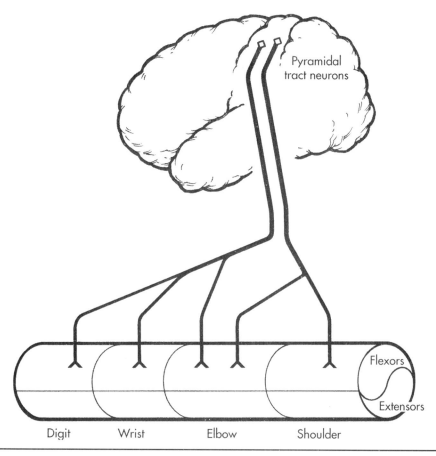

Fig. 4-8. Pyramidal tract neurons (PTNs) generally excite brain stem or spinal cord motor neuron pools of more than one muscle. One PTN will synapse on multiple synergist motor neuron pools and, via an interneuron (not pictured), inhibit antagonist motor neuron pools. (Adapted from Grillner S. Science 1985;228:143-9.)

tion to this input. It is, therefore, very responsive to afferent input and changes its output in relation to it. The influence of peripheral input to the MI can be profound. Peripheral input can excite MI cells to hundreds of action potentials per second.[146] This is actually a curious finding because most peripheral afferent information is not relayed directly from the thalamus to the MI.[121] Most peripheral afferent input to the MI is relayed to it by other cortical regions.

The MI's responsiveness to afferent input indicates its ability to operate via feedback or closed-loop mechanisms. The MI alters its output depending on its afferent input. However, because PTNs of the MI are also active before movement, they appear to contribute to the establishment of the postural set required for the desired movement. Thus the MI also operates in a feed-forward or open-loop mode.

The connections of the MI to the spinal cord, and its direct involvement in movement initiation, is only one aspect of its control over movement. The MI appears to trigger motor programs but it also modulates subcortical reflexes and sensory input.[146] It does so in a very task dependent manner. Cells within the MI, and other cortical regions as well, change their level of activity and involvement depending on several factors[50]:

1. whether the task involves a single joint or multiple joint movement,
2. the degree of speed or precision of the movement,
3. whether a memorized movement is involved,
4. the initial position of the limb,
5. whether spatial transformations are required (e.g., identifying and moving around obstacles), and
6. the individual's intent and motivation.

Within MI are multiple modules and cell columns related to different aspects of the same movement.[78] For instance, within the arm area of the MI are specialized fields or modules that control or respond to various aspects of hand control.[5,63] These modules are intracortically connected. They are also very plastic, showing changes over time and depending on use.[115,151] Other brain regions have a similar modular and columnar organization that subserve other functions. (This plastic columnar cortical organization will be discussed further in this chapter under the heading of Intrinsic Circuitry.) With regard to the MI, selected cell populations within a module might change their activity in response to changes in force, others to the direction of the force, and others to the frequency of the movement.[50,52]

Premotor areas (supplementary motor cortex and premotor cortex). Premotor areas can be subdivided into the supplementary motor cortex (SMA) and the premotor cortex (PM). Typical of newer findings, further subdivision is possible. Dr. Peter Strick and his colleagues from Syracuse, N.Y., have identified four premotor areas, each with a distinct topographic organization and specific projection pattern.[63,100] Separate functions can also be assigned to the ventral and dorsal aspects of the premotor cortex.[9,57] Functionally, evidence indicates that the PM is more directly involved in visually guided movements, whereas the SMA is more active in sequential motor tasks that are internally generated.[61] These examples should provide you an idea of the complexity and difficulty in naming brain regions. Almost certainly, additional functional areas will continue to be discovered and defined not only for the premotor area but for the entire cerebral cortex. To keep things relatively simple, the functions of the SMA and the PM will be considered collectively in subsequent paragraphs.

Premotor areas have direct projections to the spinal cord,[31] but they are not as extensive as those from the MI. Electrical stimulation of cells in this area can cause muscle contraction and movement but at much higher stimulation parameters than cells within the MI. Premotor areas, however, are vitally important for movement. Human premotor areas are six times larger than comparable areas in the macaque monkey.[146] These areas appear to be involved primarily in the preparation for movement.[74,83,146] More than the MI, premotor areas appear to be responsible for the establishment of the postural set required for a specific task. Planning and involvement in the initiation of centrally programmed motor commands are the functions most closely associated with premotor areas.

Premotor areas are involved in activities that require sequencing of goal-directed movements (e.g., typing) or a remembered sequence. They are less active during simple repetitive movements such as finger tapping on a tabletop.[55] These types of findings never cease to amaze me. In this example we have two motor acts that, to the casual observer, involve the same muscles doing the same thing, yet they involve very different cortical activations!

The connectivity of premotor areas is an ongoing study. To date, direct or indirect circuits connecting premotor areas to the MI, the primary somatosensory area, other diffuse cortical regions, the cerebellum, the striatum, the red nucleus, the reticular formation, the thalamus (motor and nonmotor nuclei), and the spinal cord have been found.[74,121,146] These areas also project back to premotor areas. The basal ganglia appear to have more projections, via the thalamus, to premotor areas than to the MI. Projections from the cerebellum to the MI and premotor areas deserve some special mention. The cerebellum, via the thalamus, appears to terminate primarily in the MI.[73,146] There appears to be one major exception to this general finding: A specific part of the dentate nucleus of the cerebellum (a very recent phylogenetic development in humans) preferentially projects to the PM.[132] This part of the cerebellum is very active during a visually guided sequential motor task. It is active regardless whether the sequential task is a mental puzzle-solving task or an actual sequential motor act. Certain cells within the PM respond to both visual input and to proprioceptive input from the upper extremities and thus are directly implicated in the control of limb movements during visually guided tasks.[57] The pathway from the dentate nucleus of the cerebellum to premotor areas might be vitally important for motor learning of proprioceptively or visually guided tasks. This has implications for training techniques such as guided imagery.

Guided imagery is often used by athletes to visualize their performance. A downhill slalom ski racer might visualize the course and mentally practice the weight shifts necessary for successful completion of the course. Apparently, the premotor areas are fully engaged during this type of activity. Cells within the premotor areas are active regardless whether a movement is real or imagined.[78,146] Cells within the MI typically are not active during visualization of a motor task. This is worth noting, because the premotor areas are involved in a cascade of connections that modulate input into the MI and ultimately control voluntary muscle contraction. How well or how often an athlete transfers information from the PM to the MI might theoretically influence performance. Similarly, a patient with a lesion involving this circuitry might not benefit from guided imagery exercises.

At least one potentially important distinction must be made between the SMA and the PM. Both are active during learning of a motor task,[26] but the PM appears to be more involved with movements that rely on sensory inputs from the environment (such as vision) and body (proprioception). The SMA appears to be more involved with internally generated motor commands.[61] The SMA is particularly active in skills that require planning several movements ahead.[134] It is active during any task that requires temporal ordering of proximal and distal movements[139] and organizational sequences that are performed without peripheral afferent guidance. In contrast, the premotor area changes its activity in direct response to changes in sensory input occurring during a complex movement or during perturbations to that movement.

Primary somatosensory area. Most MI cells become active before the start of movement. In contrast, most cells within the primary somatosensory area (SI) fire after movement starts.[37,112,121] This suggests that cells within the SI are responding to sensory feedback signals generated by the movement. Sensory perception is the function most widely attributable to the SI. Somatosensory information does not arrive directly to the SI. Sensory information first projects to specific nuclei within the thalamus. The thalamus, in turn, reciprocally connects with the SI.

Within the SI are multiple sensory fields. Each field responds in a particular way to a particular sensory input. Some fields might preferentially respond to light touch, whereas others respond to muscle stretch (Fig. 4-9). Other fields respond more like PTN cells of the MI and send efferent projections to the brain stem and spinal cord. And similar to other regions of the brain, each field within the SI is richly interconnected.

Four major fields or subdivisions of the SI include Brodman areas 3a, 3b, 1, and 2. Most thalamic inputs that convey somatic sensations terminate in areas 3a and 3b. Proprioceptive and muscle spindle input preferentially terminate in area 3a and cutaneous input to area 3b.[47,108,111] Area 3 neurons, in turn, primarily project to areas 1 and 2, where additional sensory processing takes place. Areas 1 and 2 receive their own distinct sensory input via the thalamus. Area 1 receives projections from rapidly adapting cutaneous receptors and area 2 from joint receptors.[103]

The SI connects with the MI, although not necessarily directly (Fig. 4-10). Most of the output from the SI is to parietal sensory fields[146] and premotor cortical areas.[83] By nature of these connections, sensory input arriving via the *medial lemniscal system* (a major spinal cord projection system conveying sensory information from the body) is processed before being conveyed to the MI. The majority of sensory input

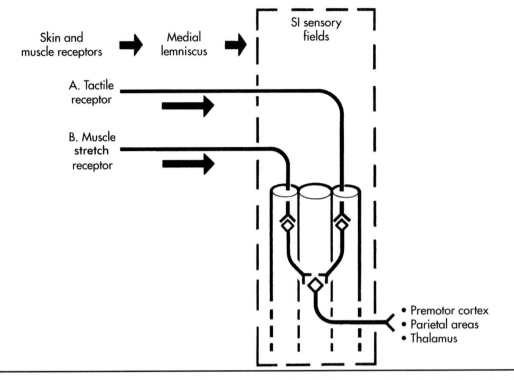

Fig. 4-9. The primary somatosensory area (SI) is composed of multiple sensory fields. Each field preferentially responds to a particular sensory input. Other cells within the SI integrate sensory input and send efferent projections out to other cortical areas, the brain stem, and spinal cord.

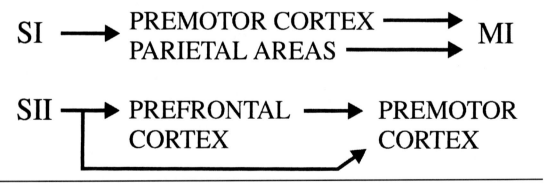

Fig. 4-10. Connections between the SI and the MI are not necessarily direct. Processing of sensory information arriving in the SI occurs before its relay to the MI. Many SII projections appear to differ from SI projections.

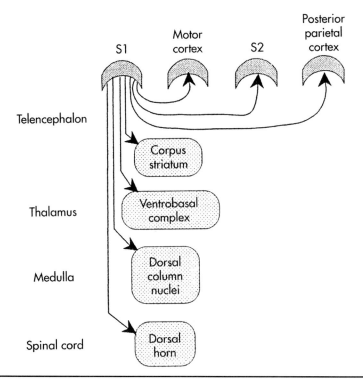

Fig. 4-11. SI cortical and subcortical projections. (From Butler AB, Hodos W. Comparative vertebrate neuroanatomy. New York: Wiley-Liss, 1996.)

to the MI is regulated by the SI. The SI also projects to the spinal cord, brain stem, and thalamus and thus has other means by which to potentiate or inhibit sensory inflow to the cerebral cortex (Fig. 4-11).

The SI must process sensory input from a multitude of sources and determine, by its intrinsic mechanisms and circuitry, where to send its signal. The integration of sensory input allows us to move gracefully and in a manner that is task specific and context appropriate. This is perhaps best exemplified by the convergence of vestibular input with somatic proprioceptive input. Cells within the SI receive convergent input from the vestibular system in addition to afferents contributing to proprioception.[150] The SI then processes this information to relate changes in head position to limb proprioceptive information. This action probably contributes to righting reactions and head-eye-hand coordination. Perhaps the SI also contributes to setting the priorities of sensory input. In one situation you might want to rely more on vestibular input than on proprioceptive input. Although the idea is conjectural, the SI may play a role in this determination. Equally plausible, however, is that posterior parietal, premotor, and prefrontal cortical areas are also involved in prioritizing different sensory inputs.

Cells within the SI also show task specificity. Some SI cells are active during reaching in a memorized task but not during reaching elicited by a visually triggered task.[50] Once again we see that cortical cells not only have a preferred stimulus to which they respond, but they also have context specificity of function.

Secondary somatosensory area. The secondary somatosensory area (SII) connects reciprocally with the SI, the MI, and the prefrontal cortex.[17,83] It also projects to the insular cortex (a cortical region that also receives somatic sensory input) and to the posterior parietal cortex.

Cells within the SII respond to somatic sensations relayed from the thalamus. Similar to the SI, cells respond to sensory input from a specific receptive field. Unlike the SI, some of the receptive fields don't exhibit strict somatotopy. In the SI each finger has its own cortical representation. In the SII some receptive fields overlap, so that the same cortical area within the SII might respond to sensory input from several fingers from the same or both hands.[17] SII cells are also very active during exploratory movements made by the hands.[7]

Lesions to the SII result in loss of abilities to discriminate an object's texture and shape. After injury, misjudgments regarding the location and intensity of an applied stimulus also occur. Ascribing these functions solely to cells within the SII is difficult, however, because the SII is so richly connected with the SI. Therefore, lesions to the SII also involve SI projections. SII cells have a totally separate somatotopy and a different connectivity organization than SI cells, but a definitive separate role for the SII with regard to sensory processing and motor control has yet to be determined.

Posterior parietal cortex (areas 5 and 7). Posterior parietal areas, comprised of Brodman's areas 5 and 7, are usually regarded as an associational sensory area. Areas 5 and 7 are located caudal to the primary sensory cortex and appear to subserve some rather unique functions that dramatically affect motor control. In very general terms, area 5 of the posterior parietal cortex is involved primarily with somatic sensory processing and area 7 is primarily involved with visual input processing. These are broad generalizations and, similar to other brain regions, both areas 5 and 7 can be further subdivided into more discrete functional units.

These functional subunits are richly interconnected with each other and with the sensorimotor cortices. Reciprocal connections exist with premotor areas of the cortex. Area 7 receives a dense projection from the SII. Area 7, in turn, has indirect projections to the cerebellum (via the pons) and thus provides a pathway by which visual input might influence movement.[121] Area 5 receives a dense projection from sensory area 2 and projects back to premotor areas. The posterior parietal cortex receives input from visual, auditory, tactile, and vestibular projections as well as projections from the limbic system.[131] The projections from the limbic system might help explain the relationship between motivation and memorization of spatial relationships exhibited by posterior parietal cells.

Experiments with monkeys have shown that some cells in the posterior parietal cortex are active only when the animal is paying attention to a stimulus. Experiments with humans have indicated that parietal areas participate in motor imagery.[25] Thus, the posterior parietal cortex might be involved in attention and memory to spatial aspects of sensation such as those involved in the visual or tactile manipulation of objects.[83] Paying closer attention to a sensory stimulus or associations between stimuli might enhance or strengthen the involved synapses and contribute to memory of spatial tasks.[131] Areas other than the parietal areas also are involved in spatial memory.

The hippocampus, a specialized area located deep within the temporal lobes, has long been known to be involved in memory. Parietal regions interact with the hippocampus during memory tasks that involve spatial orientations.[46] Interestingly, the ability of the hippocampus to form an internal representation of external spatial characteristics depends on movement.[46] If an animal is restricted in its ability to move, cells within the hippocampus are silent and the animal is unable to form a relationship between its body and its external surroundings. Considering these data, one can hypothesize that connections between parietal areas and the hippocampus are vital for visuomotor memory.

Further evidence for this idea is provided by findings that show that many posterior parietal areas are active only during the active phase of learning a task. They become silent once the task is learned.[118]

Another cortical area, the prefrontal cortex, is involved in motor learning and not surprisingly shares connections with the posterior parietal cortex.

Prefrontal cortical area. The prefrontal cortex is the black box of the black box. Located in the frontal lobe, it is a recent phylogenetic development. Frontal lobe functioning is typically associated with goal setting, cognitive skills, delayed gratification, and other presumably unique human social traits. Prefrontal motor functions include cognitive aspects of movement such as short-term motor memory, visual motor tasks, and motor planning.

The prefrontal cortex might originate memorized movements and may be involved with the storage of motor memories. Experiments have shown that prefrontal cortex cells are active during retrieval of remembered spatial cues,

In some studies, monkeys were trained to move their arms in a specific direction in response to a flash of light.[7] If the light was presented to the right visual field, the monkey had to move the arm to the right. If the light occurred in the left visual field, the monkey had to move its arm to the left. A food reward was given only if the appropriate behavior occurred. A select group of cells (i.e., not all cells responded similarly) within the prefrontal and posterior parietal cortical areas were active during these tasks. These findings indicate a close association between posterior parietal and prefrontal areas, especially with regard to visuomotor transformations and motor learning tasks.

The prefrontal cortex and posterior parietal cortex are densely interconnected. Both cortical areas also project to similar cortical and subcortical structures.[83] For instance, the premotor areas receive inputs from prefrontal and posterior parietal areas.

Certain areas within the prefrontal cortex also appear to be involved in the decision making process. Evidence indicates that certain cells within the prefrontal cortex are active only with self-initiated movement and do not respond during the same movements triggered by an external stimulus (e.g., animals trained to move the arm in response to a light stimulus).[135] Other cells within the prefrontal cortex were active during learning of a motor task but became inactive once the movement was learned. This is very similar to findings within the posterior parietal cortex.[118]

The orbitofrontal cortex, which is part of the prefrontal cortex, is considered part of the limbic system. The limbic system is involved with human emotion and motivation. One can hypothesize, therefore, that prefrontal areas attach significance to motor acts and are involved in the process of deciding whether motor sequences are stored in memory. We know that certain cells within the basal ganglia are active only when an animal is motivated to learn a task or when the task is important to the animal. The basal ganglia and prefrontal cortex share indirect connectivity. Somehow, it would appear that our *desire* to learn, via input from the limbic system, affects the functioning of the prefrontal cortex and the basal ganglia and thus contributes to our actual *ability* to learn.

Intrinsic circuitry

Horizontal laminar organization. The words *cerebral cortex* are often used to refer to the whole brain. In reality, *cortex* refers only to the outermost few millimeters of brain tissue. This outermost layer consists of gray matter (cell bodies). In humans, 90% of the cortex has six layers (neocortex). In submammalian vertebrates almost all of the cortex has three layers. Humans have retained a three-layered cortex known as the archicortex. This area is largely devoted to olfactory functions but also contains the hippocampus and dentate gyrus and is thus involved with the limbic system and memory.

The horizontal laminar organization of the neocortex is largely determined by genetic factors.[71] Different cell types are located in each layer. The pattern of projections to and from each layer is quite different. Having some familiarity with the laminar organization provides considerable insight into brain functioning. The six layers can be subdivided as follows (Fig. 4-12):

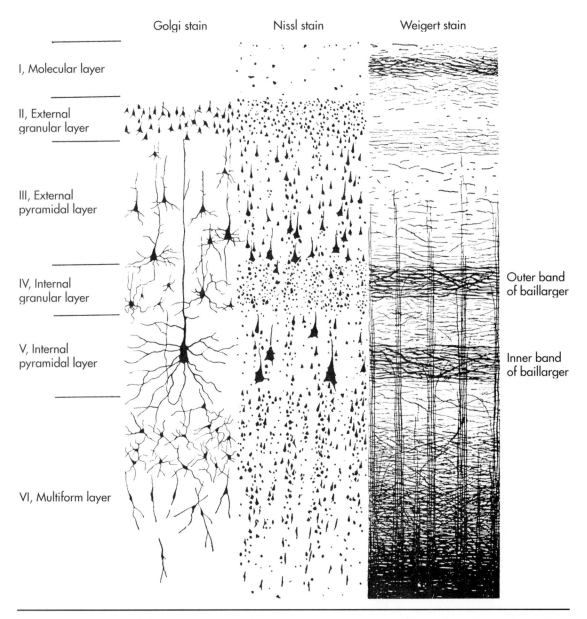

Fig. 4-12. The six-layered neocortex. Each layer has specific cell types and a specific pattern of connectivity. (From Ranson SW, Clark SL. The anatomy of the nervous system, ed 10. Philadelphia: WB Saunders, 1959.)

    I. Molecular layer: The outermost layer of the cortex. This layer does not contain many cells. Rather, it consists largely of dendrites and axons from all cell types of the inner five layers.

   II. External granular layer: This layer contains many small granular and pyramidal neurons. Many of these cells do not project out of the cortex but serve to interconnect cells from different laminae and cortical areas.

III. External pyramidal layer: This layer contains medium and large pyramidal cells.

IV. Internal granular layer: This layer contains closely packed granular cells.

V. Internal pyramidal layer: This layer contains large pyramidal cells.

VI. Multiform (fusiform) layer: This layer contains smaller nonpyramidal cells. Dendrites ascend to upper layers and axons descend into white matter (corona radiata).

Not all neocortical areas have a typical six-layered appearance. Atypical areas are referred to as being *heterotypic*. The primary motor cortex (MI; Area 4) is termed an agranular heterotypic cortical area because of the relative lack of granular cells. Within MI, layers III and V contain large pyramidal cells, with layer V containing the largest of the pyramidal cells, the Betz cells. Primary sensory areas (striate visual cortex and the SI) are termed granular heterotypic cortex because of densely packed granule cells in laminae II and IV. Most afferents to cortical areas terminate in granular layers. Most efferents arise from pyramidal layers. Cortical afferent and efferent projections do not occur randomly. Rather, general organizational schemes are apparent. Most thalamic afferents terminate in layer IV. Fibers from the cortex to the thalamus originate predominately in layer VI. Thalamic afferents give off collaterals to layer VI on their way to layer IV and connectivity also exists between layers IV and VI. Pyramidal neurons in layer V project directly to the brain stem and spinal cord and indirectly to the cerebellum. Layer III contains many cells that connect one cortical area with another. Cells within each cortical layer can be classified depending on the location of their predominant projections.

Projection neurons transmit impulses to subcortical areas such as the thalamus, brain stem, basal ganglia, and spinal cord.

Association neurons form connections with neurons in the same cortical hemisphere. The human cortex is rich with association neurons. Their organization is such that cortical neurons that control synergistic muscles (e.g., wrist and hand) share rich connectivity. Cortical neurons that tend not to act as synergistically do not share similar connectivity (e.g., head and leg).

Commissural neurons send axons to the contralateral hemisphere. The corpus callosum is the largest tract system that connects the two hemispheres, but other commissures also connect the two hemispheres.

Instrinsic neurons connect the layers within one cortical area. They do not project out of their cortical area of origin.

Being classified as one type of neuron does not mutually exclude a cell from also belonging in another category. For instance, some neurons have both an associational projection and a callosal projection.[125]

Vertical columnar organization. The neocortex is organized into both horizontal and vertical dimensions (Figs. 4-12 and 4-13). Unlike the horizontal laminations, vertical columnar organization exhibits more plasticity and its organization is more susceptible to epigenetic factors such as experience, learning, and injury.[97,115,151] Vertical columns expand or shrink depending on individual life experiences.

Columnar organization appears to be a general functional organizational scheme throughout the cortex. The SI is a good example of the functional significance of these vertical columns. Within SI are specific regions (1, 2, 3a, and 3b). Each of these regions contains its own somatotopic representation of the body surface. Each region receives input from a multitude of sensory modalities, although each region appears to receive a predominant input. All six layers (laminae) within a vertical column respond to the same type of receptor.[99] Within the cortical representation of a single body part, multiple modality representations are located in close proximity to each other (Fig. 4-13). This arrangement permits parallel processing of sensory input by different cortical areas. Each area has a slightly different projection scheme and thus sensory input can be processed by divergent pathways.

As mentioned, these vertical columns are plastic. Experiments in nonhuman animals have shown that amputation of one digit causes the cortical sensory receptive field of the adjacent digit to expand.[96] Some evidence also indicates that these columns are plastic in humans as well. Early musical training appears to expand associated cortical areas.[35] Evidence also suggests that after cortical damage, some reorganization occurs within the cerebral cortex.[15,39,104]

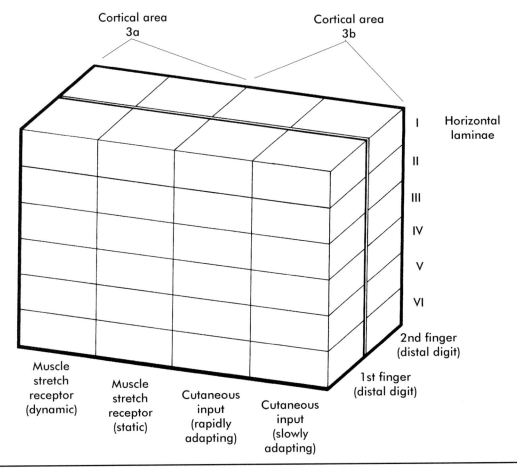

Fig. 4-13. Cortical columnar organization. Within the cortical representation of a body part in the SI (includes areas 3a, 3b, 1, and 2), multiple columns represent specific parts of the body. Each column receives predominant input from one or two sensory modalities.

■ DEVELOPMENT
All humans exhibit critical periods of immaturity
Why is it that perinatal damage to the human brain has such different consequences with regard to motor control than similar damage occurring in an adult? In a nutshell, it is because infant and adult brains are not the same. From conception onward, the cells and circuits that comprise the human brain are in a constant state of flux. Change and adaptation within the human brain and nervous system continue throughout life, but never are they as great as during early development. The following paragraphs outline some of the major changes that occur during perinatal development.

The cerebral cortex and other CNS structures mature at different rates and exhibit slightly different developmental characteristics. *Critical periods* are times during development when a neural structure or its afferent and efferent projections are in an immature state. The critical period generally represents a transformation from multiconnectivity to a more focused projection scheme. Typically, at this stage of development the structure and its circuitry are particularly vulnerable to epigenetic influences. Every CNS structure appears to have its own unique critical period. Damage occurring to a brain structure before or during a critical period of development will have very different behavioral and neural consequences than similar damage occurring after this time.[11-13,53,54] Not only is the stage of development of the damaged area important, but the stage of development of surviving pathways is equally critical to behavioral outcome.[54,117] A brief discussion of some of the neural events involved with cortical maturation will illustrate the tremendous amount of change taking place within the infant's brain and why damage occurring before or after critical periods of neural development has a different impact on motor control.

Cell migration

All neurons within the human cerebral cortex are located in the outermost few millimeters of the cerebrum. These neurons weren't born there, however. All neurons are migrants, having immigrated to the cortex from another location. Neurons begin life deep within the brain and must travel outward to the cortex. During embryonic development, cortical cells migrate from ventricular zones (gray matter that surrounds the lateral ventricles) to their final destination in the cortex. Although cortical neurons are migrants, they cannot be credited with being pioneers. Radial glial cells and subplate neurons migrate before cortical neurons and appear to provide a physical scaffolding and chemical pathway for neurons to follow.[95,115] Cell migration occurs in an inside-out pattern. Those neurons that will occupy the deepest cortical layers (lamina VI) migrate first and those in the most superficial layers migrate last. The type of cell the neuron is to become and its laminar destination within the cortex appear to be genetically predetermined.[115] Axonal and dendritic projections, columnar organization, synapse formation, and even the cell's survival or death appear to depend on or are greatly influenced by epigenetic and experiential events.[10,72,115,128]

Interaction between cortical neurons and their environment begins before the cells arrive at their final location within the cortex. At approximately 8 weeks of gestation in the human, cortical cells arrive at a subcortical location, the cortical plate.[115] Thalamic projections, having already arrived, have anxiously awaited the arrival of cortical neurons. A sensory lovefest ensues. Thalamic sensory inputs attach themselves to the migrating cortical neurons and travel outward with them to the cortex. Among other things, this process allows for appropriate sensory-motor matching. Interestingly, at about 8 weeks of age the first human fetal movements can be detected.[113]

The thalamocortical/corticothalamic matching is not totally dependent on genetic factors. Selective exposure to particular afferent input can increase the number of cortical cells that respond to this input.[128] For instance, cortical cells can be made to respond preferentially to a specific direction, but only if that cell was genetically predetermined to respond to directional cues. Its sensory input during a critical period of development influences to which direction it will respond. This type of interaction between genetic and epigenetic factors appears to be a general organizational scheme used by all areas of the cerebral cortex.

Human cortical cell migration is completed before birth.[115] Cell migration within the human cerebellum is considerably more protracted than that for the cerebral cortex. Cerebellar cell migration and differentiation continues well after birth[28] and thus remain very vulnerable to epigenetic factors. Not just cell migration is vulnerable to outside influences. Other aspects of neonatal neural development are actually influenced to a much larger degree by the environment and experience.

Youthful exuberance

The title of this section says it all. Infants and kids are exuberant in all aspects of their lives. They are all over the place, flitting from one activity to the next, always searching for a new experience and new sensory input. The biological correlate to this wild behavior is *neural exuberance*. During certain critical periods of development, many cortical cells have broader and more diverse projections than exist in the mature brain. An excess of cell numbers can also contribute to neural exuberance. The corticospinal,[1,6,105,130] corticorubral,[87] and corticothalamic[87] tracts; cortical callosal projections[69,87]; and corticocortical synapses[152] all exhibit developmental periods of exuberance. Neonates also have a wider distribution of cells within the cortex that contribute to the corticospinal tract.[130] Neural exuberance is not confined to the cerebral cortex. Some peripheral afferents and motor neurons also exhibit periods of exuberance.[43,114]

Exuberance provides a certain amount of redundancy within the CNS and thus might contribute to greater plasticity and adaptive capabilities after early brain damage. However, it also results in neural circuitry that lacks precision. Exuberance, like infatuation, does not last forever. Other neural maturation processes, including regressive events, follow the period of neonatal neural exuberance. Regressive events literally trim, tame, and temper the exuberance of the neonatal nervous system. These biochemical, physiological, and neuroanatomical processes give order and refinement to the nervous system. What we lose in redundancy and neural plasticity we gain in precision and efficiency.

Regressive events

Regressive events include cell death, loss of axonal projections, and synapse loss. These processes might sound grim, but they are a necessary part of development.

An overproliferation of neurons appears to be a general feature of CNS development. Estimates are that most brain structures so far studied lose approximately 50% of their neurons during early life.[24] Cells might be preprogrammed to die, or they might die secondary to not receiving appropriate afferent input, or to not establishing a strong efferent projection to an appropriate target. Trophic substances, such as nerve growth factor, are important for cell survival. Target areas and support cells contain different trophic factors that attract specific inputs as well as provide essential elements for cell survival.

Axon and synaptic retraction are sometimes referred to as *pruning*. The pruning of axonal projections is an important process that contributes to effective synapse formation and formation of discrete CNS connectivity. Although this chapter deals with the cerebral cortex, the neuromuscular junction is perhaps a more easily understood example of axon exuberance and subsequent retraction.

Early in development, single muscle fibers are innervated by multiple motor axons.[114] One axon usually innervates more muscle fibers than it will in the mature animal (Fig. 4-14). Over time, axons retract so that a single muscle fiber is innervated by one motor axon. Concomitant with axon retraction is an increase in the number of presynaptic terminals from the surviving axon (Fig. 4-14). The surviving axon, therefore, has a stronger input to the muscle fiber than during an earlier period of development, when it had fewer synapses onto the fiber. The mechanisms that contribute or dictate axon retraction and strengthening of surviving synapses are not completely understood. Several explanations have been forthcoming. Trophic substances appear to be important. Growth cones (extensions of growing axons), target areas, and cells within the extracellular matrix secrete chemical messengers that appear to guide axon growth.[71] Axons that don't receive necessary trophic substance don't survive. A second mechanism that contributes to pruning involves activity within the neural pathway.

The importance of early activity

Increasingly, investigators are finding that activity within a neural pathway is important for that pathway's survival.[10,77,101,114,128] Activity within a synapse strengthens the synapse and eases transmission along the pathway. If a neural pathway is not used, the synapse will weaken and possibly lead to the presynaptic axon's retraction. These findings appear to be consistent across species and throughout the CNS. They also have potentially important clinical and educational implications.

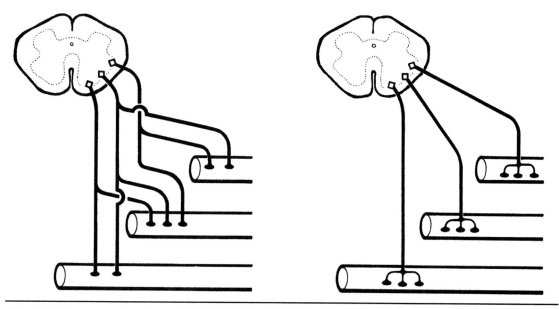

Fig. 4-14. The maturation of the neuromuscular junction. **A,** Early in development each muscle fiber might receive input from multiple motor neurons and each motor neuron synapses on multiple muscle fibers (more than in the mature animal). **B,** Via regressive events such as axon retraction and cell death, the mature neuromuscular junction has one motor neuron innervating one muscle fiber. The mature motor neuron increases its number of synapses onto the muscle fiber.

Early intervention is a therapeutic concept that emphasizes the early treatment of infants with neurological disorders or who are at risk of developing motor delays. This concept has received considerable misgivings from some clinicians. The misgivings center around the costs involved, family commitment, and lack of studies showing the effectiveness of early intervention. Data that indicate the important role of activity in CNS maturational processes, however, should remove any doubt that epigenetic factors, such as movement and sensory exploration, are important to consider. Findings with regard to the importance of activity to the development of visual centers within the brain are already being used by ophthalmologists. Surgical corrections for certain childhood visual deficits, that in the past were delayed, are now being performed as early as possible in an attempt to restore appropriate sensory input as soon as possible.

Not just the health professions can benefit from an awareness of the biological importance of early activity and experience. Educators and parents, especially those with interests in music, physical education, and the language arts, need to be aware of the potential benefits of early exposure to these activities. For example, a child might be born with a genetic aptitude for music, but if he doesn't receive early exposure, brain areas that would potentially contribute to his talent might not develop fully.[35]

Neural Darwinism
Genetics, activity-dependent changes within neural pathways, and trophic factors are important developmental organizational determinants. They do not, however, explain why some active neural pathways still

do not survive to maturity. Nor can these factors totally explain the unique and plastic nature of functional vertical columnar cortical organization. Other factors and mechanisms must exist by which each of us achieves neural diversity. Although the structure of the nervous system is very similar between individuals, a vast amount of individual variation exists with regard to connectivity.[32] The human genome alone cannot explain the connectional complexity of the nervous system or the unique characteristics that contribute to our individuality. A theory consistent with available data has been proposed to explain this mystery.

Dr. Gerald Edelman, a neuroscientist, won the Nobel Prize for Physiology and Medicine in 1972. In 1987 he published a book outlining his theory of neuronal group selection. The theory is an attempt to identify an organizational principle that explains why some neural pathways survive while others do not. It is based on the idea of natural selection not unlike that proposed by Charles Darwin to explain species variation and evolutionary change. In fact, the title of Dr. Edelman's book is "Neural Darwinism." The key element to both Edelman's and Darwin's theories is competition.

Within the nervous system, and especially during ontogeny, a great deal of overlap and redundancy exists among neural pathways. These pathways, for many reasons, respond differently to afferent input. Those pathways that receive sufficient and appropriate input and have better response characteristics are selected for survival. Synapses are strengthened and maintained by activity.[128] Neurons that fire synchronously tend to become wired together and thus enhance their rate of survival. Only those connections that are frequently coactivated become consolidated over time.[128] In other words, neural networks are formed. Any neuron that participates in an active network is likely to survive. The concept of competition is very apparent in the development of the human brain. The number and size of vertical columns, which form functional subunits of brain activity, are modified by afferent input.[115] Not just afferent activity is important for competitive survival. During critical periods of development, certain cells are more vulnerable to damage by malnutrition, alcohol abuse, hormone imbalances, and ischemia[10] and thus are at a competitive disadvantage. In the final analysis, active neural pathways that receive input necessary for physiological functioning are selected over others.[32]

A multitude of other changes occur in the developing nervous system. Axons continue to grow and dendritic arbors enlarge dramatically (Fig. 4-15). Considerable neurophysiological changes occur.[58,126] For instance, membrane conductance changes during development help to refine reflexes and make a neuron more or less susceptible to input.

Some of these neural events are not restricted to fetal and neonatal development. Competition for synaptic sites, synaptic strengthening, activity-dependent changes, axon proliferation, and cell death are processes that continue throughout life. Some of the processes that contribute to developmental plasticity also appear to be intimately involved with learning and memory and perhaps recovery from damage to the nervous system. Chapter 7 focuses on some of these neural mechanisms currently thought to underlie motor learning.

■ THE MOTOR CORTEX AND LOCOMOTION

Cats and other vertebrates are capable of treadmill locomotion after total spinal cord transections.[44,116,119] These animals retain the ability to step over obstacles and change their gait in response to changes in the speed of the treadmill.[45,120] Surgical removal of the motor cortex does little to affect the basic locomotor synergy.[2,86] Stimulation of subcortical brain stem nuclei causes rhythmical locomotor activity.[127] Taken together, these data would appear to indicate that locomotion occurs independent of, or without the need of, the motor cortex. Why then, do motor cortical neurons, including PTNs, fire phasically during treadmill locomotion[30] and respond to perturbations to the gait cycle[2]? Furthermore, as even the most casual clinical observation reveals, individuals with damage to motor cortical areas of the brain do not have a normal gait pattern. Lesions to motor areas of the brain cause disordered coordination between the knee

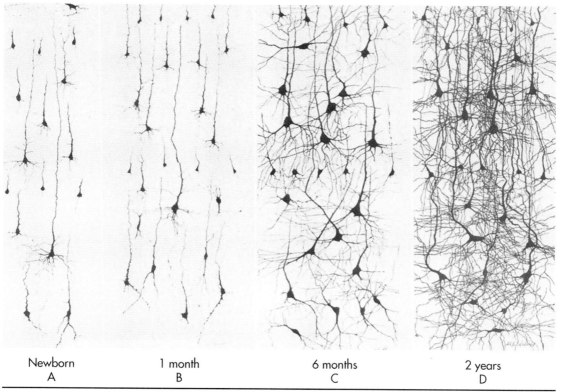

Newborn
A

1 month
B

6 months
C

2 years
D

Fig. 4-15. Axonal and dendritic growth within the cerebral cortex are hallmarks of development. (From Conel JL. The postnatal development of the human cerebral cortex. Cambridge, Mass: Harvard University Press: **A**, Vol I, 1939; **B**, vol II, 1941; **C**, vol IV, 1951; **D**, vol VI, 1959.)

and ankle,[143] altered electromyographic responses,[81,107] paresis,[81,107] excess muscle cocontraction,[88] and disordered modulation of alpha motor neuron firing.[89,138] Clearly the motor cortex is involved in some aspects of human locomotion. The following paragraphs attempt to define the potential role of the motor cortex in the initiation, generation, and modulation of the human gait cycle.

Among the problems encountered when attempting to determine the potential role of the human motor cortex in the control of locomotion are huge species differences in brain organization and in biomechanical aspects of locomotion. The cat has been the animal typically used for many studies examining the relationships between cortical function and locomotion. Cortical representations of movement in the cat are not the same as in humans, and obviously their quadrupedal gait is distinct from our preferred mode of locomotion—a plantigrade (heel-toe), bipedal gait. Considerable care must be exerted when applying data obtained from nonhuman species to generalizations about the possible role of the motor cortex or other cortical areas to human locomotion. Having said this, it is equally important to remember that during the course of mammalian evolution, most neural organizational schemes are maintained and rarely does the functioning of one neural pathway assume that of another.[19,124] Many neural organizational principles that apply to the cat or other mammals and vertebrates also apply to humans.

The concept of spinal cord–generated central pattern generators (CPGs) for locomotion was presented in Chapter 2. Beyond doubt, CPGs generate the locomotor rhythm for quadrupedal locomotion. In my opinion, the evidence for a completely autonomous spinal locomotor CPG in humans[18,27] is not convincing. In fact, a considerable body of evidence suggests that although spinal CPG circuitry exists in humans, it is not autonomous and has become increasingly dependent on supraspinal input.[34,140,145] Perhaps CPG functioning depends on tonic excitatory descending input or perhaps the increased fractionation of movement required for bipedal gait necessitates an increased role for the motor cortex.

Four major descending supraspinal pathways monosynaptically synapse on spinal cord motor neurons. These pathways originate from the motor cortex, the red nucleus, vestibular nuclei, and brain stem reticular neurons.[92] Each makes its own unique contribution to human movement and locomotion. Supraspinal locomotor control is mediated via spinal neurons. Although these supraspinal centers have monosynaptic connections with motor neurons, most supraspinal input is onto spinal cord interneurons. These interneurons, which could be part of a CPG network, integrate peripheral and central inputs and, in all likelihood, help to determine the neural output required for various aspects of human locomotion.[92,106] Only projections from the motor cortex will be considered during the subsequent discussion. You should realize, however, that other supraspinal structures and pathways, in addition to projections from the motor cortex, contribute to the control of locomotion. For instance, maintaining equilibrium during bipedal locomotion would not be possible without a contribution from vestibular nuclei.

Studies in nonhuman animals have shown that motor cortical cells were active before and during locomotion.[3,30] These cells changed their activity depending on the phase of the gait cycle and depending on sensory afferent feedback occurring during locomotion.[3] The cells were most active when the animal had to attend to its environment, such as when crossing a horizontally placed ladder or when stepping over obstacles of different heights and widths.[30] Crossing the ladder was not an automatic act but required precise placing of the limbs using visual and tactile cues.

These studies and others have led investigators to suggest that the motor cortex is involved in the following aspects of human locomotion: (1) Modulation of the stepping rhythm, (2) regulation of electromyographic output to meet demands, and (3) "skilled" locomotion-fitting movements to an environmental context.[3] The motor cortex might also be involved in setting relative levels of motor neuron excitation.[14,65] This apparently can be done proactively or in reaction to a stimulus. Motor cortical cells activate differently during self-initiated movements than during reactions to an external stimulus.[41,51] Therefore, the motor cortex appears to be involved in both voluntary movements and automatic reactions.

The pattern of corticospinal projections supports the idea that the sensorimotor cortex is involved in the sequential ordering of muscle activations. The CST does not just synapse on one local motor neuron pool. Rather, its projections collateralize and synapse on various motor neuron pools that innervate synergistic muscles (see Figs. 2-22 and 4-8). Intrinsic connections within the motor cortex are also consistent with control of synergist muscle activity.

Cortical neurons controlling different muscles that often act synergistically are richly interconnected.[100,111] For instance, cortical neurons representing knee musculature are richly connected with ankle areas. These intrinsic connections probably mediate coordinated multijoint movements. Refer to the section in this chapter on the role of the cerebral cortex in upper extremity control to review additional mechanisms by which cells within the MI contribute to multijoint movements. These events include cell population coding and preferential cell activity to movement characteristics such as limb velocity, force, and direction.

The role of the MI does not appear to be restricted to muscle activation. Muscle spindle response characteristics change during the step cycle.[90] These changes in spindle activity occur independent of changes in muscle length or velocity of muscle stretch. It appears to be under supraspinal control and is part of the motor program that presets motor neuron (inclusive of fusimotor neurons) activity to the demands of a task. Although whether the MI is the supraspinal center of origin for spindle control is not known, we do know that alpha and gamma motor neurons (which innervate muscle spindles) are often under parallel control from the MI.[93]

Other studies have shown that sensory feedback to the SI is modified during the gait cycle.[23] This gating of sensory input to the SI depends on the situational context in which it occurs.[22] Some have speculated that the gating of sensory input to the SI originates in the motor cortex.[22,23]

Studies to date suggest that the motor cortex in humans is, at the very least, involved in the modulation of the timing and intensity of muscle contractions during locomotion. It also appears that the MI contributes to the modulation of sensory input being relayed back to subcortical circuitry and cortical sensory areas and thus input back to itself.

Nonneural factors that are not directly attributable to activity within the motor cortex contribute to human locomotion. Factors such as somatotype,[67] strength,[136] mechanical interactions between joints,[82] changes in muscle length,[21] and tendon elasticity[109,110] all contribute to the uniqueness of individual gait patterns and of human bipedal gait. Somehow the MI must be aware of these nonneural constraints and integrate this information before exerting its efferent influences.

■ CONTRIBUTIONS OF THE CEREBRAL CORTEX TO UPPER EXTREMITY CONTROL
Visuomotor transformation

It is summertime. With the summer come memories of childhood and my experiences with visuomotor transformations. Actually, the memories are of spending endless hours chasing bugs or "fishing" in the local stream in pursuit of minnows, crayfish, water spiders, or anything else that moved.

Visuomotor transformation is exactly what the above childhood activities were all about. For me to have been successful with my hunts, my central nervous system had to convert the sensory input of a moving target (minnows, crayfish) into an appropriate motor response that involved reaching and grasping. The primary visual pathway for perceiving objects is in the occipital lobe (striate cortex) located in the most caudal pole of the cerebral cortex. The MI, generally thought to be the major player in the actual execution of muscle contraction and movement, is located quite some distance away in the frontal lobe. Obviously something unique must happen in between these two cortical areas, located in opposite poles of the brain, that allows all of us to transform visual cues into a precisely controlled motor act. Although neuroscientists do not know exactly how this transformation takes place, a general scheme is starting to emerge. The scheme (and a lot of it is conjectural at this stage) involves sensory processing by multiple cortical areas, neural networks, motor equivalency, multijoint synergistic muscle actions, convergent and divergent neural pathways, and cell population coding.

Let's consider the example of reaching out and grasping a moving target. First, we need to detect the movement. Humans are one of the few species that can actually see nonmoving objects. We cannot, however, identify an object when it is perceived by our peripheral visual field. We can detect peripheral motion. A reflex will move our eyes in response to movement occurring peripherally so that the object is brought into the center of our visual field. Only then can we identify it. For us to touch or grasp this moving object, we must be able not only to identify the object, but also to gauge its speed and direction. The detection of motion and the speed of a moving object appear to involve different cortical pathways than the perception of color and form.[76] Object movement information is conveyed to parietal and temporal cortices. Visual information is processed further in these areas by discrete cell modules. These cortical modules perform different functions and project to divergent cortical areas. It is not only visual information that arrives in parietal and temporal cortical areas. Information from multiple sources converge in these areas. Cells that respond to visual motion, eye movement, and head movement are located in close proximity to each other.[137] As presented earlier in this chapter, posterior parietal areas project to the SII and the PM cortical areas. These projections and the interaction of cell clusters within these cortical areas appear to be essential for the transformation of visual sensory information into the motor sequence that initiates reaching toward a moving object.

The premotor cortex appears to be directly involved with preparation and guidance of upper extremity movements, especially those that are directed by visual input. Cells in the premotor cortex respond to tactile information originating from the hand and arm. These cells also respond to a very specific type of visual stimulation.[56,57] Certain premotor cells respond only to visual stimulations that occur within the visual field that is located adjacent to the arm and hand. Experiments have shown that a visual stimulus presented away from the upper extremity did not evoke any cell activity in this area. The same visual stimulus presented in close proximity to the arm and hand caused an increased frequency of cell firing! As the arm moved, so did the visual field that elicited premotor cell activity. These cells appear to help us to judge the relationships between objects and our bodies. They are a vital link in the visual control of reaching.[57] For completeness, it should be noted that the putamen (a basal ganglia component) also contains cells that respond similarly. The putamen and the PM share similar cortical inputs.[57]

The premotor cortex projects to the MI. The MI is directly involved in initiating muscle contractions. It is tempting to say that the pathways from visual cortex to posterior parietal areas to the SII to premotor areas to the MI form a logical cascade of connectivity that results in subsequent activation of the muscles necessary for upper extremity reaching and grasping of a moving target. This does not appear to be the case exclusively, however. A tremendous amount of parallel processing, reciprocal connectivity, and extensive interconnections occurs within cortical areas. The MI receives direct sensory input, and areas other than the MI project to the spinal cord, red nucleus, and pons.[75] Each cortical area might be involved to various degrees in the planning and execution of various aspects of a reaching movement. No one cortical area appears to have sole responsibility for any one function, and the functioning of any cortical area is tremendously influenced by activity within the other cortical areas. This is where the concepts of cell assemblies and neural population vectors enter into the picture.

Cortical cell assemblies and neural population vectors: contributions to the control of reaching

Let us say you have visually identified the moving object and now want to generate the command to move your upper extremity in its direction. The MI now becomes a major player in the transformation from the detection and identification of an object to the generation of muscle activity to move the upper extremity in its direction. Cells within the MI become active before any electromyographic activity in the upper extremity is detected.[37] An ensemble of cells within the MI become active—all to different degrees of intensity and all very dependent on the direction of your arm movement. Cells within the MI appear to have a preferred direction for activation.[52] For instance, a particular cell might be quiet before reaching toward the right but increases its activation for movements toward the left. This is not an all-or-none phenomenon. As movement approximates the cell's preferred direction, it will gradually increase its frequency of firing. This can be interpreted as creating a preferred movement vector. A *vector* is defined as the magnitude of the cell's discharge rate in relation to a specific angle or direction of movement. Apparently the assembly or collective firing of multiple cells within a cluster determines the final arm trajectory[52,102] (Fig. 4-16). Although some disagreement exists with this concept,[123] substantial evidence indicates that neural population vectors within the MI can predict directional tendencies of the neural ensemble.[91] It remains to be determined how, or even if, the CNS makes use of the concept of vectors.

Furthermore, the firing rate frequencies of cortical neurons from different cortical areas synchronize during certain movements.[40,102] Perhaps this is one physiological mechanism by which associations and coordination between cortical regions are obtained. Perhaps visual cell population vectors indicate target location and proprioceptive vectors inform about limb position with regard to the object. These bundled

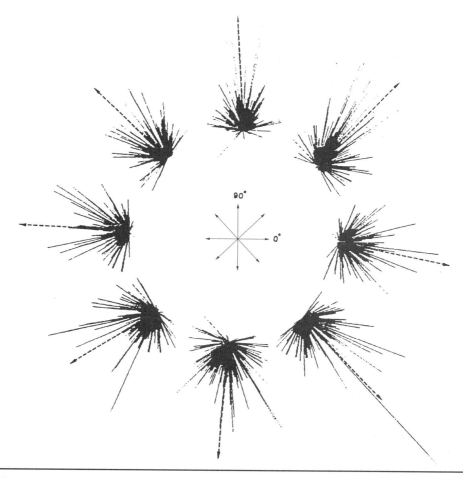

Fig. 4-16. Recordings made from 241 motor cortex cells during upper extremity movement in eight different directions. The longer the spike, the more active a particular cell during the movement. Direction of movement (dashed arrow) is dictated from the sum of the vectors of all active cells. (From Georgopoulos AP et al. J Neurosci 1982;2:1527-37.)

sensory inputs converge on motor areas to assist with the establishment of a situationally appropriate movement vector.[40]

Inherent to this explanation or model of visuomotor transformation is the concept that the net output from any cortical area does not contain information from a single cell. Each cell has a preferential firing frequency to different movement parameters such as direction or force. Each cell has a unique frame of reference that changes depending on its individual afferent input and the situational context of that input.[75] The net output reflects the summation of the predominant activity of the cell clusters.

Although all the above information has supportive scientific data, it still remains largely conjectural. And, as complicated as it all seems, we still aren't finished. Possible mechanisms by which you identify and reach for a moving object have been presented, but the cortical contribution to the actual grasping of the object has not yet been addressed.

Cortical control of grasping

The fingers begin to adapt to the size and shape of an object during arm movement and before any contact with the object is made. Therefore, the size and shape of an object is recognized before grasping, and this information is conveyed to specific cortical areas to initiate appropriate hand and finger movements. As previously discussed, visual input (especially from visual fields adjacent to the upper extremity) determines the relative positions of the hand to the desired object.

The SII and the premotor areas appear to be the cortical areas most directly involved in transforming visual input into appropriate hand activity.[70] In all probability, the pathways connecting these areas are leaky and involve considerable parallel processing. PET and fMRI studies in humans show that movements of even a single finger are controlled by networks of neurons.[5] Refer to Chapter 5 for a more in-depth discussion of the role of the cerebral cortex in grasping. Grasping is intimately connected with reaching and hand-eye coordination. It involves complicated and diffuse cortical interactions. Perhaps the best insight into the contributions of various cortical areas to grasping and other movements can be obtained from human brain lesion studies.

■ CLINICAL MANIFESTATIONS OF DAMAGE TO MOTOR AREAS

Much of what we know about the functioning of various areas within the cerebral cortex has been derived from brain lesion studies. Precise brain lesions and subsequent behavioral analysis made in nonhuman animals have revealed how the absence of certain cortical areas impact movement and sensory processing. Careful clinical observations of human patients have been equally informative, although the precise location of the lesion is rarely known when the observations are made. Bear in mind, however, that these types of studies are not without inherent interpretive error. Determining whether the effects of a lesion are secondary to damage directly related to the area or rather to the afferent or efferent projections within the lesioned area is extremely difficult. And, as is becoming increasingly defined, cortical areas do not function in isolation. An intact cortical area might behave differently when deprived of input from an area that has been lesioned. With these caveats in mind, the following paragraphs summarize some of the clinical and experimental repercussions of damage to cortical areas involved in motor control.

Primary motor area

Because of the large projection from the MI to the spinal cord and directly to motor neurons, damage to the MI classically results in muscle paresis, spasticity, and difficulties with multijoint movements on the side of the face and body contralateral to the lesion. The MI is necessary for the fractionation of movement. *Fractionation* is the ability to isolate movement to a single muscle or limb. After MI lesions, fractionation of movement is lost. Rather, all movements tend to be influenced by obligatory synergies. The individual with damage to the MI loses his or her movement repertoire. Perhaps the patient cannot flex the elbow without also flexing the shoulder or, in the lower extremity, flexion of the knee occurs concomitantly with hip flexion.

Functional loss and decreased fractionation of movement after damage to the MI is especially profound in the fingers and hands. Precision grip is almost always lost after MI or pyramidal tract lesions. Finger movements become slow and coordination is lost.

Fractionation can be lost after other cortical lesions as well. Muscles are not controlled solely by the MI. The pattern of activity within populations of cells from different cortical fields contributes to the movement parameters that permit movement fractionation.[8,112] Therefore, damage to other areas that project to the MI can also result in loss of fractionation as well as other movement impairments.

The MI is especially important in the control of complex, multijoint movements. Most functional movements performed on a daily basis involve multiple joints and muscles. Learning to control these multiple degrees of freedom after MI damage is a challenge to both patients and therapists. Some interesting experimental data have been found with regard to the retraining of complex movements after its damage.

Monkeys with MI lesions exhibit deficits in motor control similar to humans. Hand and finger movement fractionation and upper extremity control are lost. One study examined whether monkeys with MI lesions could be retrained to use their involved extremities. Monkeys with lesions to the MI could be retrained, but a specific training strategy appeared necessary. The monkeys were trained to restrict their movements to a single joint and a single plane of movement. They were trained to move one joint and then the next to achieve the desired movement goal.[65] Diagonal movements involving action at two or more joints were impossible for the monkeys to perform. The monkeys appeared incapable of coordinating the control of two joints. By restricting movement to one joint at a time, however, the investigators limited the need for the monkeys to control multiple degrees of freedom and thus increased the functioning of the limb.

Premotor area

Damage to the PM can result in a muscle paresis contralateral to the lesion similar to that seen after MI lesions. The distribution of the weakness, however, tends to involve the proximal musculature, especially the hips and shoulders.[141]

Motor planning skills are also affected. A person with a lesion to the PM might be able to physically reach out for an object but will be unable to manipulate around an obstacle. Or, the person might be unable to solve simple motor planning problems. For example, a person might be physically capable of carrying objects with either hand and of opening a car door. But when presented with the problem of carrying objects in both hands and being asked to open a car door, he might not be able to accomplish this task. The person will not think to put both objects in one hand or to put one object down to free the other hand to open the door.

Bilateral activities seem to be particularly affected after PM lesions. A temporal uncoupling of bilateral arm movements occurs. Any activity that requires the two hands to work together will likely be compromised.[142] This is especially apparent when the movements rely on vision.

Supplementary motor cortex

SMA lesions will also affect bimanual coordination,[141] but the problems are most apparent *not* during visually guided movements, but rather during movements that are made based on memorized movement patterns or sequences.[60] Individuals with SMA involvement appear unable to generate sequenced movements.

Correlates to a loss in the ability to generate internal motor commands are lengthened response latencies to a reaction time task. Response latencies increase with the complexity of the task, the more joints that are involved, or the more response choices available. Individuals with SMA lesions appear unable to decide on the most appropriate motor response to a given situation. They do much better when they are told what to do and their movement options are minimized.

After SMA damage a general akinesis of movement occurs. Deficits in movement preparation (e.g., activation of postural muscles before a reaching task) and disruption in the timing of movements are also common. Many of these deficits overlap with those associated with PM lesions. The major difference appears to be that the SMA is more involved with internally generated movement sequences, whereas the PM is more directly influenced by ongoing peripheral afferent feedback such as vision. One study reported the inability of patients with SMA damage to generate rhythmic hand movements from memory.[60] The impairment was most noticeable when both hands needed to be used in an alternate manner.

Primary somatosensory area

The typical impairment associated with damage to the SI is contralateral sensory loss. Loss can involve various degrees of deficits in the ability to distinguish sharp and dull sensations, position sense in the limbs, tactile localization, and perhaps *stereognosis* (the ability to perceive an object's nature through touch). Posterior parietal lesions can also result in a loss of stereognosis. The causes for the loss of stereognosis, however, differ between the two types of damage. The person with SI damage does not perceive accurate sensory feedback from the manipulation of an object and therefore cannot appropriately identify it. After posterior parietal lesions, the person can typically perceive sensory input but cannot appropriately interpret the input and place functional significance to it. These impairments contribute to an inability to discriminate size, texture, and shapes of objects. Therefore, grip and load force synergies tend to be disrupted with either SI or posterior parietal lesions. Because limb position sense can be affected after SI damage, a type of sensory ataxia can result. The patient appears uncoordinated during attempted limb movements. This is secondary to an inability to perceive accurately afferent sensory feedback subsequent to the movement.

Secondary somatosensory area

Lesions to the SII can cause impairments similar to those described for the SI. These two areas are richly interconnected and separating their functions is difficult. Removal of the SII results in an animal's failure to learn associations between hand movements and object sizes. They also cannot adapt grip force to changes in the texture of objects. Some children with cerebral palsy exhibit similar deficits presumably secondary to perinatal damage involving the SI or the SII.[36]

Prefrontal cortex

In addition to their connections with motor areas of the brain, prefrontal areas also receive input from the limbic system and frontal lobes. Thus, lesions here will affect emotional reactions and cognitive functions. Deficits in these areas will, in turn, affect motor behavior.

Individuals with prefrontal lesions exhibit a lack of foresight and deficits in short-term memory. They will often inappropriately persevere on a task. Others will show increased distractibility and a decrease in goal-directed behaviors.[129] Motivation to practice motor skills is often lacking.

Spatial memory is also affected in subjects with prefrontal lesions. Experiments with monkeys have helped to elucidate this concept. Monkeys were shown a piece of food being placed under a container. Typically the monkeys with prefrontal lesions could reach under the container to obtain the food. If, however, a delay was introduced between when the food was hidden and when the monkeys were allowed to reach for it, they were unable to remember where the food was placed. Spatial memory is of course used in many motor tasks. Individuals with prefrontal lesions can be expected to have difficulties remembering visual cues in their environment.

Posterior parietal cortex

The motor deficits most commonly associated with posterior parietal lesions involve deficits of the contralateral hand and arm. Reaching and grasping are affected probably secondary to a loss of visual and tactile placing abilities. *Placing* is the ability to place the limb accurately in response to either visual or tactile input. If I reach out to hold your hand but instead just stroke the lateral border of your hand, you will be able to orient your hand to the stimulus to find and grasp my hand. An individual with a posterior parietal lesion will not be able to do this. Not only does such a person lose placing reactions, but there is a general paucity of hand movements and the hands cannot adapt grip force to object size.

Other perceptual dysfunctions are associated with posterior parietal lobe lesions. A loss of stereognosis is common, especially if area 5 is affected. This is not due to a loss of sensory input as in lesions to the SI, but rather to an inability to associate sensory input with a memory of the object. Some individuals with posterior parietal lobe lesions might be able to name an object but cannot associate a function with it. As an example, an individual with posterior parietal damage, when presented with a toothbrush, can verbally identify it but does not associate a tube of toothpaste with it and cannot mimic the motor act of brushing the teeth when asked to demonstrate an activity associated with the toothbrush.

A loss of visually guided movement is usually associated with area 7. This results in misreaching and poorly timed limb movements, especially when attempting to reach for a moving object.[75]

A *hemianopia* (ignorance of one side of the body) might also be evident after posterior parietal lobe damage that damages visual pathways. The person with this type of damage ignores not only one side of the body, but also the entire half of the visual field. Imagine walking down a hallway and only seeing the right side of the hall. When you turn around to come back, because you are now seeing the opposite side of the hall, it will be as if you are in an entirely different place. In milder forms of hemianopia, individuals have difficulties learning tasks that require a knowledge of the body in space.[83]

Subtle, and rather bizarre, perceptual problems that reflect the contextual importance in which an object is seen might also be apparent. One report indicated that an individual with a posterior parietal lobe lesion was unable to grasp and hold small plastic cylinders, yet was able to grasp similarly shaped objects that were familiar to her. Although unable to grasp small objects, she was able to grasp cylinders of lipstick[70]!

Disruption of different visual pathways that connect with parietal areas can cause a variety of visual deficits. Object identification difficulties result from interruption of pathways connecting the striate cortex (primary visual cortex) with parietal areas whereas spatial discrimination problems are more typical of interruption of pathways connecting prestriate areas (visual associational areas) with parietal areas.[70] Dysfunction of cortical areas that include the posterior parietal cortex has also been implicated in an impairment in detecting visual motion that contributes to a reading disorder known as dyslexia.[33]

Differences in affected behaviors also happen depending on which hemisphere is involved. With a posterior parietal lesion of the dominant hemisphere (usually the left), speech is also commonly affected. Not just the posterior parietal lobes exhibit differences in hemispheric functions. Throughout the cerebral cortex one finds asymmetries with regard to function. Some of these asymmetries have a direct impact on motor control.

■ DIFFERENTIAL ROLES FOR THE RIGHT AND LEFT HEMISPHERES: IMPLICATIONS FOR MOTOR CONTROL

The most often-cited difference between the right and left hemispheres of the human cerebral cortex involves language functions. In the vast majority of people (even left-handers), language centers are located in the left hemisphere. Damage to the left hemisphere can result in any number of language disorders (*aphasias*). Various types of expressive (inability to verbally express thoughts) and receptive (inability to understand spoken or written words) aphasias have been described. Damage to similar areas in the right hemisphere most typically impact the emotional aspects of speech. In addition to differences in language capabilities, other differences exist between the two hemispheres.

The right hemisphere appears to be preferentially activated during certain cognitive tasks, such as visuospatial information processing, face recognition, and musical skills.[149] Of these, visuospatial processing has the most impact on motor control skills.

Movement takes place within a situational context. For movement to occur with precision, detection and interpretation of spatial cues are essential. The right hemisphere appears to be more directly involved in spatial perceptions. This might involve activities as divergent as puzzle solving and dressing. Any activity that requires a motor response to visual input, such as visually tracking and reaching for an object, seems preferentially to activate the right hemisphere. Patients with damage to the right hemisphere are slow to respond to visual cues. Patients with right parietal lobe damage perform fewer *saccades* (rapid eye movements) and thus do not scan their surroundings as well as nondisabled individuals. They can generally move with some accuracy to a visual target. However, they have considerable difficulty relating the object to its surrounding environment[42] or in making immediate use of sensory processing.[144] As a result, they require extra time to process spatial information.

Damage to the right hemisphere might also result in an inability to relate body parts to spatial cues in the environment. In severe cases of right hemisphere damage, the individual might totally neglect the left side of the bodies. Because the right hemisphere receives its visual input from the left visual field, the person might neglect any visual stimulus coming from that side. Not atypically, individuals with right hemisphere damage tend to have an indifference to or a lack of an awareness of their disability. This behavior has more to do with emotional affect and is not necessarily due to sensory loss. The right hemisphere, however, does appear to play a rather unique role in tactile sensory processing.

The right and left hemispheres appear to respond similarly to tactile input. Both hemispheres are equally adept at identifying tactile information and precisely locating the point on the body where the tactile stimulus was applied. If some time is allowed to elapse between the time of stimulus application and the time the individual is asked to point to its location on the body, however, the right hemisphere is consistently more accurate.[149] It would appear that the right hemisphere has a role to play in remembering sensory input. This role, of course, has an impact on motor control and motor learning.

The left hemisphere, in addition to its language capabilities, seems preferentially active during tasks that have a temporal or sequential ordering of events. It is said to be more involved in making causal inferences and interpreting sensory stimuli.[49] For instance, left hemisphere damage can result in an ideomotor apraxia. Patients with this syndrome, despite sufficient strength and sensation, are unable to produce movements in response to verbal or visual cueing. When asked to make a movement to simulate combing the hair, they are unable to do so. The left hemisphere appears to be preferentially involved in the programming of sequenced movements.[42,79,144]

The left hemisphere is also not without its emotional component. Damage to the left hemisphere does not result in ignorance of the problem, but often results in emotional depression.[83]

No doubt, asymmetry of function and division of labor exist between the hemispheres. Findings, however, have often been misinterpreted by the lay public and have led to some misconceptions regarding hemispheric specializations. Some of these misconceptions include the beliefs that the hemispheres function independently of each other and that each hemisphere has unique functions not duplicated by the other.[149] These ideas are not consistent with existing scientific literature.

Studies that have examined the functioning of the two hemispheres have often assumed that the two hemispheres, although richly connected by the corpus callosum and commissural systems, can operate independently of each other. This is actually not the case. The two hemispheres are dependent on each other to create a fully functioning whole.[49,64,83] Removing input from one hemisphere alters the functioning of the intact hemisphere. Several studies with patients with adult-onset brain damage have shown bilateral deficits after unilateral brain damage.[59,80] This could be due to removal of one hemisphere's influence over the other or a certain amount of bilateral control from one hemisphere. Some evidence indicates that the right hemisphere has a larger role to play in bilateral upper extremity movements during spatial tasks.[79,80] Other studies have shown that the left hemisphere has a predominant role to play in fast, bilateral alternating movements.[98,148] Neither task, however, is performed as well after damage to either hemisphere.

SUGGESTED READINGS

Abbott LF, Varela JA, Sen K, Nelson SB. Synaptic depression and cortical gain control. Science 1997;275:220-4.

Adams RD, Victor M. Principles of neurology, 5th ed. New York: McGraw-Hill, 1993.

Ashe J, Taira M, Smyrnis N, et al. Motor cortical activity preceding a memorized movement trajectory with an orthogonal bend. Exp Brain Res 1993;95:118-30.

Barbeau H, Rossignol S. The effects of serotonergic drugs on the locomotor pattern and on cutaneous reflexes of the adult chronic spinal cat. Brain Res 1990;514:55-67.

Barbeau H, Rossignol S. Initiation and modulation of the locomotor pattern in the adult chronic spinal cat by noradrenergic, serotonergic and dopaminergic drugs. Brain Res 1991;546:250-60.Bawa P. Dorsal root reflexes in kittens. Dev Brain Res 1988;39:145-8.

Bradley NS, Smith JL. Neuromuscular patterns of stereotypic hindlimb behaviors in the first two postnatal months. I. Stepping in normal kittens. Brain Res 1988;38:37-52.

Brunt D, Lafferty MJ, McKeon A, Goode B, Mulhausen C, Polk P. Invariant characteristics of gait initiation. Am J Phys Med Rehabil 1991;70:206-12.

Burleigh AL, Horak FB, Malouin F. Modification of postural responses and step initiation: evidence for goal-directed postural interactions. J Neurophysiol 1994;72:2892-2902.

Conradi S, Ronnevi LO. Spontaneous elimination of synapses on cat motoneurons after birth. Do half of the synapses on the cell bodies disappear? Brain Res 1975;92:505-10.

Day BL, Rothwell JC, Thompson PD, et al. Motor cortex stimulation in intact man. 2. Multiple descending volleys. Brain 1987;110:1191-1209.

Eccles RM, Shealy CN, Willis WD. Patterns of innervation of kitten motoneurones. J Physiol (Lond) 1963;165:392-402.

Farde L. The advantage of using positron emission tomography in drug research. Trends Neurosci 1996;19:211-4.

Feldman JL, Grillner S. Control of vertebrate respiration and locomotion: a brief account. Physiologist 1983;26:310-6.

Fetz EE, Finochio DV. Operant conditioning of specific patterns of neural and muscular activity. Science 1971;174:431-5.

Georgopoulos AP. Neural networks and motor control. Neuroscientist 1997;3:52-60.

Georgopoulos AP, Ashe J, Smyrnis N, Taira M. Motor cortex and the coding of force. Science 1992;256:1692-5.

Georgopoulos AP, Caminiti R, Kalaska JF, Massey JT. Spatial coding of movement: a hypothesis concerning the coding of movement direction by motor cortical populations. Exp Brain Res 1983;7:327-36.

Georgopoulos AP, Taira M, Lukashin A. Cognitive neurophysiology of the motor cortex. Science 1993;260:47-52.

Gerfen CR. The neostriatal mosaic: striatal patch-matrix organization is related to cortical lamination. Science 1989;246:385-8.

Glial signalling: special issue. Trends Neurosci 1996;19:305-69.

Grillner S. Neurobiological bases of rhythmic motor acts in vertebrates. Science 1985;228:143-9.

Grillner S, Deliagina T, Ekeberg O, et al. Neural networks that co-ordinate locomotion and body orientation in lamprey. Trends Neurosci 1995;18:270-9.

Gur RC, Mozley LH, Mozley PD, et al. Sex differences in regional cerebral glucose metabolism during a resting state. Science 1995;267:528-31.

Holzreiter SH, Kohle ME. Assessment of gait patterns using neural networks. J Biomech 1993;26:645-51.

Ikeda A, Luders HO, Burgess RC, Shibasaki H. Movement-related potentials recorded from supplementary motor area and primary motor area. Brain 1993;115:1017-43.

Innocenti GM. Exuberant development of connections, and its possible permissive role in cortical evolution. Trends Neurosci 1995;18:397-402.

Iriki A, Pavlides C, Keller A, Asanuma H. Long-term potentiation in the motor cortex. Science 1989;245:1385-8.

Jeng S, Holt KG, Fetters L, Certo C. Self-optimization of walking in nondisabled children and children with spastic hemiplegic cerebral palsy. J Motor Behav 1996;28:15-27.

Kawashima R, Fukuda H. Functional organization of the human primary motor area: an update on current concepts. Rev Neurosci 1994;5:347-54.

Kawashima R, Roland PE, O'Sullivan BT. Fields in human motor areas involved in preparation for reaching, actual reaching, and visuomotor learning: a positron emission tomography study. J Neurosci 1994;14:3462-74.

Light KE, Purser JP, Giuliani CA. Motor programming deficits of patients with left versus right CVAs. Proc Neurol Section Am Phys Ther Assoc 1992;4:2-6.

Lim SH, Dinner DS, Pillay PK, et al. Functional anatomy of the human supplementary sensorimotor area: results of extraoperative electrical stimulation. Electroencephalogr Clin Neurophysiol 1994;91:179-93.

Lundberg A, Norrsell U, Voorhoeve P. Pyramidal effects on lumbo-sacral interneurones activated by somatic afferents. Acta Physiol Scand 1962;56:220-9.

Mah CD, Hulliger M, Lee RG, O'Callaghan IS. Quantitative analysis of human movement synergies: constructive pattern analysis for gait. J Motor Behav 1994;26:83-02.

Martin JH, Ghez C. Differential impairments in reaching and grasping produced by local inactivation within the forelimb representation of the motor cortex in the cat. Exp Brain Res 1993;94:429-43.

Neshige R, Luders H, Shibasaki H. Recording of movement-related potentials from scalp and cortex in man. Brain 1988;111:719-36.

Northcutt RG, Kaas JH. The emergence and evolution of mammalian neocortex. Trends Neurosci 1995;18:373-9.

O'Leary DDM. Do cortical areas emerge from a protocortex? Trends Neurosci 1989;12:400-6.

O'Leary DDM, Stanfield BB, Cowan WM. Evidence that the early postnatal restriction of the cells of origin of the callosal projection is due to the elimination of axonal collaterals rather than to the death of neurons. Dev Brain Res 1981;1:607-17.

Oberg R, Divac I. Levels of motor planning: cognition and the control of movement. In: Evarts EV, Wise SP, Bousfield D, eds. The motor system in neurobiology. Amsterdam: Elsevier, 1985:284-7.

Okamoto T, Goto Y. Human infant pre-independent and independent walking. In: Kondo S, ed. Primate morphophysiology, locomotor analyses and human bipedalism. Tokyo: University of Tokyo Press, 1985:25-45.

Orlovsky GN. Activity of rubrospinal neurons during locomotion. Brain Res 1972;46:99-112.

Orlovsky GN. The effect of different descending systems on flexor and extensor activity during locomotion. Brain Res 1972;40:359-72.

Pellizzer G, Sargent P, Georgopoulos AP. Motor cortical activity in a context-recall task. Science 1995;269:702-5.

Pons TP, Garraghty PE, Ommaya AK, Kaas JH, Taub E, Mishkin M. Massive cortical reorganization after sensory deafferentation in adult macaques. Science 1991;252:1857-60.

Pritzel M, Markowitsch HJ. Organization of cortical afferents to the prefrontal cortex in the bush baby (galago senegalensis). Brain Behav Evol 1982;20:43-56.

Purves D. Neural activity and the growth of the brain. Cambridge: Cambridge University Press, 1994.

Purves D, Riddle DR, LaMantia AS. Iterated patterns of brain circuitry (or how the cortex gets its spots). Trends Neurosci 1992;15:362-8.

Roberton MA, Halverson LE. The development of locomotor coordination: longitudinal change and invariance. J Motor Behav 1988;20:197-241.

Rothwell JC, Gandevia SC, Burke D. Activation of fusimotor neurones by motor cortical stimulation in human subjects. J Physiol (Lond) 1990;431:743-56.

Rothwell JC, Thompson PD, Day BL, et al. Motor cortex stimulation in intact man. 1. General characteristics of EMG responses in different muscles. Brain 1987;110:1173-90.

Scholz JP, Kelso JAS. A quantitative approach to understanding the formation and change of coordinated movement patterns. J Motor Behav 1989;21:122-44.

Schwartz AB, Kettner RE, Georgopoulos AP. Primate motor cortex and free arm movements to visual targets in three-dimensional space. I. Relations between single cell discharge and direction of movement. J Neurosci 1988;8:2913-27.

Talbot JD, Marrett S, Evans AC, Meyer E, Bushnell MC, Duncan GH. Multiple representations of pain in human cerebral cortex. Science 1991;251:1355-8.

Tanaka H, Mori S, Kimura H. Developmental changes in the serotonergic innervation of hindlimb extensor motoneurons in neonatal rats. Dev Brain Res 1992;65:1-12.

Tanaka S. Hypothetical joint-related coordinate systems in which populations of motor cortical neurons code direction of voluntary arm movements. Neurosci Lett 1994;180:83-6.

Thorstensson A, Carlson H, Zomlefer MR, Nilsson J. Lumbar back muscle activity in relation to trunk movements during locomotion in man. Acta Physiol Scand 1982;116:13-21.

Thorstensson A, Nilsson J, Carlson H, Zomlefer MR. Trunk movements in human locomotion. Acta Physiol Scand 1984;121:9-22.

Ungerleider LG. Functional brain imaging studies of cortical mechanisms for memory. Science 1995;270:769-75.

Vejsada R, Hnik P, Payne R, Ujec E, Palecek J. The postnatal functional development of muscle stretch receptors in the rat. Somatosensory Res 1985;2:205-22.

Warach S. Mapping brain pathophysiology and higher cortical function with magnetic resonance imaging. Neuroscientist 1995;1:221-35.

Wickelgren I. For the cortex, neuron loss may be less than thought. Science 1996;273:48-50.

Wickens J, Hyland B, Anson G. Cortical cell assemblies: a possible mechanism for motor programs. J Motor Behav 1994;26:66-82.

Yumiya H, Ghez C. Specialized subregions in the cat motor cortex: anatomical demonstration of differential projections to rostral and caudal sectors. Exp Brain Res 1984;53:259-76.

REFERENCES

1. Alisky JM, Swink TD, Tolbert DL. The postnatal spatial and temporal development of corticospinal projection in cats. Exp Brain Res 1992;88:265-76.

2. Amos A, Armstrong DM, Marple-Horvat DE. Responses of motor cortical neurones in the cat to unexpected perturbations of locomotion. Neurosci Lett 1989;104:147-51.

3. Armstrong DM. The supraspinal control of mammalian locomotion. J Physiol (Lond) 1988;405:1-37.

4. Armstrong E. A comparative review of the primate motor system. J Motor Behav 1989;21:493-517.

5. Barinaga M. Remapping the motor cortex. Science 1995;268:1696-8.

6. Bates CA, Killackey HP. The emergence of a discretely distributed pattern of corticospinal projection neurons. Brain Res 1984;13:265-73.

7. Batuev AS, Shaefer VI, Orlov AA. Comparative characteristics of unit activity in the prefrontal and parietal areas during delayed performance in monkeys. Behav Brain Res 1985;16:57-70.

8. Bennett KMB, Lemon RN. Corticomotoneuronal contribution to the fractionation of muscle activity during precision grip in the monkey. J Neurophysiol 1996;75:1826-42.

9. Boussaoud D. Primate premotor cortex: modulation of preparatory neuronal activity by gaze angle. J Neurophysiol 1995;73:886-90.

10. Bower AJ. Plasticity in the adult and neonatal central nervous system. J Neurosurg (Br) 1990;4:253-64.

11. Bradley NS, Smith JL. Neuromuscular patterns of stereotypic hindlimb behaviors in the first two postnatal months. II. Stepping in spinal kittens. Brain Res 1988;38:53-67.

12. Bregman BS, Goldberger ME. Anatomical plasticity and sparing of function after spinal cord damage in neonatal cats. Science 1982;217:553-5.13.

Bregman BS, Kunkel-Bagden E, McAttee M, O'Neill A. Extension of the critical period for developmental plasticity of the corticospinal pathway. J Comp Neurol 1989;282:355-70.

14. Brooke JD, Collins DF, McIlroy WE. Human locomotor control, the Ia autogenic spinal pathway, and interlimb modulations. In: Swinnen S, Hever H, Massion J, Casaer P, eds. Interlimb coordination: neural, dynamical, and cognitive constraints. New York: Academic Press, 1994:127-46.

15. Brouwer B, Ashby P. Do injuries to the developing human brain alter corticospinal projections? Neurosci Lett 1990;108:225-30.

16. Brouwer B, Ashby P. Corticospinal projections to lower limb motoneurons in man. Exp Brain Res 1992;89:649-54.

17. Burton H, Kopf EM. Ipsilateral cortical connections from the second and fourth somatic sensory areas in the cat. J Comp Neurol 1984;225:527-53.

18. Bussel B, Roby-Brami A, Yakovleff A, Bennis N. Late flexion reflex in paraplegic patients. Evidence for a spinal stepping generator. Brain Res Bull 1989;22:53-6.

19. Butler AB, Hodos W. Comparative vertebrate neuroanatomy. New York: Wiley-Liss, 1996.

20. Caramia MD, Cicinelli P, Zarola F, Bernardi G, Rossini PM. Motor tract excitability changes in spastic patients: studies with non-invasive brain stimulation. New Trends Adv Tech Clin Neurophysiol Electroencephalogr (suppl) 1990;41:286-91.

21. Carrier DR, Heglund NC, Earls KD. Variable gearing during locomotion in the human musculoskeletal system. Science 1994;265:651-3.

22. Chapin JK, Woodward DJ. Somatic sensory transmission to the cortex during movement: gating of single cell responses to touch. Exp Neurol 1982;78:654-69.

23. Chapin JK, Woodward DJ. Somatic sensory transmission to the cortex during movement: phasic modulation over the locomotor step cycle. Exp Neurol 1982;78:670-84.

24. Cowan WM, Fawcett JW, O'Leary DDM, Stanfield BB. Regressive events in neurogenesis. In: Abelson P, ed. Neuroscience. Washington, DC: American Association for the Advancement of Science, 1985:13-29.

25. Crammond DJ. Motor imagery, never in your wildest dream. Trends Neurosci 1997;20:54-7.

26. Deiber M-P, Passingham RE, Colebatch JG, Friston KJ, Nixon PD, Frackowiak RSJ. Cortical areas and the selection of movement: a study with positron emission tomography [abstract]. Exp Brain Res 1991;84:393-402.

27. Dietz V, Colombo G, Jensen L, Baumgartner L. Locomotor capacity of spinal cord in paraplegic patients. Ann Neurol 1995;37:574-82.

28. Dobbing J, Sands J. Quantitative growth and development of human brain. Arch Dis Child 1973;48:757-67.

29. Drew T. Discharge patterns of pyramidal tract neurones in motor cortex during a locomotion task requiring a precise control of limb trajectory. Presented at the Annual Meeting of the Society for Neuroscience, 1987, abstract no 71.17.

30. Drew T. Motor cortical cell discharge during voluntary gait modification. Brain Res 1988;457:181-7.

31. Dum RP, Strick PL. Cingulate motor areas. In: Vogt BA, Boston GM, eds. Neurobiology of cingulate cortex and limbic thalamus: a comprehensive treatise. Boston: GM Birkhauser, 1993:415-41.

32. Edelman GM. Neural Darwinism. New York: Basic Books, 1987.

33. Eden GF, VanMeter JW, Rumsey JM, Masiog JM, Woods RP, and Zeffiro TA. Abnormal processing of visual motion in dyslexia revealed by functional brain imaging. Nature 1996;382:66-9.

34. Eidelberg E, Walden JG, Nguyen LH. Locomotor control in macaque monkeys. Brain 1981;104:647-63.

35. Elbert T, Pantev C, Wienbruch C, Rockstroh B, Taub E. Increased cortical representation of the fingers of the left hand in string players. Science 1995;270:305-7.

36. Eliasson AC, Gordon AM, Forssberg H. Basic coordination of manipulative forces in children with cerebral palsy. Dev Med Child Neurol 1991;33:661-70.

37. Evarts E. Pyramidal tract activity associated with a conditioned hand movement in monkey. J Neurophysiol 1966;29:1011-27.

38. Evarts EV, Tanji J. Reflex and intended responses in motor cortex pyramidal tract neurons of monkey. J Neurophysiol 1976;39:1069-80.

39. Farmer SF, Harrison LM, Ingram DA, Stephens JA. Plasticity of central motor pathways in children with hemiplegic cerebral palsy. Neurology 1991;41:1505-10.

40. Fetz EE. Cortical mechanisms controlling limb movement. Curr Opin Neurobiol 1993;3:932-9.

41. Fetz EE, Cheney PD. Post-spike facilitation of forelimb muscle activity by primate corticomotoneural cells. J Neurophysiol 1980;44:751-72.

42. Fisk JD, Goodale MA. The effects of unilateral brain damage on visually guided reaching: hemispheric differences in the nature of the deficit. Exp Brain Res 1988;72:425-35.

43. Fitzgerald M, Butcher T, Shortland P. Developmental changes in the laminar termination of a fibre cutaneous sensory afferents in the rat spinal cord dorsal horn. J Comp Neurol 1994;348:225-33.

44. Forssberg H, Grillner S, Halbertsma J. The locomotion of the spinal cat. I. Coordination within a hindlimb. Acta Physiol Scand 1980;108:269-81.

45. Forssberg H, Grillner S, Rossignol S. Phasic gain control of reflexes from the dorsum of the paw during spinal locomotion. Brain Res 1977;132:121-39.

46. Foster TC, Castro CA, McNaughton BL. Spatial selectivity of rat hippocampal neurons: dependence on preparedness for movement. Science 1989;244:1580-1.

47. Fromm C, Evarts EV. Pyramidal tract neurons in somatosensory cortex: central and peripheral inputs during voluntary movement. Brain Res 1982;238:186-91.

48. Gahr M. How should brain nuclei be delineated? Consequences for developmental mechanisms and for correlations of area size, neuron numbers and functions of brain nuclei. Trends Neurosci 1997;20:58-62.

49. Gazzaniga MS. Organization of the human brain. Science 1989;245:947-52.

50. Georgopoulos AP. New concepts in generation of movement. Neuron 1994;13:257-68.

51. Georgopoulos AP, Kalaska JF, Caminiti R, Massey JT. On the relations between the direction of two-dimensional arm movements and cell discharge in primate motor cortex. J Neurosci 1982;2:1527-37.

52. Georgopoulos AP, Schwartz AB, Kettner RE. Neuronal population coding of movement direction. Science 1986;233:1416-9.

53. Goldberger ME, Murray M. Recovery of function and anatomical plasticity after damage to the adult and neonatal spinal cord. In: Cotman CW, ed. Synaptic plasticity. New York: Guilford Press, 1985:77-110.

54. Goldman-Rakic PS. Development of cortical circuitry and cognitive function. Child Dev 1987;58:601-22.

55. Gordon AM, Flament D, Lee JH, Ugurbil K, Kim SG, Ebner TJ. Functional MRI of cortical motor areas during sequential typing movements. Presented at the Annual Meeting of the Society for Neuroscience, 1995:1422.

56. Graziano MSA, Gross CG. How the brain represents space near the body. J Natl Health Inst Res 1995;7:48-9.

57. Graziano MSA, Yap GS, Gross CG. Coding of visual space by premotor neurons. Science 1994;266:1054-6.

58. Hakamada S. Development of the monosynaptic reflex pathway in the human spinal cord. Dev Brain Res 1988;42:239-46.

59. Halaney ME, Carey JR. Tracking ability of hemiparetic and healthy subjects. Phys Ther 1989;69:342-8.

60. Halsband U, Ito N, Tanji J, Freund HJ. The role of premotor cortex and the supplementary motor area in the temporal control of movement in man. Brain 1993;116:243-66.

61. Halsband U, Matsuzaka Y, Tanji J. Neuronal activity in the primate supplementary, pre-supplementary and premotor cortex during externally and internally instructed sequential movements. Neurosci Res 1994;20:149-55.

62. Hari R, Lounasmaa OV. Recording and interpretation of cerebral magnetic fields. Science 1989;244:432-6.

63. He SQ, Dum RP, Strick PL. Topographic organization of corticospinal projections from the frontal lobe: motor areas on the medial surface of the hemisphere. J Neurosci 1995;15:3284-306.

64. Hellige JB. Hemispheric asymmetry. Cambridge: Harvard University Press, 1993.

65. Hoffman DS, Strick PL. Effects of a primary motor cortex lesion on step-tracking movements of the wrist. J Neurophysiol 1995;73:891-5.

66. Humphrey DR, Tanji J. What features of voluntary motor control are incoded in the neuronal discharge of different cortical motor areas? In: Humphrey DR, Freund HJ, eds. Motor control: concepts and issues. Chichester: John Wiley, 1991:413-44.

67. Hurov JR. Rethinking primate locomotion: what can we learn from development. J Motor Behav 1991;23:211-8.

68. Ingram DA. Central motor conduction in neurologic disorders: studies with electrical and magnetic brain stimulation. In: Anonymous. Non-invasive stimulation

of brain and spinal cord: fundamentals and clinical applications. Philadelphia: Alan R Liss, 1988: 207-18.

69. Ivy GO, Killackey HP. Ontogenetic changes in the projections of neocortical neurons. Neuroscience 1982;2:735-43.

70. Jeannerod M, Arbib MA, Rizzolatti G, Sakata H. Grasping objects: the cortical mechanisms of visuomotor transformation. Trends Neurosci 1995;18:314-20.

71. Jessell TM. Cell migration and axon guidance. In: Kandel ER, Schwartz JH, Jessell TM, eds. Principles of neural science, 3rd ed. Norwalk, Conn: Appleton & Lange, 1991:908-28.

72. Jessell TM. Neuronal survival and synapse formation. In: Kandel ER, Schwartz JH, Jessell TM, eds. Principles of neural science, 3rd ed. Norwalk, Conn: Appleton & Lange, 1991:929-44.

73. Jones EG. Connectivity of the primate sensory-motor cortex. In: Jones EG, Peters A, eds. Cerebral cortex. New York: Plenum Press, 1986:113-83.

74. Jurgens U. The efferent and afferent connections of the supplementary motor area. Brain Res 1984;300:63-81.

75. Kalaska JF, Crammond DJ. Cerebral cortical mechanisms of reaching movements. Science 1992;255:1517-23.

76. Kandel ER. Perception of motion, depth, and form. In: Kandel ER, Schwartz JH, Jessell TM, eds. Principles of neural science, 3rd ed. Norwalk, Conn: Appleton & Lange, 1991:440-66.

77. Kandel ER, Jessell T. Early experience and the fine tuning of synaptic connections. In: Kandel ER, Schwartz JH, Jessell TM, eds. Principles of neural science, 3rd ed. Norwalk, Conn: Appleton & Lange, 1991:945-73.

78. Keller A. Intrinsic synaptic organization of the motor cortex. Cereb Cortex 1993;3:430-41.

79. Kimura D. Left-hemisphere control of oral and brachial movements and their relation to communication. Philos Trans R Soc Lond B Biol Sci 1982;298:135-49.

80. Kimura D, Archibald Y. Motor functions of the left hemisphere. Brain 1974;97:337-50.

81. Knutsson E, Richards C. Different types of disturbed motor control in gait of hemiparetic patients. Brain 1979;102:405-30.

82. Kuhtzbuschbeck JP, Boczekfuncke A, Illert M, Weinhardt C. X-ray study of the cat hindlimb during treadmill locomotion. Eur J Neurosci 1994;6:1187-98.

83. Kupfermann I. Localization of higher cognitive and affective functions: the association cortices. In: Kandel ER, Schwartz JH, Jessell TM, eds. Principles of neural science, 3rd ed. Norwalk, Conn: Appleton & Lange, 1991:823-38.

84. LaMantia AS, Rakic P. Axon overproduction and elimination in the corpus callosum of the developing rhesus monkey. J Neurosci 1990;10:2156-75.

85. Lavoie BA, Cody FWJ, Capaday C. Cortical control of human soleus muscle during volitional and postural activities studied using focal magnetic stimulation. Exp Brain Res 1995;103:97-107.

86. Leonard CT, Goldberger ME. Consequences of damage to the sensorimotor cortex in neonatal and adult cats. I. Sparing and recovery of function. Dev Brain Res 1987;32:1-14.

87. Leonard CT, Goldberger ME. Consequences of damage to the sensorimotor cortex in neonatal and adult cats. II. Maintenance of exuberant projections. Dev Brain Res 1987;32:15-30.

88. Leonard CT, Hirschfeld H, Forssberg H. The development of independent walking in children with cerebral palsy. Dev Med Child Neurol 1991;33:567-77.

89. Leonard CT, Moritani T, Hirschfeld H, Forssberg H. Deficits in reciprocal inhibition in children with cerebral palsy as revealed by H reflex testing. Dev Med Child Neurol 1990;. 32:974-84.

90. Loeb GE, Duysens J. Activity patterns in individual hindlimb primary and secondary muscle spindle afferents during normal movements in unrestrained cats. J Neurophysiol 1979;42:420-40.

91. Lukashin AV, Georgopoulos AP. Directional operations in the motor cortex modeled by a neural network of spiking neurons. Biol Cybern 1994;71:79-85.

92. Lundberg A. The significance of segmental spinal mechanisms in motor control. Proceedings of the Fourth Biophysics Congress, Moscow, 1972.

93. Lundberg A. Control of spinal mechanics from the brain. In: Tower DB, ed. The nervous system. New York: Raven Press, 1975:253-65.

94. Martin JH, Brust JCM, Hilal S. Imaging the living brain. In: Kandel ER, Schwartz JH, Jessell TM, eds. Principles of neural science, 3rd ed. Norwalk, Conn: Appleton & Lange, 1991:309-28.

95. McConnell SK, Ghosh A, Shatz CJ. Subplate neurons pioneer the first axon pathway from the cerebral cortex. Science 1989;245:978-86.

96. Merzenich MM, Kaas JH, Wall J, Nelson RJ, Sur M, Felleman D. Topographic reorganization of somatosensory cortical areas 3B and 1 in adult monkeys following restricted deafferentation. Neuroscience 1983;8:33-55.

97. Merzenich MM, Sameshima K. Cortical plasticity and memory. Curr Opin Neurobiol 1993;3:187-96.

98. Meudell PR, Mills VM, DiGenio M. Functional differences in patients with left or right cerebrovascular accidents. Phys Ther 1983;63:481-5.

99. Mountcastle VB, Darian-Smith I. Neural mechanisms in somesthesia. In: Mountcastle VB, ed. Medical physiology. St Louis: Mosby-Year Book, 1968:1372-1423.

100. Muakkassa KF, Strick PL. Frontal lobe inputs to primate motor cortex: evidence for four somatotopically organized 'premotor' areas. Brain Res 1979;177:176-82.

101. Muir GD, Steeves JD. Sensorimotor stimulation to improve locomotor recovery after spinal cord injury. Trends Neurosci 1997;20:72-7.

102. Nicolelis MAL, Baccala LA, Lin RCS, Chapin JK. Sensorimotor encoding by synchronous neural ensemble activity at multiple levels of the somatosensory system. Science 1995;268:1353-8.

103. Nolte J. The human brain. St Louis: Mosby-Year Book, 1988.

104. Nudo RJ, Wise BM, SiFuentes F, Milliken GW. Neural substrates for the effects of rehabilitative training on motor recovery after ischemic infarct. Science 1996;272:1791-4.

105. Oudega M, Varon S, Hagg T. Distribution of corticospinal motor neurons in the postnatal rat: quantitative evidence for massive collateral elimination and modest cell death. J Comp Neurol 1994;347:115-26.

106. Pearson KG. Interneurones and locomotion. In: Evarts EV, Wise SP, Bousfield P, eds. The motor system in neurobiology. Amsterdam: Elsevier, 1985:52-7.

107. Peat M, Dubo HI, Winter DA, Quanbury AO, Steinke T, Grahame R. Electromyographic temporal analysis of gait: hemiplegic locomotion. Arch Phys Med Rehab 1976;57:421-5.

108. Phillips CG. Motor apparatus of the baboon's hand. Proc R Soc Lond [Biol] 1996;173:141-74.

109. Pollock CM, Shadwick RE. Allometry of muscle, tendon, and elastic energy storage capacity in mammals. Am J Physiol 1994;266(part 2):R1022-31.

110. Pollock M, Shadwick RE. Relationship between body mass and biomechanical properties of limb tendons in adult mammals. Am J Physiol 1994;266(part 2):R1016-21.

111. Porter LL. Intrinsic functional organization of the motor cortex. 1994. Presented at the Neural Control of Movement meeting, Maui, Hawaii, April 1994.

112. Porter R, Lemon R. Corticospinal function and voluntary movement. New York: Oxford University Press, 1993.

113. Prechtl HFR. Ultrasound studies of human fetal behaviour. Early Hum Dev 1985;12:91-8.

114. Purves D, Lichtman JW. Elimination of synapses in the developing nervous system. Science 1980;210:153-7.

115. Rakic P. Specification of cerebral cortical areas. Science 1988;241:170-6.

116. Robinson GA, Goldberger ME. The development and recovery of motor function in spinal cats. I. The infant lesion effect. Exp Brain Res 1986;62:373-86.

117. Rodier P. Chronology of neuron development. Dev Med Child Neurol 1980;22:525-45.

118. Roland PE, Seitz RJ. Mapping of learning and memory functions in the human brain. In: Ottoson D, ed. Visualization of brain functions. London: Stockton Press, 1989:141-51.

119. Rossignol S, Barbeau H, Julien C. Locomotion of the adult chronic spinal cat and its modification by monoaminergic agonists and antagonists. In: Goldberger ME, Gorio A, Murray M, eds. Development and plasticity of the mammalian spinal cord. New York: Fidia Research Series, 1984:323-45.

120. Rossignol S, Drew T. Phasic modulation of reflexes during rhythmic activity. In: Grillner S, Forssberg H, Stein PSG, Stuart D, Herman RM, eds. Neurobiology of vertebrate locomotion. London: Macmillan, 1986:517-34.

121. Rothwell J. Control of human voluntary movement, 2nd ed. London: Chapman & Hall, 1994.

122. Sanes JN, Donoghue JP, Thangaraj V, Edelman RR, Warach S. Shared neural substrates controlling hand movements in human motor cortex. Science 1995;268:1775-77.

123. Sanger TD. Theoretical considerations for the analysis of population coding in motor cortex. Neural Comput 1994;6:29-37.

124. Sarnat HB, Netsky MG. Evolution of the nervous system. London: Oxford University Press, 1974.

125. Schwartz ML, Goldman-Rakic PS. Single cortical neurones have axon collaterals to ipsilateral and contralateral cortex in fetal and adult primates. Nature 1982;299:154-5.

126. Seebach BS, Mendell LM. Postnatal maturation of frequency-dependent behavior of rat Ia-motoneuron synapses. Presented at the Annual Meeting of the Society for Neuroscience, 1994:789.

127. Shik ML, Severin FV, Orlovsky GN. Control of walking and running by means of electrical stimulation of the mid-brain. Biofizika 1966;11:659-66.

128. Singer W. Development and plasticity of cortical processing architectures. Science 1995;270:758-64.

129. Singh J, Knight RT. Frontal lobe contribution to voluntary movements in humans. Brain Res 1990;531:45-54.

130. Stanfield BB. The development of the corticospinal projection. Prog Neurobiol 1992;38:169-202.

131. Stein JF. The representation of egocentric space in the posterior parietal cortex. In: Cordo P, Harnad S, eds. Movement control. Cambridge: Cambridge University Press, 1994:89-100.

132. Strick PL, Hoover JE, Mushiake H. Evidence for "output channels" in the basal ganglia and cerebellum. In: Mano N, Hamada I, Delong MR, eds. Role of the cerebellum and basal ganglia in voluntary movement. Amsterdam: Elsevier, 1996:171-80.

133. Swanson LW. Mapping the human brain: past, present, and future. Trends Neurosci 1995;18:471-4.

134. Tanji J, Shima K. Role for supplementary motor area cells in planning several movements ahead. Nature 1994;371:413-6.

135. Tanji J, Strick P, Hikosaka O, Joseph JP. Neural control of sequential limb movements [abstract]. Proceedings of the Neural Control of Movement Meeting, 1994.

136. Thelen E, Fisher D, Ridley-Johnson R. The relationship between physical growth and a newborn reflex. Infant Behav Dev 1984;7:479-93.

137. Thier P, Erickson RG. Convergence of sensory inputs on cortical area MSTl during smooth pursuit. In: Berthoz A, ed. Multisensory control of movement. Oxford: Oxford University Press, 1993:112-27.

138. Toft E, Sinkjaer T. H-reflex changes during contractions of the ankle extensors in spastic patients. Acta Neurol Scand 1993;88:327-33.

139. Tokuno H, Tanji J. Input organization of distal and proximal forelimb areas in the monkey primary motor cortex: a retrograde double labeling study. J Comp Neurol 1993;333:199-209.

140. Vilensky JA. Locomotor behavior and control in human and non-human primates: comparisons with cats and dogs. Neurosci Biobehav Rev 1987;11:263-74.

141. Wiesendanger M, Wicki U, Rouiller E. Are there unifying structures in the brain responsible for interlimb coordination? In: Swinnen S, Hever H, Massion J, Caesar P, eds. Interlimb coordination: neural, dynamical, and cognitive constraints. New York: Academic Press, 1994:179-207.

142. Wiesendanger M, Wise SP. Current issues concerning the functional organization of motor cortical areas in nonhuman primates. Adv Neurol 1992;57:117-34.

143. Winstein CJ, Garfinkel A. Qualitative dynamics of disordered human locomotion: a preliminary investigation. J Motor Behav 1989;21:373-91.

144. Winstein CJ, Pohl PS. Effects of unilateral brain damage on the control of goal-directed hand movements. Exp Brain Res 1995;105:163-74.

145. Winter DA. Biomechanics of normal and pathological gait: implications for understanding human locomotor control. J Motor Behav 1989;4:337-55.

146. Wise SP, Evarts EV. The role of the cerebral cortex in movement. In: Evarts EV, Wise SP, Bousfield D, eds. The motor system in neurobiology. Amsterdam: Elsevier, 1985:307-15.

147. Wolpaw JR, McFarland DJ, Neat GW, Forneris CA. An EEG-based brain-computer interface for cursor control. Electroencephalogr Clin Neurophysiol 1991;78:252-9.

148. Wyke M. Effect of brain lesions on the rapidity of arm movements. Neurology 1967;17:1113-20.

149. Young AW. Functions of the right cerebral hemisphere. London: Academic Press, 1983.

150. Zarzecki P, Blum PS, Bakker DA, Herman D. Convergence of sensory inputs upon projection neurons of somatosensory cortex: vestibular, neck, head, and forelimb inputs. Exp Brain Res 1983;50:408-14.

151. Zecevic N, Bourgeois JP, Rakic P. Changes in synaptic density in motor cortex of rhesus monkey during fetal and postnatal life. Dev Brain Res 1989;50:11-32.

152. Zecevic N, Rakic P. Synaptogenesis in monkey somatosensory cortex. Cereb Cortex 1991;1:510-23.

Neural Control of Human Locomotion

The Ontogenetic Development of Human Locomotion
The Neurology of Human Locomotion
The Neuropharmacology of Human Locomotion
The Clinical Analysis of Human Gait

Vera had developed a bit differently from her peers. Her legs and pelvis appeared misshaped. Her pelvis was shorter and wider, and had an excessive forward angle. This placed her legs in a seemingly awkward and physically striking position. Her lower leg bone, the tibia, was straighter and thicker than that of her peers, and her foot was clearly not the same. But apart from physical appearances, she did not appear to be handicapped in any way. She matured and gave birth to a son, who shared her peculiar physical characteristics.

Presently, she was living life as a single mother in Africa. She was not, however, raising her son alone. Her "tribe" of friends and relatives spent their days together socializing and watching their offspring play among the dense forest canopy that grew along the lakes and rivers that traversed the African savanna. Despite being born with slightly misshaped legs, Vera was one of the most athletic of her tribe and would often show off her abilities by climbing to the top of the tree canopy. There she would balance precariously and walk to the ends of the smallest branches. Somehow her unique legs, or equally unique attitude, provided her with some sort of an advantage in this activity because her friends were never able to imitate her bold acts. She loved being able to show off her skills, and over time her hip extensor and calf musculature hypertrophied and grew strong. It was her athleticism that prepared her for an unforeseen event that would thrust her to center stage in a play that would forever alter the fate of the human species.

Although we know less about this remarkable woman and the events that changed the destiny of a planet than we would like, scientists believe that she was a member of the *Australopithecus afarensis*, *Australopithecus anamensis*, or *Ardipithecus ramidus* tribes that lived about 4 million years ago. One of these tribes, or one not yet uncovered by paleoanthropologists, led to the elite club known as *Homo sapiens*.[67,72,127,131] Her tribe likely led both an arboreal and terrestrial existence.[20] Most of their time was spent among tree arbors because the ground held dangers of predation by saber-toothed cats, bears, and perhaps other tribes. The trees, however, held only so much food and space for the ever-expanding population. Periodically the tribe had to make forays across the open savanna in search of food and shelter.

One day, while crossing a particularly open exposure in search of more fertile feeding grounds, a pack of wolflike animals descended on Vera's group. It was quadruped vs. quadruped. The tribe was no match for the swifter and more vicious wolves. Thus, in a matter of minutes, the massacre was complete, and the tribe ceased to exist. Except, that is, for two members. In a moment of sheer terror, Vera had grabbed her infant with one arm, and before she was capable of giving it any conscious thought, she threw a rock at a would-be predator with her free arm, rose onto her two back legs, and ran to climb the nearest tree to safety.

These events or other very different and less violent scenarios, such as a need to stand upright in shallow water to make river crossings to more fertile foraging territory, quite possibly gave rise to bipedalism and began what many consider to be the most significant characteristic of hominid development: bipedal locomotion. Among other things, an upright, bipedal posture freed the hands to develop increased object manipulation skills. These types of hand manipulative skills can result in brain expansion.[31,58,70,85,99] Considerable evidence indicates that a bipedal gait predated hominid cortical development.[20,72,117,128] Anatomical changes of the pelvis and leg, tubercle formations indicative of hypertrophied gluteal and calf musculature, and a more forwardly placed *foramen magnum* (the opening in the skull that connects the spinal cord to the brain; a more forward position indicates a species with an upright posture) occurred before any significant change in the size of the cranial vault.[9,36,72,117,120] The famous fossilized Laetoli footprints of Tanzania prove that *A. afarensis* was bipedal 3.6 million years ago.[25,128] Indications are that these footprints were made by an adult walking hand-in-hand with a youngster, thereby indicating a relationship between bipedal gait and social interaction.

It can easily be argued that bipedalism was the primary hominid adaptation that separated us from the great apes millions of years ago. Walking upright freed the hands for tool use, infant carrying and play, food gathering, and perhaps increased socialization. All of these could result in cortical enhancement and further evolutionary changes that ultimately yielded a species we now see when we look in the mirror or interact with our neighbors. The evolutionary acquisition of bipedalism is quite possibly the root of our humanity. Do you really need any better incentive to read further to learn more about this uniquely human trait?

Genetic accidents combined with forced-use adaptations likely led to biomechanical changes that fostered the development of bipedal gait. These biomechanical changes could not have occurred without concomitant neural adaptations. The limb and muscle coordination needed for bipedal gait is considerably different than that required for quadrupedal locomotion. An upright posture imposes additional challenges to equilibrium. Postural muscles and vestibular organs must, therefore, be increasingly coordinated with limb control. Coordination is the domain of the nervous system. Interestingly, however, biomechanical changes appear to have occurred first and thus directed changes in the brain rather than vice versa. This is our first indication that biomechanics doesn't just necessarily place constraints upon which the nervous system must work, but, in some instances, it directs neural adaptations and operations.

Controlling bipedal locomotion is not an easy task. The central nervous system (CNS) somehow must generate the locomotor pattern; generate appropriate propulsive forces; modulate changes in center of gravity; coordinate multilimb trajectories; adapt to changing conditions and changing joint positions; coordinate visual, auditory, vestibular, and peripheral afferent information; and account for the viscoelastic properties of muscles. It must do all of this within milliseconds and usually in conjunction with coordinating a multitude of other bodily functions and movements. The human infant faces a daunting challenge.

■ THE ONTOGENETIC DEVELOPMENT OF HUMAN LOCOMOTION

Reflexive movements of the human fetus begin at about 8 weeks' gestation.[106] Infants with *anencephaly* (a total lack of cerebral cortex development) also exhibit some ability to move their legs in a coordinated, steppinglike manner.[125] These data would seem to support the idea that the human locomotor pattern is reflexive and, therefore, innate. Whether human locomotion is the result of innate, genetically prede-termined neural wiring or is a learned behavior has been a contentious scientific issue. According to the innate circuitry view, any change in afferent input brought about by a changing environment or goal-directed behavior merely serves to modulate a preexisting pattern. This theory assumes that the necessary machinery to carry out human locomotion is contained within the spinal cord and brain stem centers. Studies with nonhuman animals add considerable support to the innate, hard-wired theory of human locomotion.

Cats with totally transected spinal cords still maintain the ability to ambulate and coordinate limb movements.[110] They lose righting and equilibrium responses, but maintain the ability to walk and to alter limb positions appropriately for avoiding obstacles.[41] A collection of neurons contained within the spinal cord termed central pattern generators (CPGs) is responsible for generating the locomotor rhythm.[51]

The limited research in humans that is available, however, suggests that spinal cord CPGs might not have the same primacy of control in humans as in other species. The role of higher brain centers, such as the cerebral cortex, may be considerably different in humans than it is in other species. Data from humans, in fact, suggest that learning plays a critical role in the attainment of an adultlike, bipedal, *plantigrade* (heel-toe) gait pattern. Examination of the development of independent locomotion in children provides some evidence for this.

Although stepping movements are present at birth in the human infant, this behavior ceases to exist or becomes increasingly difficult to elicit at about 2 months of age. Stepping behavior reappears as goal-directed ambulation at approximately 10 months. During the next few months, childrens' biomechanical and muscle activity patterns exhibit considerable intra- and intersubject variability.[77,95] This variability cannot be explained by a species-specific, hard-wired reflexive model of walking. Rather, this interval of time in a child's life appears to reflect a period of trial and error in the attainment of walking. Learning also occurs in adults. Adults maintain the ability to change their ambulation pattern. For instance, individuals with lower extremity amputations learn to modify ambulation patterns to optimize prosthetic use.[129]

Although the point remains debatable, I believe that a great deal of the circuitry required for the generation of rhythmic activities, such as bipedal locomotion, is the result of genetically predetermined wiring. CPGs almost certainly play a role in human locomotion. Differences between humans and other mammalian species with regard to CPG functioning provide clues, however, that learning plays a large role in the attainment and maturation of human bipedal locomotion. The fact that learning is involved in the acquisition of bipedal gait is reflected in the differences between the gait patterns of human infants and adults.

The locomotor pattern of a human infant differs considerably from that of a mature adult[37,77,95,123] (Figs. 5-1 to 5-3). Muscle activation patterns are dissimilar,[37,42,77] reciprocal arm swing does not develop until sometime between 18 months and 3 years of age, heel strike (plantigrade gait) is not performed consistently until about 1.5 years of age, and the shock-absorbing knee yield phase at the beginning of stance is not mature until 3 to 7 years of age.[121,122] Many biomechanical and somatic changes contribute to these changes. An intriguing question is whether the neural substrate for locomotion actually changes over time and whether these neural changes can account for the biomechanical and behavioral changes. Nonhuman animal studies have indicated that the neural substrate for certain reflexes and motor behaviors does indeed change over time.[47,75,108]

In the cat, a reflex known as low threshold placing is initially controlled at a segmental level, but very quickly after birth this reflex becomes dependent on an intact sensorimotor cortex.[1,74] Although no direct evidence exists that the neural substrate for human locomotion changes with development, experimental evidence suggests that, similar to certain motor behaviors of other mammalian species, human locomotion is first controlled segmentally and then becomes progressively more dependent on supraspinal systems. Human newborns exhibit stepping behaviors immediately after birth even though descending projections are not fully developed or completely myelinated.[37,103] As mentioned previously, infants with anencephaly also exhibit stepping movements.[125] Apparently, the cerebral cortex is not necessary for early infant stepping. Yet, brain damage occurring later in life has a profound effect on the gait pattern.[69,102]

In the 1960s, researchers suggested that "encephalization" was responsible for the transition from the infant stepping pattern to an adult pattern of locomotion.[103] Infant stepping was regarded as a reflex that later became inhibited by descending systems. It was further believed that the original circuits that generated reflexive stepping were not used in the adult. More recently it has been suggested that spinal cord CPGs generate the basic locomotor rhythm[51] and supraspinal systems serve to initiate and drive the CPGs.[38] Experimental evidence suggests that neither explanation adequately addresses the enhanced involvement of supraspinal centers in the generation and control of human locomotion.

The progression to a mature gait pattern involves a transition from a stereotyped, synergistic pattern to one in which anticipatory postural changes and precise, fractionated movements replace fixed synergistic movements.[37,77,95,123] The corticospinal tract fractionates movement in the upper extremity.[105] Similarly, it may serve to fractionate the locomotor pattern so that a coordinated, energy-efficient gait is obtained. Individuals who have suffered perinatal damage to the cerebral cortex, internal capsule, periventricular white matter, or the pyramids never develop a mature gait pattern.[26,77] Rather, they continue to exhibit many characteristics of early reflexive stepping. This finding provides additional indirect evidence that supraspinal pathways, and specifically corticofugal pathways, are necessary for the attainment of a mature gait pattern. That supraspinal centers supersede CPGs is unlikely. Rather more probable, descending systems integrate with existing spinal cord circuitry to fractionate lower extremity movement and provide greater adaptability to changing afferent conditions.

Whether these developmental "plastic" changes in the human infant's nervous system reflect learning or are genetically controlled is not known. The physiological mechanisms involved in CNS plasticity during development or after injury are actually very similar to those involved in motor learning. Activity within a neural pathway and competition for synaptic sites help to shape neural connectivity. These mechanisms will be discussed in greater detail in Chapter 7.

Changes in the neural substrates subserving movement during development have considerable clinical relevance with regard to the effects of brain damage. After perinatal brain damage, the stage of development of surviving pathways, as well as pathways that have been damaged, contribute to functional outcomes.[47,75] The nature and degree of the integration of different neural structures responsible for locomotion is the subject of the next section.

■ THE NEUROLOGY OF HUMAN LOCOMOTION

Chapters 2 and 3 introduced various neural structures, their connectivity, and their physiological functioning. In this section, I will again present many of the same structures and physiological principles, but they are now presented within a specific context: human locomotion. What follows is a synthesis of the contributions of various neural components, physiological functions, and pharmacological mechanisms to human locomotion.

Neural convergence

Principles of convergence and divergence, which have been introduced previously, greatly enhance the relative activity and influence of any given neuron. *Convergence* refers to multiple afferent input onto a single neuron or nucleus. *Afferent input* refers to signals providing incoming information to the target neu-

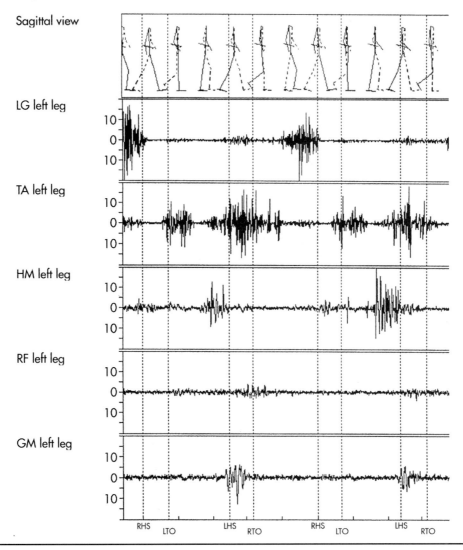

Fig. 5-1. A, Electromyographic recordings from five leg muscles of a nondisabled adult woman during overground locomotion. *(continued on facing page)*

ron (includes descending as well as peripheral sensory input). *Divergence* refers to the multiple outputs of a neuron or nucleus. Divergence greatly increases the realm of influence of a neuron (see Fig. 3-3).

Convergence occurs at every level of the CNS. Segmentally (i.e., within the spinal cord), interneurons and motor neurons receive multiple inputs (see Fig. 2-5).[56] The complexity increases in supraspinal centers. Determining which input has greater relative influence is a difficult task. The difficulty of the task is increased by the fact that the relative influences of afferent inputs change within a situational context,[32-34,49] the position of the limbs,[10] weight-bearing status,[101] and anticipatory motor set.[33]

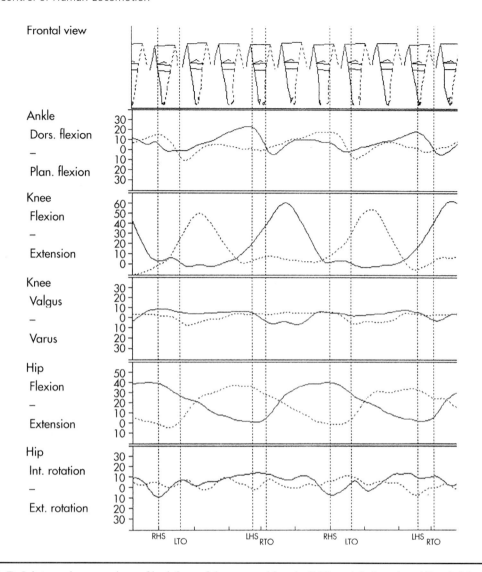

Fig. 5-1. B, Joint angular excursions of both legs of the same subject (*solid line*, right leg; *dotted line*, left leg). *LG,* Lateral gastrocnemius; *TA,* tibialis anterior; *HM,* biceps femoris: *RF,* rectus femoris; *GM,* gluteus maximus; *RHS,* right heel strike; *LTO,* left toe off; *LHS,* left heel strike; *RTO,* right toe off. (Data and graphs generated by a three-dimensional, computerized, four-camera, 200 Hz, VP-320 Motion Analysis System from The Motor Control Research Laboratory, The University of Montana.)

Convergence is an important concept to bear in mind during subsequent paragraphs of this chapter. I will be discussing inputs and outputs of various neural structures and attempting to summarize function based on connectivity. This is useful for a global understanding of the neural influences on locomotion. Because of the complexity introduced by convergence, divergence, and neuromodulation, however,

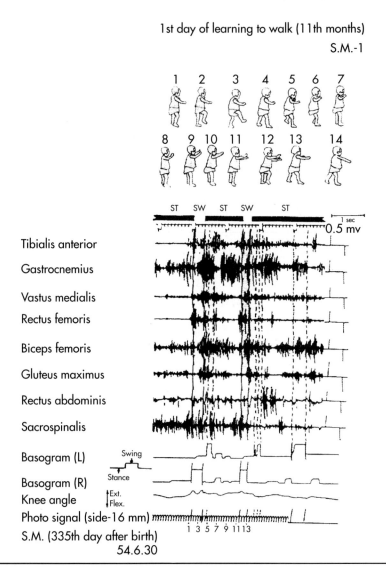

Fig. 5-2. Electromyographic and kinematic data obtained from an infant during the very early stages of developing independent locomotion. Note the lack of sequential EMG patterns, the high degree of muscle cocontraction, and the synchronous joint movements. (From Okamoto T, Goto Y. In: Kondo S, ed. Primate morphophysiology, locomotor analyses and human bipedalism. Tokyo: University of Tokyo Press, 1985.)

descriptions of neural connectivity alone may not be able accurately to determine what initiates, generates, and maintains locomotion. Always have in the back of your mind concepts such as: convergence, presynaptic inhibition and facilitation, neuromodulation, and long-term potentiation (refer back to Chapters 2 and 3 as needed).

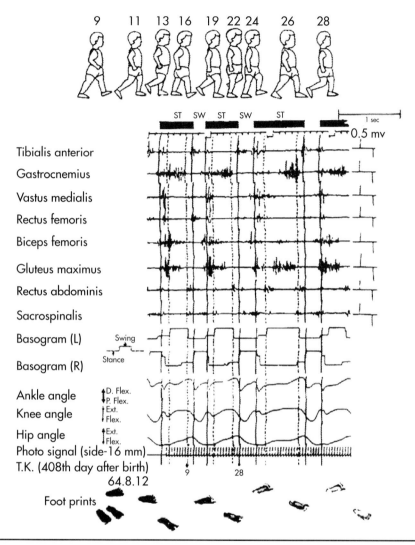

Fig. 5-3. Electromyographic and kinematic data obtained from an infant after having been walking independently for a little over a month. Note how the pattern has changed from Fig. 5-2. Although still not a mature gait pattern, as the child matures and gains more equilibrium, the pattern will very quickly assume adult characteristics. (From Okamoto T, Goto Y. In: Kondo S, ed. Primate morphophysiology, locomotor analyses and human bipedalism. Tokyo: University of Tokyo Press, 1985.)

Central pattern generators

CPGs refer to a grouping of neurons or neural circuits that can generate coordinated movements autonomously (see Fig. 3-11). CPGs for locomotion have been identified in the vertebrate spinal cord.[65,79]

CPGs can generate coordinated locomotor movements even in the absence of all movement-related afferent feedback.[53,55] Although CPGs form an innate neural network that can independently activate coordinated stepping, this does not imply that the network, or its output, is invariant. CPGs can change output depending on speed requirements[39,118] and in response to obstacle avoidance.[2,40] Although CPGs can operate without afferent input, CPG activity is constantly modified by available sensory input.[51] CPG activations are also constantly modified by ongoing internal and external sensory changes.

At any given moment or phase of a step cycle, the importance and consequences of various afferent inputs change. For instance, during the transition from stance to swing, hip flexor stretch receptors might be the primary sensory input that initiates change in CPG output.[54] During other stages and conditions, other sensory input, such as weighting and unweighting of the limb or input from other muscles, might be of primary importance.[100,101] These findings have yielded the concept of command neurons. *Command neurons* are defined as those neurons that respond to sensory input and initiate CPG activity. Different movements or different conditions might activate different command neurons. Command neurons, in turn, activate specific neural discharge sequencing within the CPG. Command neurons are probably not at all unique, but rather represent any neuron within the CPG. Future work might show that afferent input can gate the CPG, and therefore exert specific influences during various phases of the gait cycle via access to any neuron within the network. Thus, different movements are possible depending on which neurons are activated and which afferent input is having the most influence within the network at a given moment (see Fig. 3-13).

Clinicians often make use of this scientific principle. For instance, if a patient is having difficulty initiating a movement, therapists change the afferent input or position of the limb. This often enhances the patient's abilities.

Activity within the CPG, and the patterns of movement that result from CPG activation, appear to be influenced primarily by three factors:
1. Supraspinal center input
2. The type and degree of afferent feedback, and
3. The influences of limb and body position on afferent feedback.

CPG models of locomotion will continue to be modified as new information becomes available. Clearly the nervous system processes more information than was previously thought. Neural outputs change depending on joint angle and interjoint positions.[10,11] Weight-bearing status of a limb also affects neural transmission of some neurons.[101] Perhaps changes in the body's center of gravity are recognized within the CNS by unique processing of multisensorial afferent input or by peripheral receptors yet to be defined. These additional factors will have to be considered in any future analysis of CPG functioning in human locomotion. The role, or even the existence, of CPGs in human locomotion remains a debatable issue.

There is little doubt that spinal CPGs exist in many, if not all, vertebrate species. To date, however, scientists have been unable to provide evidence for an autonomously functioning spinal cord CPG in humans or other mature primates.[30] Some data suggest the existence of spinal CPGs in humans,[15] but this work has failed to provide conclusive evidence for autonomous spinal cord CPG functioning. Unlike lower mammalian species, the CPG, if it does exist in adult humans, appears unable independently to generate coordinated rhythmic locomotion. If CPGs in humans functioned as they do in cats, for instance, we could place someone with a total spinal cord transection on a motorized treadmill to elicit walking. Although this is not the case, innovative work combining pharmacological agents with forced treadmill use has shown some enhanced locomotor activity of individuals with spinal cord injuries[7] (Fig. 5-4).

Strictly from a logical point of view, it would be surprising if CPGs did not exist in some form in humans. Entire neural pathways are rarely lost during evolutionary development.[16,112] Not surprisingly, however, the role and organization (in terms of underlying circuitry) of the CPG in generating locomotion has changed with phylogenetic development. Quadrupedal locomotion requires the coordination of four independently moving limbs. Human bipedal locomotion has halved this complexity. Bipedal loco-

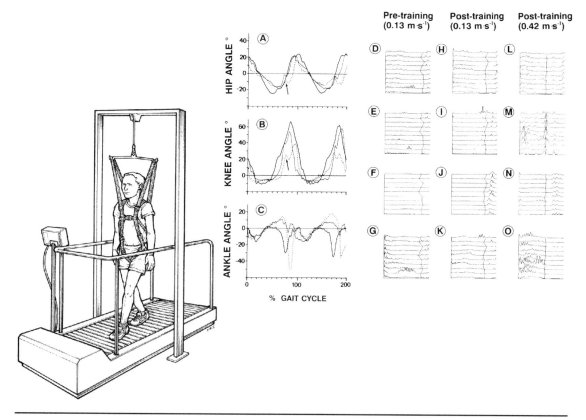

Fig. 5-4. *Insert*: **A-C**, Kinematic data and **D-O**, electromyograhic (EMG) data from a subject with spastic paresis secondary to a cervical spinal cord injury. Data were taken while the subject was walking on a treadmill and show the combined effects of drug intervention with locomotor training. Postmedication graphs show general activation of locomotor pattern after administration of cyproheptadine or clonidine. Posttraining graphs show increased activation plus a more orderly temporal sequence of muscle activations. **A-C**, *Dotted line*, Pretraining evaluation; *thin line*, posttraining evaluation at 0.13 msec; *thick line,* posttraining evaluation at 0.42 msec; **D, H, L**, medial hamstring EMG; **E, I, M**, vastus lateralis; **F, J, N**, tibialis anterior; **G, K, O**, gastrocnemius. *Solid line* across EMG data indicates stance-swing transition. (Insert from Barbeau H, Fung J. In: Forssberg H, Hirschfeld H, eds. Movement disorders in children. Basel: Karger, 1992.)

motion, however, results in increased equilibrium demands. Equilibrium control is, to a large degree, a supraspinal function. Neuroanatomical data indicate that humans have more extensive descending supraspinal pathways than any other species. The autonomous nature of spinal cord CPGs could be lost in preference for the added influences of descending systems. Thus, conceivably, in humans the spinal cord CPG for locomotion (defined as the minimum network capable of generating a rhythmic locomotor pattern) may be more distributed and include circuitry in the brain stem or higher centers.

Peripheral receptors and afferents

The generation of locomotion depends on sensory input, and the act of locomoting, in turn, results in a wide array of sensory changes. Sensory afferent information derived from the muscles can be considered among the most important. Control of bipedal locomotion requires constant monitoring of muscle length and tension. This monitoring is provided by muscle spindles, which are sensitive to changes in muscle length, and Golgi tendon organs (GTOs), which are responsive to muscle tension. Refer to Chapters 2 and 3 for a review of the basic physiology of these receptors.

Muscle spindles are sensitive to changes in muscle length. Primary spindle afferents respond to the rate of change in muscle length, whereas secondary spindle afferents respond mainly to absolute length changes. Although this spindle physiology has long been accepted, recent studies have questioned whether the spindle actually does accurately monitor changes in whole muscle length during certain movements.[60] Locomotion might be one such movement, but additional work is needed before any conclusions can be made.

Spindles are innervated by gamma motor neurons. The gamma motor neuron determines the sensitivity of the spindle to stretch. The sensitivity of the spindle changes with the requirements of the movement. Dynamic changes in muscle length occur during the human gait cycle. Therefore, the spindle not only serves as a feedback receptor, but also as a feed-forward mechanism during human locomotion. Gamma and alpha motor neurons are to some extent controlled in parallel from supraspinal centers.[80] Several descending pathways, however, have been identified that appear to provide selective control of gamma motor neurons, especially of dynamic gamma efferents.[64,107] Stretch of a muscle, such as a hip flexor at the end of stance phase, activates spindles and initiates transmission in the Ia afferent. One result of Ia afferent activation is monosynaptic excitation of the stretched muscle and its synergists. This excitation assists in the motor unit recruitment of hip flexors needed to initiate swing phase. Hip flexor Ia afferents also synapse on an interneuron, the Ia inhibitory interneuron, which inhibits muscles antagonistic to the hip flexors. The Ia afferent also gives off collaterals that ascend in the dorsal columns of the spinal cord to higher brain centers.[6] It is hypothesized that these ascending projections inform higher brain centers (e.g., cerebellum, cerebral cortex) of changing conditions. Higher brain centers can then modify gamma and alpha motor neuron discharge to meet the requirements of the changing condition. For instance, the neural drive and motor unit recruitment needed for running is different from that required during walking.[52,92,93] And the sequencing of muscle contractions and relative propulsive forces required of certain muscles differs during an uphill climb versus walking on level ground. Spindles, together with other receptors such as GTOs, constantly inform higher centers of peripheral conditions and constantly modulate their input into the segmental circuitry to alter the bias of reflexive responses.

GTOs are contraction-sensitive mechanoreceptors that are innervated by fast-conducting Ib afferent fibers. Their speed of conduction is only slightly less than the Ia fibers that innervate muscle spindles. GTOs have been hypothesized to play a role in locomotion.[22,101] GTOs are thought to alter the force output of different muscles constantly to meet the requirements of ongoing movement.[113] The timing of the locomotor rhythm is strongly influenced by group I afferents.[22] Input from Ib afferents inhibits flexors during the stance phase of gait.[101] Apparently, then, changes in group I afferent activity might play a role in regulating the stance to swing transition in gait. Considering the extensive multisensorial convergence onto Ib interneurons and Ib supraspinal projections, the group I afferent system seems to have an important role in the control of locomotion.

Flexor reflex afferents

Flexor reflex afferents (FRAs) refer to a multisensorial and interneuronal reflex system that appears to be at least partially responsible for the generation of locomotion.[83] The afferents included in this reflex pathway include mechanoreceptors, cutaneous afferents, nociceptors, joint afferents, and muscle afferents.[113] These various afferents were initially grouped together because their stimulation caused the same motor response: limb flexion. This is not always true, however. For instance, during stance, light mechanical stimulation of the skin will result in limb extension. Stimulation of nociceptors during stance will result in flexion of the limb. Sensory afferents and neurons that contribute to FRA circuitry, therefore, can initiate variable motor responses during different phases of locomotion. FRAs exert either an inhibitory or excitatory effect on the motor neuronal pool of a limb. Activity in one motor neuronal pool generally results in inhibition of antagonist pools. Alternating activity between various motor neuronal pools forms the basis for rhythmic locomotor activity.[113]

FRAs send projections to higher brain centers and receive input from descending supraspinal centers. During locomotion, stimulation of FRAs results in differing motor outputs. For example, a cutaneous stimulation applied during limb extension in the cat will result in limb flexion. Applying the same cutaneous stimulation during limb flexion will result in extension of the limb.[111] This finding and others[10] show that reflex activity can be altered based on the position of the limb. Knowledge of the effects of these types of motor responses to sensory input potentially have some clinical usefulness. For instance, application of a cutaneous electrical stimulation to the sole of the foot can assist in the initiation of the swing phase of individuals who have had a stroke.[44]

Brain stem locomotor regions

Electrical stimulation of neural centers located in the nonhuman mammalian midbrain and brain stem causes spontaneous locomotion.[96,98,115] Three such centers are the mesencephalic locomotor region (MLR), the pontine locomotor region (PLR), and the subthalamic locomotor region (SLR). These centers receive and process diverse descending and afferent input. Their efferent output is to spinal CPGs. Although stimulation of any of these centers in nonhuman vertebrates elicits coordinated locomotion, the effects of lesioning the centers, or their projections, are somewhat different. The primary role of each center in an intact animal, therefore, is likely to be different.

The MLR receives afferent input from the basal ganglia, the limbic system, and the sensorimotor cortex.[13] It connects with spinal circuitry via the reticulospinal tract.[97] The MLR appears to be an important relay station between cortical limbic drives and CPGs. By nature of the sympathetic inputs to the limbic system, the MLR may be the center by which the "flight" component of the "fight or flight" sympathetic response becomes manifest.

The PLR is located caudal to the MLR and may actually be contiguous with it. Some have suggested that a pontomedullary locomotor strip extends from the MLR to the upper cervical spinal cord.[116] Stimulation of this area changes postural tone and alters firing within the MLR.[87]

Electrical stimulation of the SLR, located in close proximity to the subthalamus, also elicits locomotion. If this region is disconnected from cortical centers in the cat, the animal can ambulate spontaneously but loses all ability to avoid obstacles. The SLR, therefore, appears to be necessary for the modulation of the locomotor pattern. A lesion immediately caudal to the SLR in cats will result in the disappearance of all spontaneous locomotion.[50]

These brain stem locomotor regions receive input from sensorimotor regions of the cerebral cortex. We can imagine that a signal or signals emanating from cells in the brain trigger a set of neurons within the brain stem locomotor regions that, in turn, synapse on neurons within the spinal cord CPGs. In this way, the cerebral cortex does not have to encode all the postural and volitional movements needed for a certain motor behavior or situational context.

Cerebellum

It is hypothesized that the cerebellum compares motor commands emanating from the cerebral cortex with the resultant afferent consequences of the movement.[12] No doubt the cerebellum is essential for the smooth execution of voluntary movement. Some regions of the cerebellar cortex are active before a movement and appear to preset the body for the intended movement. Other regions of the cerebellum are not active before a movement. Rather, they become active during the movement and reflect the afferent result. The cerebellum encodes reaction times of intended movement and the patterns of muscles used.[13] In other words, it contributes to coordination of muscle activity. The cerebellum is also important for our ability to adapt to a changing environment. Despite years of experimental work, the way the cerebellum accomplishes its putative computational tasks remains an enigma. As a working hypothesis, however, let's assume that the cerebellum contributes to optimal movement solutions. By constantly comparing the afferent consequences of a particular movement sequence with the desired outcome, an optimal movement solution is developed. With repetitive trials, adaptation will yield to learning. Motor learning takes place when adaptations provide the desired outcome to a specific stimulus. Many CNS structures are involved in motor learning, but the cerebellum is absolutely essential in developing selective associations.[126] The cerebral cortex provides insights into motor outcome, but the cerebellum is necessary for the development of smooth motor responses that result from the learning of a motor task. Combining these general statements regarding cerebellar functioning with what has been discussed previously in this chapter regarding the ontogeny of human locomotion, the cerebellum has an integral role in the development and ongoing refinement of human locomotion and other learned motor tasks. However, to design experiments that directly assess cerebellar functioning during human locomotion is extremely difficult. Much of what we know has been derived from studies in nonhuman animals. Research involving people with cerebellar damage, however, has supported many of the findings from nonhuman animal studies.[8,61,124]

The cerebellum receives somatotopically organized input from the cerebral cortex (motor areas 4 and 6, visual and auditory cortices), brain stem nuclei such as vestibular nuclei, and the midbrain.[13] The ventral and dorsal spinocerebellar tracts relay information from the peripheral muscle spindles, GTOs, and joint afferents to the cerebellum during movement. These tracts relay somewhat dissimilar information. Both tract systems are phasically active during locomotion. The dorsal tract appears to convey information about the activity of individual muscles. The ventral tract receives more diffuse input and may be involved in comparing the descending copy of the motor program for locomotion with the resultant changes in the periphery.[4,5] Cerebellar output indirectly affects spinal cord interneurons and motor neurons and the motor cortex. Its effect on spinal cord circuitry is via its initial connections with vestibular nuclei and the red nucleus. Its influence over the motor cortex is via its input to the thalamus. Because the comparative anatomy and physiology of the cerebellum differs among species and because humans are the only species with a bipedal plantigrade gait, making unequivocal statements regarding cerebellar functioning based solely from studies in nonhumans is difficult. Clinical observations have contributed equally important insights into the cerebellar control of locomotion.

Cerebellar lesions result in the decomposition of movement. Muscles that normally act synergistically lose their ability to do so. Errors in direction, muscular force, and velocity are common. Intentional tremors and *nystagmus* (aberrant eye movements) often result. Lesions that affect the vestibular component of the cerebellum result in a wide-based staggering gait and an inability to make correct postural adjustments to movement. Individuals may be able to compensate somewhat for cerebellar dysfunction by an increased reliance on vision, but the movements are slow, clumsy, and require much concentration. All fluidity and grace of movement are lost after lesions of the cerebellum. Damage to the anterior lobe of the cerebellum also seems to impair an individual's ability to alter postural responses appropriately based on prior experience.[61] Again, this is evidence that the cerebellum is intimately involved in the neural processes required for motor learning.

To summarize current working concepts briefly, the cerebellum coordinates movement, assimilates parameters necessary for motor learning, creates something analogous to motor programs for specific movements, establishes an internal model of expected afferent consequences of a motor act, provides ongoing comparisons of descending motor commands with changing peripheral and internal conditions, preprograms alpha and gamma motor neurons, and integrates vestibular reflexes. It appears to be involved in any activity, motor or cognitive, that depends on temporal sequencing of events.

Basal ganglia

The basal ganglia play an important role in human locomotion. Although this role cannot be precisely defined, diseases of the basal ganglia provide insights into the tremendous importance of the basal ganglia with regard to locomotion and other movements. Diseases that affect the basal ganglia include Huntington's chorea, athetosis, and Parkinson's disease. These disorders result in disruption of motor control and lead to serious motor disabilities. Observations of patients with athetosis provide a clinical example of the importance of the basal ganglia for locomotion. Patients with *athetosis* are unable to control limb movements and have fluctuating muscle tone and poor stabilization of the trunk musculature. Other clinical disorders of the basal ganglia include *akinesia,* a loss of voluntary movement; *extrapyramidal dyskinesia*, a difficulty in performing movement accompanied by involuntary, unsuppressible movements; and *bradykinesia,* a slowness of movement.

The functions of the basal ganglia with regard to movement and locomotion remain a mystery. The basal ganglia are thought to process afferent information from the periphery and the cerebral cortex and somehow impact motor planning. They play a role in the initiation and termination of movement. Some basal ganglia neurons fire before movement, whereas others fire after movement and after neurons within the sensorimotor cortex have already finished firing.[21] Neurons within the basal ganglia respond to sensory input, but only if the sensory input is related to movement. To complicate our understanding further, some neurons that respond to a given sensory stimulus will only be activated in a given situational context.[21] The basal ganglia appear to process sensory stimuli and determine which stimuli will be used by the CNS to impact movement. They not only integrate sensory information, but also appear to attach situational and emotional significance to it.

Cerebral cortex

Many supraspinal centers have obvious roles in human locomotion. Known functions of the cerebral cortex with regard to locomotion include cognitive aspects of motor control, visuomotor coordination, and motor planning. Cortical neurons often are activated before movement onset, and typically fire phasically during locomotion.[3,32,35] The possible role of the cerebral cortex in the generation and coordination of human locomotion remains controversial. The existence of locomotor activity in nonhuman animals after spinal cord transection argues against a role for the cerebral cortex in the generation of locomotion. The neural circuitry required for quadrupedal and other forms of vertebrate locomotion, however, may be entirely different from that required for bipedal locomotion. Bipedal, plantigrade gait is a uniquely human activity. In addition to increased equilibrium demands, bipedal gait involves increased anticipatory muscle activations, the functional stretch reflex, and bodily responses to the unweighting of a limb and single leg stance.[18] All of these functions rely on cerebral centers.[28] Sir John Eccles, one of the most noted neuroscientists of all time, states that, "The rhythmic movements of human walking are not explicable by spinal mechanisms, and only imperfectly by lower cerebral levels such as the vestibular inputs to the reticulospinal and vestibulospinal pathways... Undoubtedly a bipedal gait had entailed a drastic reorganization of the central nervous system..."[28] Part of this reorganization undoubtedly involves the cerebral cortex.

Reciprocal inhibition, the neural mechanism that inhibits an antagonist muscle during an agonist contraction, serves as a possible example of Sir John's insight. In quadrupeds, reciprocal inhibition of antagonist muscles in the lower leg is a spinal cord reflex. In humans, this reciprocal inhibition is lost after damage to sensorimotor cortical pathways.[78] Thus, proper functioning of reciprocal inhibition in humans, which still involves spinal cord circuitry, appears reliant on input from the cerebral cortex.

To begin to understand the potential role of the cerebral cortex with regard to locomotion, it is advantageous to understand something of its organization. These concepts are discussed in Chapters 2, 3, and 4. The following paragraphs briefly summarize points that were made in these chapters that bear direct relevance to human locomotion.

Neurons within functionally related cerebral cortical cell columns hypothetically transform afferent sensory stimuli into a generalized motor plan. Direction, amplitude, velocity, and the final desired outcome of the intended movement can be prescribed. Subcortical regions, such as brain stem locomotor regions, further refine the response by taking into account joint positions and interjoint degrees of freedom. The cerebral cortex appears able to modulate activity within all neural structures either directly or indirectly. Supraspinal centers determine the "motor set" required for a certain movement by altering segmental reflex responses. Via long-loop transcortical reflex pathways (Chapter 3), the cerebral cortex is able to modulate and shape the simplest of spinal cord reflexes. Shaping of segmental reflex activity is vitally important for anticipatory reactions. Locomotion is an example of a motor act that incorporates anticipatory reactions to loading and unloading of the limb.

Long-loop reflexes alter segmental reflexes and thus can contribute to a desired motor output.[34,35,63,86] For instance, they inhibit segmental reflexes if the segmental reflex response opposes a desired movement. Conversely, they enhance segmental reflex activity if the reflex assists in a desired movement.[91] These modulations and other segmental mechanisms are disrupted after damage to the sensorimotor cortex or its projections in humans.[13,19,62,78] Thus, the cerebral cortex appears to be more intimately involved in the generation of coordinated locomotion in humans than it is with other species.

■ THE NEUROPHARMACOLOGY OF HUMAN LOCOMOTION

Knowledge of the connectivity of various neural systems that contribute to the control of locomotion is a necessary step toward understanding the neural basis of human locomotion. Equally important are events that occur at a molecular level. Neurochemical processes that underlie synaptic transmission have as much of a role to play in final behavioral outcome as actual physical connectivity between neurons. Transmission changes that occur pre- or postsynaptically can dramatically modulate activity within any given neural pathway. An understanding of some of the neurotransmitters and postsynaptic membrane receptors involved in locomotion enhances our abilities to understand the mechanisms involved, aids our understanding of the affects of diseases or chemical imbalances on locomotion, and is the first step toward developing drug therapies designed to ameliorate motor disorders.

Postsynaptic receptor physiology

The postsynaptic membrane contains highly specialized membrane proteins called *receptors*. These receptors respond in a certain way to specific neurotransmitters. The way in which a receptor responds determines whether the postsynaptic neural membrane becomes more permeable to sodium, potassium, calcium, or chloride. This, in turn, determines whether the neurotransmitter will have an excitatory or inhibitory effect on the postsynaptic neuron. Different neurons contain different membrane receptors. A single neuron may have receptors for a variety of neurotransmitters. Therefore, each neuron responds differently to any given stimulus. For instance, norepinephrine might be excitatory at some receptor sites and inhibitory at others. The interaction between neurotransmitters and receptor sites increases the diversity available within any given pathway.

Neurotransmitters

To be classified as a neurotransmitter, a substance must meet certain pharmacological criteria. A simplified definition of a *neurotransmitter* is any substance that is released synaptically by a neuron and has an affect on another neuron or organ. The tremendous growth in identifying neurotransmitters is evident when reviewing the literature. In 1981, nine substances were tentatively identified as neurotransmitters.[114] Today the number of putative neurotransmitters or neuroactive peptides is about 90 (Dr. Craig Johnston, neuropharmacologist; personal communication). Following is a brief discussion of some transmitters known to be involved in motor control and human locomotion.

Acetylcholine. Acetylcholine (Ach) was the first neurotransmitter to be identified. It remains the only transmitter that has been convincingly shown experimentally to fit all the criteria of a neurotransmitter.[94] It is the transmitter of the neuromuscular junction. Ach is released by alpha and gamma motor neurons, thereby controlling extrafusal and intrafusal muscle contraction. It is not just found at the neuromuscular junction. The reticular formation and the striatum are rich in cells containing Ach. Any pathway that uses Ach as its neurotransmitter is said to be a *cholinergic* pathway. The parasympathetic component of the autonomic system is also referred to as a cholinergic system because it uses Ach as its primary transmitter.

Interestingly, the physiological action of Ach differs somewhat between the peripheral nervous system and CNS.[94] In the peripheral nervous system it is excitatory and its action is very short lived. In the CNS, the action of ACh is slow and diffuse.[94] This speaks to the importance of the receptor site in determining excitatory or inhibitory effects of a given neurotransmitter. Cholinergic neuron projections include the hippocampus, thalamus, and cerebral cortex. Considering these projections, clearly ACh has effects on locomotion, and other neural functions, in addition to neuromuscular transmission. For example, ACh decreases dramatically in individuals diagnosed with Alzheimer's disease.[94] Patients with this disease not only exhibit mental deterioration, but motor deterioration as well.

Glutamate and aspartate. The role of glutamate and aspartate in the CNS is analogous to the role of Ach in the peripheral nervous system. These neurotransmitters cause brief, point-to-point excitation within the CNS. Glutamate tends to be a bit more potent than aspartate in its ability to cause neural excitation.[84] Excess accumulation of glutamate can be toxic to neurons. This condition is known as *excitotoxicity*.[94]

One of the contributing factors to cell death and dysfunction after a stroke is glutamate excitotoxicity. Cortical neurons are rich in glutamate. As a consequence of a stroke or trauma to the brain, many cortical neural membranes are damaged and leak glutamate. This excess glutamate is toxic to neighboring neurons and a cascade of cortical damage results. The development of glutamate antagonists and enzymes that deactivate glutamate is a very promising area in stroke research.

Don't be overly alarmed, but some reports indicate that consumption of large amounts of the artificial sweetener Aspartane, which is structurally related to aspartate, causes subtle symptoms that could be related to excitotoxicity. Monosodium glutamate, a food preservative and flavor enhancer, has caused similar effects.[84]

Glutamate most likely is one of the primary transmitters used by the corticospinal tract. Glutamate tends to have excitatory effects on the postsynaptic membrane of cells within the spinal cord, but its net effect is often inhibition. How is this possible? Most corticospinal tract projections terminate on interneurons. These interneurons can be excitatory or inhibitory. Glutamate, therefore, either has excitatory or inhibitory effects on spinal cord circuitry depending on what type of interneuron receives its input. Many glutamate and aspartate receptors are found within the cerebral cortex, yet no neural pathway has yet been associated with these receptor sites. Glutamate and aspartate are also found in high concentrations in the mammalian hippocampus, amygdala, cerebellum, red nucleus, striatum, and thalamus. Glutamate is also the neurotransmitter used by the endings of primary afferents.[84]

Gamma-aminobutyric acid. Gamma-aminobutyric acid (GABA) is the major transmitter for point-to-point inhibition in the CNS. Similar to glutamate, it can be found in the cerebral cortex and the spinal cord, in addition to other structures concerned with motor control such as the cerebellum and the basal ganglia.[90]

Two main types of receptors are receptive to GABA. Many subtypes of GABA receptors have also been identified. GABA(A) receptor sites are postsynaptic receptors and are responsible for mediating postsynaptic inhibition. The GABA(B) sites are on presynaptic autonomic and central nerve terminals. GABA(B) receptors reduce the outflow of excitatory neurotransmitters such as glutamate and norepinephrine. They therefore serve a modulatory function.[84]

Many clinically administered drugs interact with GABA. Its inhibitory effects, therefore, can be manipulated somewhat. Benzodiazpines (such as diazepam), which are prescribed to decrease anxiety and spasticity, facilitate GABA binding and therefore increase its inhibitory effects. Baclofen, also used to control spasticity, is a GABA(B) agonist.[84] Therefore, its administration mimics the inhibitory effects of GABA. Bicuculline is a GABA(A) antagonist. It inhibits the inhibitory effects of GABA and thereby causes disinhibition (disinhibition results in relative excitation). Bicuculline has been used to enhance the ambulation of animals with spinal cord injuries.[109]

Glycine. Glycine is an inhibitory neurotransmitter that is used by spinal cord inhibitory interneurons.[90] It is also found in the cerebral cortex and cerebellum. The actions of glycine at the spinal level are similar to those of GABA. However, the effects of these two transmitters are affected quite differently by different substances. Strychnine will block the action of glycine but not GABA. Bicuculline will block GABA but not glycine. This type of drug interaction specificity may one day be used by neuropharmacologists to develop drug therapies for various neurological disorders. Because different pathways subserve different functions and use different transmitters, it should be possible to develop drugs to enhance the functioning of a specific pathway and thereby affect a particular behavior.

■ THE CLINICAL ANALYSIS OF HUMAN GAIT

Many excellent texts and journal articles address clinical issues related to human gait. The purpose of the following paragraphs is not to review the mechanics of gait analysis, but rather to show how clinical gait analysis can be used to obtain information about the neural and biomechanical control of human locomotion. Because bipedal, plantigrade gait is so uniquely human and involves interactions between the nervous system, muscular mechanics, and kinesiology, its study can be revealing and yield insights into impairments and pathologies that remain elusive to other methods of investigation. The development and ongoing refinement of three-dimensional computerized motion analysis systems have been extraordinary aids to gait analysis. Combined with electromyographic (EMG) analyses to assess various aspects of muscle function during gait, three-dimensional analysis is an even more powerful tool. Today, most research studies—and increasingly many clinical evaluations—make use of these technologies. Clinical and intellectual interest in human gait, however, predates computerized technology.

Historical perspective

Eadweard Muybridge, a late nineteenth century artist and engineer, was perhaps the first to document photographically the dynamic aspects of human gait. My guess is that he was not unlike the computer artists of today. His work actually began as a horse wager. As the story goes, a wealthy benefactor was engaged in a disagreement with a colleague concerning whether, during a full gallop, all four legs of a horse were ever simultaneously off the ground. Muybridge was hired to settle the debate. Ingeniously he set up a series of cameras on tripods that were triggered as the horse passed directly in front of the camera (Fig. 5-5). In this way Muybridge was able to collect a series of still photographs that captured the motion of the horse at various phases of the gallop. Intrigued, he then analyzed the movements of many different

Continued on page 167

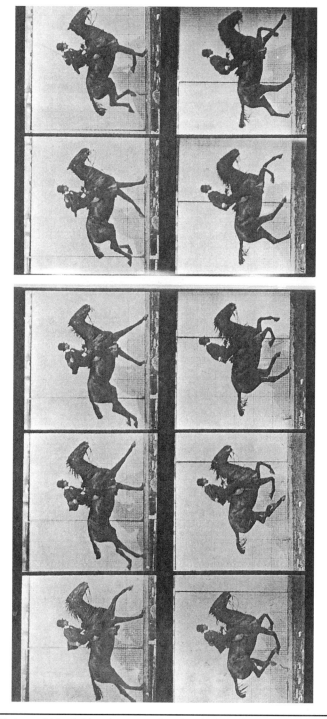

Fig. 5-5. A photograph by Eadweard Muybridge demonstrating that during a full gallop, all four limbs of the horse are indeed off the ground simultaneously. (From Brown LS, ed. Animals in motion: Eadweard Muybridge. New York: Dover Publications, 1957.).

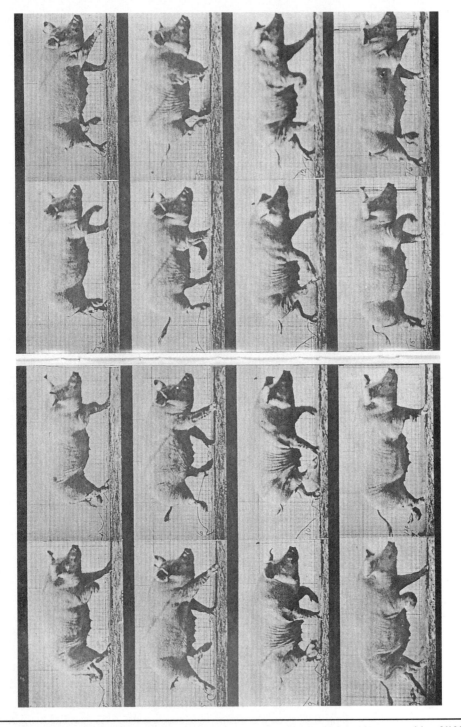

Fig. 5-6. A photograph by Eadweard Muybridge demonstrating that not all quadrupeds are capable of lifting all four limbs off the ground simultaneously. (From Brown LS, ed. Animals in motion: Eadweard Muybridge. New York: Dover Publications, 1957.)

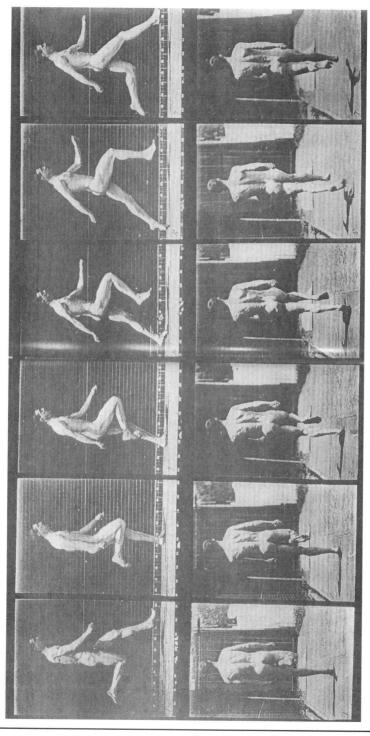

Fig. 5-7. A human figure running, photographed by Eadweard Muybridge. (From Brown LS, ed. *Animals in motion: Eadweard Muybridge*. New York: Dover Publications, 1957.)

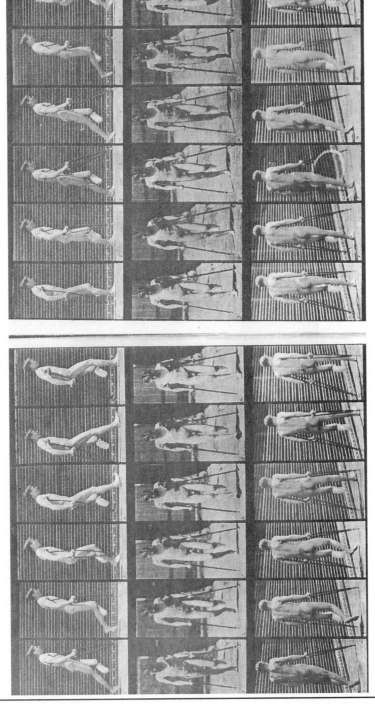

Fig. 5-8. Person with a left below-the-knee amputation walking with a crutch, photographed by Eadweard Muybridge (From Brown LS, ed. Animals in motion: Eadweard Muybridge. New York: Dover Publications, 1957.)

domestic and wild animals. Fig. 5-6 illustrates the species-specific nature of gait characteristics. From this work, he perfected his technique and engaged himself in examining humans during various activities such as walking, running (Fig. 5-7), jumping, falling, and balancing. He did not limit his interests to nondisabled adults. He also examined crutch walking (Fig. 5-8), ambulation after amputation, and child ambulation. For a real visual treat, obtain the books containing Muybridge's photographs listed at the end of this chapter.[88,89] Other historical figures have contributed to present knowledge of human gait characteristics.

Dr. G.B. Duchenne in his book, "The Physiology of Motion," was perhaps the first to treat human gait from an intellectual and medical perspective. Many of Dr. Duchenne's clinical descriptions are still used today to assist in the diagnosis of movement disorders.

EMG assessment of muscle activity did not exist in 1920, but this did not stop Dr. Scherb from documenting the onset and duration of muscle activity during gait. He placed subjects on a treadmill and used muscle palpation skills to determine the phasic activity of walking. It is surprising how closely his temporal estimations of muscle contraction onset and durations compare with present-day data gathered via computerized EMG techniques.

Dr. Inman, an orthopedic surgeon with degrees in mechanical engineering and anatomy, perhaps issued in the modern era of gait analysis. Working in the late 1940s after World War II, Dr. Inman worked with veterans to develop prosthetics based on biomechanical principles. He is given credit for being the first to describe the sinusoidal nature of center of gravity changes during gait. Drs. D. Sutherland and J. Perry, both students of Inman, continued his legacy and have contributed much to the human gait literature. Today, the number of investigators who examine human gait has grown exponentially. Probably more data have been collected during the past 5 years than in the previous 100. Yet, much remains to learn about an activity that started over 4 million years ago.

Computerized gait analysis

Figs. 5-1, 5-2, and 5-3 show computer printouts of some of the kinematics and muscle activation patterns of the human step cycle. These data provide information regarding muscle temporal sequencing, muscle amplitudes, duration of contractions, muscular cocontraction, joint kinematics, movement kinetics, changes in interjoint degrees of freedom, and the relationships among each variable. Most of these data would be difficult or impossible to discern with the eye alone. For all of you doubting Thomases, I refer you to Dr. Francine Malouin's intriguing chapter[82] in which she refers to Dr. David Kreb's research[71] and others showing that clinicians were unable, by use of eyes alone, to identify various variables consistently in the human gait pattern. Of particular interest was a study that showed that physical therapists rated their abilities in this area much higher than a factual analysis of their skills revealed.[82]

Information from human gait studies have been correlated with data from studies of nonhuman animals and have provided insights into the neural control of locomotion.[73,76,77,130] Gait analysis data, either alone or in conjunction with other techniques, provide an uncommon opportunity to interface and synthesize neural and biomechanical analyses. Neuroscientists are becoming increasingly aware that the biomechanics of locomotion not only place constraints on the system, but also serve to modulate neural responses.[10,29] For instance, alpha motor neurons change their levels of activation during various phases of the gait cycle,[10] changes occur in neural activity between quiet standing and the stance phase of the gait cycle that are independent of EMG activity,[17] and joint position alone appears to be capable of modulating neural output.[10,29]

Computerized gait analysis has been used most often by orthopedic surgeons and physical therapists to assist with surgical and orthotic device decisions involving patients with cerebral palsy.[45,46,104,122] Another application is the use of computerized gait analysis and surface EMG (sEMG) to quantify the relative degree to which muscle paresis (weakness), spasticity, muscle cocontraction, and muscle contracture con-

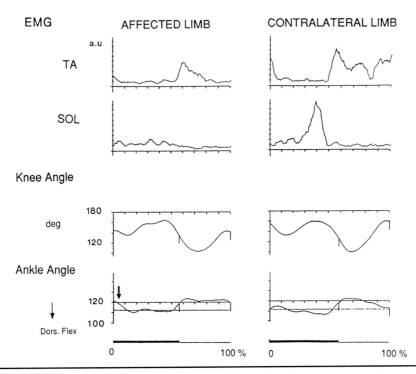

Fig. 5-9. Example of electromyographic recording from paretic tibialis anterior (*TA*) and soleus (*SOL*) muscles and the kinematic correlates. The tibialis anterior is not active on the affected side during initiation of stance. The kinematic correlate shows a lack of dorsiflexion (*arrow*). Data are from a 7-year-old child with spastic hemiplegia walking at normal speed. *Thick line*, Stance phase; *thin line*, swing phase. (From Crenna P, Inverno M, Frigo C, Palmieri R, Fedrizzi E. In: Forssberg H, Hirschfeld H, eds. Movement disorders in children. Basel: Karger, 1992.)

tribute to a disability. Drs. Crenna and Frigo from Milan, Italy, who began development in this area, refer to it as a pathophysiological profile of gait.[24] They have begun to establish criteria for determining which impairments are the most important to be addressed clinically. sEMG is not used diagnostically but rather as a way to analyze and identify the neural and nonneural basis of a disability.

To determine whether muscle paresis contributes to a gait abnormality, sEMG is used to monitor the electrical output of the muscle in question (Fig. 5-9). If the muscle generates less than 50% of the normal EMG amplitude during all phases of the gait cycle when the muscle would normally be active, the muscle is said to have a level 2 impairment. If the muscle generates less than 50% EMG amplitude but only during certain phases of the gait cycle, it is given a level 1 impairment. Other criteria exist, including that the weakness must be apparent and without the influence of antagonist muscle cocontraction, without soft tissue limitations, and with concomitant lack of joint angle changes that correlate to the lack of torque production by the contracting muscle (e.g., lack of ankle dorsiflexion during the swing phase concomitant with decreased tibialis anterior muscle EMG activity).

To determine whether spasticity is interfering with gait, the EMG record is analyzed for the presence of short-latency reflex spikes occurring simultaneously with the stretch of a muscle. The larger the EMG

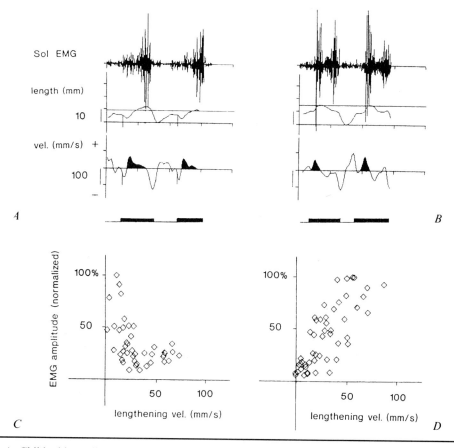

Fig. 5-10. A, Child without disability. **B,** Child with spastic hemiplegia. Electromyographic data indicate accentuated velocity-dependent activity of the soleus muscle (*Sol*) during stretching of theat muscle at stance initiation of the child with hemiplegia. **C** and **D,** Relationship between soleus muscle EMG activity and velocity of stretch to the muscle. Note the lack of relationship between stretch and EMG activity in the nondisabled child (**C**) and the linear relationship between stretch and EMG activity in the child with spasticity (**D**). *Solid bars,* stance phase. (From Crenna P, Inverno M, Frigo C, Palmieri R, Fedrizzi E. In: Forssberg H, Hirschfeld H, eds. Movement disorders in children. Basel: Karger, 1992.)

amplitude during muscle stretch, and the more closely it correlates with speed of stretch, the more influence spasticity has on the gait pattern (Fig. 5-10).

Using these data, a pathophysiological profile of the gait disorder is generated. Fig. 5-11 shows the profiles from two patients of about the same age and with the same diagnosis. Obviously their two profiles are considerably different. Equally obvious is that the medical and rehabilitation interventions should differ between these two individuals. Drs. Crenna and Frigo have found that the profiles of individual patients are not static.[24] From year to year they report changes indicating the dynamic, changing nature of these impairments. Further development of this profile should enable clinicians increasingly to focus their treatment plans and provide a means to monitor treatment effectiveness.

Drs. Manuel Hulliger and Chris Mah from The University of Calgary, Canada[81] as well as others[14,43,59,66,68,119] are working on methods of gait analysis that will enable clinicians to assess only two or three

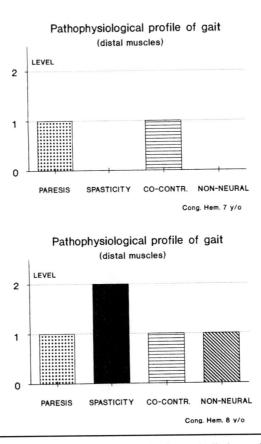

Fig. 5-11. Examples of pathophysiological profiles during gait of two similarly aged children with spastic hemiplegia. (See text for details of level determination.) (From Crenna P, Inverno M, Frigo C, Palmieri R, Fedrizzi E. In: Forssberg H, Hirschfeld H, eds. Movement disorders in children. Basel: Karger, 1992.)

gait variables (principle component analysis) to be able to predict which impairments are most limiting and what interventions would be most appropriate. Again, this holds great promise for lessening the amount of time currently needed to do a gait analysis and will take some of the guess work out of intervention strategies. These methods of analysis can also be applied to other movement dysfunctions such as reach and grasp.

These are only a few examples of the promise computerized techniques hold. Noninvasive techniques such as computerized gait analysis, sEMG, and functional scanning methodologies (positron emission tomography, functional magnetic resonance imaging, single positron emission computed tomography) are allowing investigators to glimpse views of the nervous system during human movement. Before the development of these technologies, most work had to be performed rather invasively on nonhuman animals and conjectures made regarding applicability to humans. We will likely learn more about the neural control of human movement in the next decade than we have during the "Decade of the Brain"—the title given to the present decade because of the tremendous neuroscientific advances that have occurred.

Integrating biomechanical and neurophysiological perspectives

Peripheral receptors in joints and muscles detect changes in muscle length and force, joint position, and possibly weight-bearing status of the limb. Conceptually, therefore, the nervous system is aware of at least some biomechanical aspects of movement. How it makes use of this information remains a mystery. Changes in the biomechanics of a movement alter neural responses.[10,23,27,29,48,54] The generation and control of locomotion can be roughly divided into two phases: (1) descending projections from higher brain centers signal subcortical systems to initiate movement, and (2) information relating to the subsequent movement is relayed back to the nervous system. Changes in afferent sensory information alter motor responses. In the analysis of feedback and feed-forward systems, biomechanists and engineers have contributed much to our understanding of locomotion. Their analyses provide information that includes, but is not limited to, forces acting on a limb, torque generation, relationships between torque production and joint angle changes, control of limb trajectories, descriptions of interjoint kinematics, and changes in mechanical relationships over time.[57] The control of these parameters requires feedback mechanisms.

Feedback from peripheral receptors assists in the refinement of ongoing movement. Engineers use feedback loops in robotic design. Servoregulation is a term they use to describe the process by which a feedback signal (afferent sensory discharge) is compared with the set point (desired motor output) to make necessary corrections for successful completion of the task.[57] The vocabulary may be different, but neuroscientists and engineers have been struggling with similar problems within their respective fields. The human body is governed by the same physical constraints as any other moving object. The CNS must make use of biomechanical information for the final shaping of its motor output. Similarly, neuroscientists, biomechanists, engineers, and mathematicians increasingly are making use of the knowledge base of various disciplines to decipher the intricacies of movement. This interchange will continue to elucidate the various mechanisms inherent to human locomotion.

SUGGESTED READINGS

Armstrong DM. The supraspinal control of mammalian locomotion. J Physiol (Lond) 1988;405:1-37.

Barbeau H, Rossignol S. The effects of serotonergic drugs on the locomotor pattern and on cutaneous reflexes of the adult chronic spinal cat. Brain Res 1990;514:55-67

Barbeau H, Rossignol S. Initiation and modulation of the locomotor pattern in the adult chronic spinal cat by noradrenergic, serotonergic, and dopaminergic drugs. Brain Res 1991;546:250-60.

Craik RL, Oatis CA. Gait analysis: theory and application. St. Louis: Mosby-Year Book, 1995.

Hirschfeld H, Forssberg H. Phase-dependent modulations of anticipatory postural activity during human locomotion. J Neurophysiol 1991;66:12-19.

Jeng S, Holt KG, Fetters L, Certo C. Self-optimization of walking in nondisabled children and children with spastic hemiplegic cerebral palsy. J Mot Behav 1996,28.15-27.

Muir GD, Steeves JD. Sensorimotor stimulation to improve locomotor recovery after spinal cord injury. Trends Neurosci 1997;20:72-7.

Winder DA. Biomechanics of normal and pathological gait: implications for understanding human locomotor control. J Mot Behav 1989;4:337-55.

REFERENCES

1. Amassian VE, Ross R. Development in the kitten of control of contact placing by sensorimotor cortex. J Physiol (Lond) 1972;230:55-6.

2. Andersson O, Forssberg H, Grillner S. Peripheral feedback mechanisms acting on the central pattern generators for locomotion in fish and cat. Can J Physiol Pharmacol 1981;59:713-26.

3. Armstrong DM, Drew T. Discharges of pyramidal tract and other motor cortical neurones during locomotion in the cat. J Physiol (Lond) 1984;346:471-95.

4. Arshavsky YI, Berkenblit MB, Fukson OI, Gelfand IM, Orlovsky GN. Recordings of neurons of the dorsal spinocerebellar tract during evoked locomotion. Brain Res 1972;43:272-5.

5. Arshavsky YI, Berkinblit MB, Gelfand IM, Orlovsky GN, Fukson OI. Activity of the neurones of the ventral spinocerebellar tract during locomotion. Biophysics 1972;17:926-35.

6. Baldissera F, Hultborn H, Illert M. Integration in spinal neuronal systems. In: Brooks VB, ed. Handbook of physiology: the nervous system II. Baltimore: Williams & Wilkins, 1981:509-95.

7. Barbeau H, Fung J. New experimental approaches in the treatment of spastic gait disorders. In: Forssberg H, Hirschfeld H, eds. Movement disorders in children. Switzerland: Karger, 1992:234-47.

8. Bastian JJ, Thach WT. Cerebellar outflow lesions: a comparison of movement deficits resulting from lesions at the levels of the cerebellum and thalamus. Ann Neurol 1995;38:881-92.

9. Begley S. Out of Africa a missing link. Newsweek Oct 3, 1994:56-8.

10. Brooke JD, McIlroy WE. Effect of knee joint angle on a heteronymous Ib reflex in the human lower limb. Can J Neurol Sci 1989;16:58-62.

11. Brooke JD, McIlroy WE. Vibration insensitivity of a short latency reflex linking the lower leg and the active knee extensor muscles in humans. Electroencephalogr Clin Neurophysiol 1990;75:401-9.

12. Brooks VB. The cerebellum and adaptive tuning of movements. Exp Brain Res (Suppl) 1984;7:170-83.

13. Brooks VB. The neural basis of motor control. New York: Oxford University Press, 1986.

14. Brunt D, Lafferty MJ, Mckeon A, Goode B, Mulhausen C, Polk P. Invariant characteristics of gait initiation. Am J Phys Med Rehabil 1991;70:206-12.

15. Bussel B, Roby-Brami A, Yakovleff A, Bennis N. Late flexion reflex in paraplegic patients. Evidence for a spinal stepping generator. Brain Res Bull 1989;22:53-6.

16. Butler AB, Hodos W. Comparative vertebrate neuroanatomy. New York: Wiley-Liss, 1996.

17. Capaday C, Lavoie BA, Comeau F. Differential effects of a flexor nerve input on the human soleus H-reflex during standing versus walking. Can J Physiol Pharmacol 1995;73:436-49.

18. Chan CWY, Melvill Jones G, Catchlove RFH. The "late" electromyographic response to limb displacement in man. II. Sensory origin. Electroencephalogr Clin Neurophysiol 1979;46:182-8.

19. Chan CWY, Melvill Jones G, Kearney RE, Watt DGD. The "late" electromyographic response to limb displacement in man. I. Evidence for supraspinal contribution. Electroencephalogr Clin Neurophysiol 1979;46:173-81.

20. Clarke RJ, Tobias PV. Sterkfontein member 2 foot bones of the oldest South African hominid. Science 1995;69:521-4.

21. Connor NP, Abbs JH. Sensorimotor contributions of the basal ganglia: recent advances. Phys Ther 1990;70:118-26.

22. Conway BA, Hultborn H, Kiehn O. Proprioceptive input resets central locomotor rhythm in the spinal cat. Exp Brain Res 1987;68:643-56.

23. Corcos DM, Gottlieb GL, Agarwal GC. Organizing principles for single-joint movements 2. A speed-sensitive strategy. J Neurophysiol 1989;62:358-68.

24. Crenna P, Inverno M, Frigo C, Palmeri R, Fedrizzi E. Pathophysiological profiles of gait in children with cerebral palsy. In: Forssberg H, Hirschfeld H, eds. Movement disorders in children. Switzerland: Karger, 1992:186-99.

25. Day MH, Wickens EH. Laetoli pliocene hominid footprints and bipedalism. Nature 1980;286:385-7.

26. Dubowitz L, Finnie N, Hyde SA, Scott OM, Vrbov AG. Improvement of muscle performance by chronic electrical stimulation in children with cerebral palsy. Lancet 1988;1:587-8.

27. Duysens J, Pearson KG. Inhibition of flexor burst generation by loading ankle extensor muscles in walking cats. Brain Res 1980;187:321-32.

28. Eccles JC. Evolution of the brain. London: Routledge, 1989.

29. Edamura M, Yang JF, Stein RB. Factors that determine the magnitude and time course of human H-reflexes in locomotion. J Neurosci 1991;11:420-7.

30. Eidelberg E, Walden JG, Nguyen LH. Locomotor control in macaque monkeys. Brain 1981;104:647-63.

31. Elbert T, Pantev C, Wienbruch C, Rockstroh B, Taub E. Increased cortical representation of the fingers of the left hand in string players. Science 1995;270:305-7.

32. Evarts E. Pyramidal tract activity associated with a conditioned hand movement in monkey. J Neurophysiol 1966;29:1011-27.

33. Evarts EV, Granit R. Relations of reflexes and intended movements. Prog Brain Res 1976;39:1-14.

34. Evarts EV, Tanji J. Gating of motor cortex reflexes by prior instruction. Brain Res 1974;71:479-94.

35. Evarts EV, Tanji J. Reflex and intended responses in motor cortex pyramidal tract neurons of monkey. J Neurophysiol 1976;39:1069-80.

36. Fischman J. Putting our oldest ancestors in their proper place. Science 1994;265:2011-2.

37. Forssberg H. Ontogeny of human locomotor control I. Infant stepping, supported locomotion and transition to independent locomotion. Exp Brain Res 1985;57:480-93.

38. Forssberg H. Development and integration of human locomotor functions. In: Goldberger ME, Gorio A, Murray M, eds. Development and plasticity of the mam-

malian spinal cord. Padova: Liviana Press, 1986: 53-63.

39. Forssberg H, Grillner S, Halbertsma J. The locomotion of the spinal cat. I. Coordination within a hindlimb. Acta Physiol Scand 1980;108:269-81.
40. Forssberg H, Grillner S, Rossignol S. Phase dependent reflex reversal during walking in chronic spinal cats. Brain Res 1975;85:103-7.
41. Forssberg H, Grillner S, Rossignol S. Phasic gain control of reflexes from the dorsum of the paw during spinal locomotion. Brain Res 1977;132:121-39.
42. Forssberg H, Hirschfeld H, Stokes VP. Development of human locomotor mechanisms. In: Shimamura M, ed. Neurobiological basis of human locomotion. Amsterdam: Elsevier, 1991.
43. Fung J, Barbeau H. A dynamic EMG profile index to quantify muscular activation disorder in spastic paretic gait. Electroencephalogr Clin Neurophysiol 1989;73:233-44.
44. Fung J, Barbeau H. Modulatory effects of cutaneomuscular stimulation on the soleus H-reflex in spastic paretic subjects during standing and walking. In: Woollacott M, Horak F, eds. Posture and gait: control mechanisms. Portland: University of Oregon Books, 1992:27-30.
45. Gage JE, Deluca PA, Renshaw TS. Gait analysis: principles and applications—emphasis on its use in cerebral palsy. J Bone Joint Surg [Am] 1995;77:1607-23.
46. Gage JR. Gait analysis in cerebral palsy. Oxford: MacKeith, 1991.
47. Goldman PS, Galkin TW. Prenatal removal of frontal association cortex in the fetal rhesus monkey: anatomical and functional consequences in postnatal life. Brain Res 1978;152:451-85.
48. Gottlieb GL, Corcos DM, Agarwal GC. Organizing principles for single-joint movements 1. A speed-insensitive strategy. J Neurophysiol 1989;62:342-57.
49. Grillner S. Interaction between central and peripheral mechanisms in the control of locomotion. Prog Brain Res 1979;50:227-35.
50. Grillner S. Control of locomotion in bipeds, tetrapods, and fish. In: Handbook of physiology: the nervous system II. Baltimore: Bethesda: American Physiological Society, 1981:1179-236.
51. Grillner S. Neurobiological bases of rhythmic motor acts in vertebrates. Science 1985;228:143-9.
52. Grillner S, Halbertsma J, Nilsson J, Thorstensson A. The adaptation to speed in human locomotion. Brain Res 1979;165:177-82.
53. Grillner S, Perret C, Zangger P. Central generation of locomotion in the spinal dogfish. Brain Res 1976;109:255-69.
54. Grillner S, Rossignol S. On the initiation of the swing phase of locomotion in chronic spinal cats. Brain Res 1978;146:269-77.

55. Grillner S, Zangger P. How detailed is the central pattern generation for locomotion? Brain Res 1975;88:367-71.
56. Harrison PJ, Jankowska E. Sources of input to interneurons mediating group I non-reciprocal inhibition of motoneurones in the cat. J Physiol (Lond) 1985;361:379-401.
57. Hasan Z, Enoka RM, Stuart DG. The interface between biomechanics and neurophysiology in the study of movement: some recent approaches. In: Buskirk ER, ed. Exercise and sport science. New York: American College of Sports Medicine, 1985:169-234.
58. Hata Y, Stryker MP. Control of thalomocortical afferent rearrangement by postsynaptic activity in developing visual cortex. Science 1994;265:1731-5.
59. Hatze H. Gait analysis: adequacy of current models and research strategies. J Motor Behav 1987;19:280-7.
60. Hoffer JA, Caputi AA, Pose IE. Movement of muscle fibers in cat locomotion: what do muscle proprioceptors sense? In: Woollacott M, Horak F, eds. Posture and gait: control mechanisms. Portland: University of Oregon Books, 1992:25-7.
61. Horak FB, Diener HC. Cerebellar control of postural scaling and central set in stance. J Neurophysiol 1994;72:479-93.
62. Horak FB, Esselman P, Anderson ME, Lynch MK. The effects of movement velocity, mass displaced, and task certainty on associated postural adjustments made by normal and hemiplegic individuals. J Neurol Neurosurg Psychiatry 1984;47:1020-8.
63. Horak FB, Nashner LM. Central programming of postural movements: adaptation to altered support-surface configurations. J Neurophysiol 1986;55:1369-81.
64. Hulliger M. Fusimotor control of proprioceptive feedback during locomotion and balancing: can simple lesions be learned for artificial control of gait. Prog Brain Res 1993;97:173-80.
65. Jankowska E, Jukes MGM, Lund S, Lundberg A. The effect of DOPA on the spinal cord. 5. Reciprocal organization of pathways transmitting excitatory action to alpha motoneurones of flexor and extensors. Acta Physiol Scand 1967;70:369-88.
66. Jeng SF, Holt KG, Fetters L, Ratcliffe R. A preliminary study of self-optimization in normal children and children with spastic cerebral palsy during ambulation. In: Woollacott M, Horak F, eds. Posture and gait: control mechanisms. Portland: University of Oregon Books, 1992:83-7.
67. Johanson DC, White TD. A systematic assessment of early African hominids. Science 1979;203:321-30.
68. Knutsson E. Analysis of gait and isokinetic movements for evaluation of antispastic drugs of physical therapies. In: Desmedt JE, ed. Motor control mechanisms in health and disease. New York: Raven Press, 1983:1013-35.

69. Knutsson E, Richards C. Different types of disturbed motor control in gait of hemiparetic patients. Brain 1979;102:405-30.

70. Kocsis JD. Competition in the synaptic marketplace: activity is important. Neuroscientist 1995;1:185-7.

71. Krebs D, Edelstein J, Fishman S. Reliability of observational kinematic gait analysis. Phys Ther 1985; 65:1027-33.

72. Leakey M. The farthest horizon. National Geographic Sept 1995;38-51.

73. Leonard CT. Neural and neurobehavioral changes associated with perinatal brain damage. In: Forssberg H, Hirschfeld H, eds. Movement disorders in children. Amsterdam: Karger, 1992:50-6.

74. Leonard CT, Goldberger ME. Consequences of damage to the sensorimotor cortex in neonatal and adult cats. I. Sparing and recovery of function. Dev Brain Res 1987;32:1-14.

75. Leonard CT, Goldberger ME. Consequences of damage to the sensorimotor cortex in neonatal and adult cats. II. Maintenance of exuberant projections. Dev Brain Res 1987;32:15-30.

76. Leonard CT, Hirschfeld H, Forssberg H. Gait acquisition and reflex abnormalities in normal children and children with cerebral palsy. In: Amblard B, Berthoz A, Clarac F, eds. Posture and gait: development adaptation and modulation. Amsterdam: Elsevier, 1988:33-45.

77. Leonard CT, Hirschfeld H, Forssberg H. The development of independent walking in children with cerebral palsy. Dev Med Child Neurol 1991;33:567-77.

78. Leonard CT, Moritani T, Hirschfeld H, Forssberg H. Deficits in reciprocal inhibition in children with cerebral palsy as revealed by H reflex testing. Dev Med Child Neurol 1990;32:974-84.

79. Lundberg A. Reflex control of stepping. Presented as the Nansen Memorial Lecture, October 10, 1968. Oslo: Universitetsforlaget, 1969.

80. Lundberg, A. Control of spinal mechanics from the brain. In: Tower DB, ed. The nervous system. New York: Raven Press, 1975:253-65.

81. Mah CD, Hulliger M, Lee RG, O'Callaghan IS. Quantitative analysis of human movement synergies: constructive pattern analysis for gait. J Motor Behav 1994;26:83-102.

82. Malouin F. Observational gait analysis. In: Craik RL, Oatis C, eds. Gait analysis: theory and application. St. Louis: Mosby-Year Book, 1995:112-25.

83. McCrea DA. Spinal cord circuitry and motor reflexes. In: Pandolf KB, ed. Exercise and sport science reviews, vol 14. New York: Macmillan, 1986:105-41.

84. McGeer PL, McGeer EG. Amino acid neurotransmitters. In: Siegel G, Agranoff B, Albers RW, Molinoff P, eds. Basic neurochemistry. New York: Raven Press, 1989:311-33.

85. Merzenich MM, Kaas JH, Wall J, Nelson RJ, Sur M, Felleman D. Topographic reorganization of somatosensory cortical areas 3B and 1 in adult monkeys following restricted deafferentation. Neuroscience 1983;8:33-55.

86. Moore SP, Rushmer DS, Windus SL, Nashner LM. Human automatic postural responses: responses to horizontal perturbations of stance in multiple directions. Exp Brain Res 1988;73:648-58.

87. Mori S, Kawahara K, Sakamoto T, Aoki M, Tomiyama T. Setting and resetting of postural muscle tone in the decerebrate cat by stimulation of the brainstem. J Neurophysiol 1982;48:737-48.

88. Muybridge E. The human figure in motion. New York: Dover, 1955.

89. Muybridge E. Animals in motion. New York: Dover, 1957.

90. Nagai T, McGeer PL, Araki M, McGeer EG. GABA-T intensive neurons in the rat brain. In: Bjorklund A, Hokfelt T, Kuhar MJ, eds. Classical transmitters and transmitter receptors in the CNS, part II. Handbook of chemical neuroanatomy, vol 3. Amsterdam: Elsevier, 1984:247-72.

91. Nashner LM. Adapting reflexes controlling human posture. Exp Brain Res 1976;26:59-72.

92. Nilsson J, Thorstensson A. Adaptability in frequency and amplitude of leg movements during human locomotion at different speeds. Acta Physiol Scand 1987;129:107-14.

93. Nilsson J, Thorstensson A, Halbertsma J. Changes in leg movements and muscle activity with speed of locomotion and mode of progression in humans. Acta Physiol Scand 1985;123:457-75.

94. Nolte J. The human brain. St. Louis: Mosby-Year Book, 1988.

95. Okamoto T, Goto Y. Human infant pre-independent and independent walking. In: Kondo S, ed. Primate morphophysiology, locomotor analyses and human bipedalism. Tokyo: University of Tokyo Press, 1985:25-45.

96. Orlovsky GN. Electrical activity in brainstem and descending paths in guided locomotion. Sechenov Physiol J USSR 1969;55:437-44.

97. Orlovsky GN. Connections between reticulospinal neurons and locomotor regions of the brainstem. Biofizika 1970;15:171-7.

98. Orlovsky GN. The effect of different descending systems on flexor and extensor activity during locomotion. Brain Res 1972;40:359-72.

99. Pascual-Leone A, Grafman J, Hallett M. Modulation of cortical motor output maps during development of

implicit and explicit knowledge. Science 1994;263:1287-8.

100. Pearson KG, Collins DF. Reversal of the influence of group Ib afferents from plantaris on activity in medial gastrocnemius muscle during locomotor activity. J Neurophysiol 1993;70:1009-17.

101. Pearson KG, Ramirez JM, Jiang W. Entrainment of the locomotor rhythm by group Ib afferents from ankle extensor muscles in spinal cats. Exp Brain Res 1992;90:557-66.

102. Peat M, Dubo HI, Winter DA, Quanbury AO, Steinke T, Grahame R. Electromyographic temporal analysis of gait: hemiplegic locomotion. Arch Phys Med Rehabil 1976;57:421-5.

103. Peiper A. Cerebral function in infancy and childhood. New York: Consultants Bureau, 1963.

104. Perry J. Gait analysis: normal and pathological function. Thorofare: Slack, 1992.

105. Porter R. Corticomotoneuronal projections: synaptic events related to skilled movement. Proc R Soc Lond [Biol] 1987;231:147-68.

106. Prechtl HFR. Ultrasound studies of human fetal behaviour. Early Human Dev 1985;12:91-8.

107. Prochazka A, Hulliger M, Zangger P, Appenteng K. "Fusimotor set": new evidence of alpha-independent control of gamma-motoneurones during movement in the awake cat. Brain Res 1985;339:136-40.

108. Robinson GA, Goldberger ME. The development and recovery of motor function in spinal cats. I. The infant lesion effect. Exp Brain Res 1986;62:373-86.

109. Robinson GA, Goldberger ME. The development and recovery of motor function in spinal cats. II. Pharmacological enhancement of recovery. Exp Brain Res 1986;62:387-400.

110. Rossignol S, Barbeau H, Julien C. Locomotion of the adult chronic spinal cat and its modification by monoaminergic agonists and antagonists. In: Goldberger ME, Gorio A, Murray M, eds. Development and plasticity of the mammalian spinal cord. New York: Fidia Research Series, 1984:323-45.

111. Rossignol S, Gauthier L. An analysis of mechanisms controlling the reversal of crossed spinal reflexes. Brain Res 1980;182:31-45.

112. Sarnat HB, Netsky MG. Evolution of the nervous system. London: Oxford University Press, 1974.

113. Schomburg ED. Spinal sensorimotor systems and their supraspinal control. Neurosci Res 1990;7:265-340.

114. Schwartz JH. Chemical basis of synaptic transmission. In: Kandel ER, Schwartz JH, eds. Principles of neural science. Amsterdam: Elsevier, 1981:106-20.

115. Shik ML, Severin FV, Orlovsky GN. Control of walking and running by means of electrical stimulation of the mid-brain. Biofizika 1966;11:659-66.

116. Shik ML, Yagodnitsyn AS. The pontobulbar "locomotion strip." Neurophysiol USSR 1977;9:72-4.

117. Shipman P. Climbing the family tree: what makes a hominid a hominid? J Zool (Lond) 1995;7:50-5.

118. Shurrager PS, Dykman RA. Walking spinal carnivores. J Comp Psychol 1951;44:252-62.

119. Stanhope SJ. A procedure for evaluating gait analysis system performance. Gait Post 1994;2:54.

120. Stern JT, Randall LS. The locomotor anatomy of Australopithecus afarensis. Am J Phys Anthropol 1983;60:279-317.

121. Sutherland DH. Gait analysis in cerebral palsy. Dev Med Child Neurol 1978;20:807-13.

122. Sutherland DH, Olshen RA, Biden EN, Wyatt MP. The development of mature walking. Philadelphia: MacKeith Press, 1988.

123. Sutherland DH, Olshen RA, Cooper L, Woo SY. The development of mature gait. J Bone Joint Surg [Am] 1980;62:336-53.

124. Thach WT. A cerebellar role in acquisition of novel static and dynamic muscle activities in holding, pointing, throwing, and reaching. In: Bloedel JR, Ebner TJ, Wise SP, eds. The acquisition of motor behavior in vertebrates. Cambridge, Mass: The MIT Press, 1996:223-34.

125. Thomas A, Autgaerden S. Locomotion from pre- to post-natal life. In: Thomas A, Autgaerden S, eds. Locomotion from pre- to post-natal life. London: Medical Books Ltd, 1966.

126. Thompson RF, Clark GA, Donegan DH, et al. Neuronal substrates of learning and memory: a "multiple trace" view. In: Lynch G, McGaugh JL, Weinberger NM, eds. Neurobiology of learning and memory. New York: Guilford Press, 1984:137-64.

127. White T, Suwa G, Asfan B. Australopithecus ramidus, a new species of early hominid from Aramis, Ethiopia. Nature 1994;371:306.

128. White TD. Evolutionary implications of pliocene hominid footprints. Science 1980;208:175-6.

129. Winter DA, Sienko SE. Biomechanics of below-knee amputee gait. J Biomech 1988;21:361-7.

130. Yang JF, Stein RB, James KB. Contribution of peripheral afferents to the activation of the soleus muscle during walking in humans. Exp Brain Res 1991;87:679-87.

131. Yoon CK. New hominid species was bipedal 3.9-4.2 million years ago. J NIH Res 1995;7:30-2.

Neural Control of Head, Eye, and Upper Extremity Coordination

I am not the type of parent to worry excessively about the hours and hours my son spends playing any of the apparently endless stream of computer and video games. Rather, I consider it preparation for his future and an intriguing educational resource for me. When he began playing at the ripe old age of 3, he was not able to operate the controls and had no idea of the deathly consequences of colliding with a multicolored mushroom or the benefits of leaping his cursor-driven superhero into the clouds. Neither did his father, unfortunately. Unlike his father, he persevered and now, at the age of 7, he has achieved levels of mouse mastery that surely are the equivalent of a black belt in the martial arts. To watch him play is to watch total absorption and to glimpse the future of the impending man-machine interface. I could plausibly argue that the dexterity and eye-hand coordination required to play baseball or a musical instrument pales in comparison to the subtleties of the wrist and finger coordination, the visual tracking skills, and the quickness required to master some of these computer games. It is the ultimate test of transferring visual perception into precise motor action. It is a marvel of anticipatory reactions and fine motor skills.

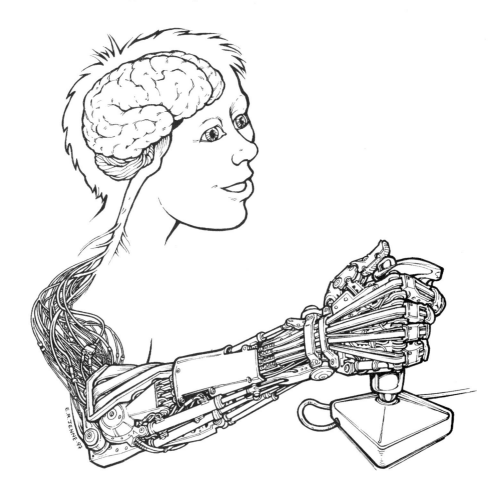

Of course, computer games aren't doing a thing for his strength, flexibility, or stamina—all attributes needed by most athletes. But my guess is that the Wired Generation will far exceed past generations' skill levels in activities that require precise fine motor skills and quick reactions. Look for a future glut of concert pianists, fighter pilots, and slight-of-hand hucksters. Keyboard operators will have to type a gazillion words per minute or find themselves another line of work. Technology is going to contribute to the next phase of human evolution: the flatlining of Fitt's Law. Fitt's Law states there is a speed/accuracy tradeoff (Fig. 6-1): the faster a movement, the less accurate it becomes. Computer games increasingly mandate faster and more accurate movements. Those of you Who still think that Tommy the Pinball Wizard represents the pinnacle of arcade game success don't stand a chance. Visual tracking and upper extremity (UE) reaching reaction speed change in relation to the speed of the target's movement.[17] The faster the moving target, the faster your movements. Thanks to computer game technology and challenges, the eye-hand speed and accuracy of the next generation will be exceptional. The human hand and UE are already genuinely special and distinctive; they are not just the rostral equivalent of the lower extremities.

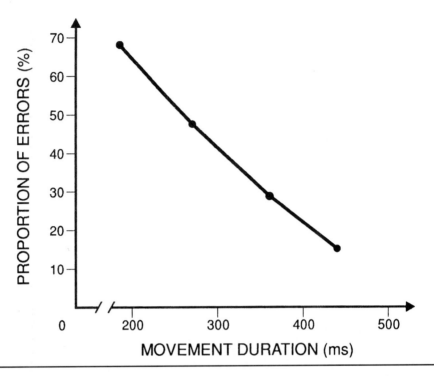

Fig. 6-1. An experimental example of Fitt's Law regarding the speed/accuracy tradeoff. Data are the percentage of errors made as a function of movement duration of subjects during a visually guided pointing task. The faster the movement, the greater the percentage of errors. (Data from Keele SW, Posner MI. J Exp Psychol 1968;77:155-8.)

Unlike the lower extremities, the UEs rarely have to support our body weight. Such grunt work is literally below the level of these unique manipulative appendages. The human UE is incredibly versatile and adaptable. In a short while I plan to take a break from writing to do a little garden work before joining some friends at the local Bitteroot crag scene for some rock climbing. Afterward I will prepare a meal, do some long-neglected sewing, and perhaps challenge my son to a game of Asterix (he will have been practicing inside all day, so my quick defeat at the hands of a 7-year-old is imminent). I, and my human brethren, are able to accomplish these diverse sets of tasks primarily because of neural and biomechanical advantages that are largely attributable to human genetics. No other primate species is quite so adaptable. Our human adaptability isn't due solely to increased human cognitive abilities. We have evolved neural circuitry to control our dexterous ambitions. Unlike the legs, which are primarily used for motor activities, the arms and hands are used as much for sensory explorations as they are for motor acts. The tips of your fingers have more cutaneous receptors than the collective receptors of the trunk and lower extremities. Only our lips and genitalia can match our fingertips for the ability to identify and respond to tactile stimulation. No other appendage is so intimately connected to the visual system, which is the human's primary mode of sensory perception. Somehow these neural connections allow us to transform sensory perception into motor action in the blink of an eye. These connections and the wonder of eye-head-hand coordination are the focus of this chapter.

■ PERCEPTUOMOTOR/VISUOMOTOR COORDINATION

Sensory perception

For the sighted person, most tasks that involve use of the UE begin with receptors far removed from the arms and hands. Retinal receptors of the eye detect changes in our environment and relay this information along the visual pathways so that we can perceive our world and respond to it. Visual pathways are numerous, complex, and fascinating. Refer to any number of excellent neuroscience texts to obtain further information about visual system connectivity and physiology. Visual pathways will not be covered in any depth in this chapter.

Although the UEs are intimately connected with visual system pathways, we can also use our UEs independently of vision. We can rely on proprioception, auditory cues, or tactile receptors to guide our movements. Accurate reaching and grasping requires processing of information about the position of the arm and hand in relation to the object and in relation to the body's position. Supraspinal input pertaining to the intention, planning, and execution of the task must be smoothly integrated with this multifarious afferent input.

Perceptuomotor coordination begins with perception. Perceptions include the receptor's actual physical response characteristics and also our cognitive interpretations of these electrochemical responses. Cognitive interpretation of receptor input is highly individualized and is based on prior experiences with your world and body. Two experiments—one with tendon vibration that alters muscle spindle feedback characteristics and one with eyeglass prisms that distort visual input—demonstrate how UE coordination is disrupted if we do not receive accurate receptor input or if we receive input that is not consistent with previous experiences.

Try the following experiment of your own reliance on muscle spindle input. The experiment is based on some classic proprioceptive illusion experiments first performed by Dr. Peter Matthews and his colleagues from Great Britain.[31] I call this particular version the "pick your nose" experiment. You will need a vibrator and a friend (perhaps the same understanding friend who assisted you with the ice pick experiment described in Chapter 2). Close your eyes and extend your arm away from the body. Now bend your elbow and touch your nose with the tip of your finger. Do this a few times to convince yourself of the ease of the task. Next, with your eyes closed and your arm extended, have your friend place the vibrator over your triceps tendon for a few moments. Now, touch your nose with the tip of your finger. If you are like most people, you will arrest your arm trajectory short of your nose. Does vibrating your triceps tendon suddenly make you think your nose has grown longer? An interesting hypothesis, but a better one exists.

Vibrating the triceps tendon primarily excites muscle spindle primary afferents. Spindle afferents usually respond to dynamic muscle stretch so that when they are activated, the nervous system interprets their input as indicating a stretch to the muscle. Through years of nose-picking experience, you have an internal map of the amount of stretch in the triceps that equates to nose location. With the excessive activation supplied by the vibrator, you think you have arrived at your nose when in reality you have not. How you respond to this sensory discrepancy is equally interesting. You cognitively recognize that you are not touching your nose because tactile receptors in the tips of your finger and nose inform you that no contact has been made. So, after some delay, you continue to bend your elbow against all muscle spindle logic. Some people will experience a very bizarre sensation at this point. It will actually feel as if you are putting your finger through your head! I kid you not; give it a try.

Just how quickly the nervous system adapts to altered sensory input is amazing. If you continue with the above experiment, in only a few trials you will lose the discomforting feeling and be equally accurate with your finger placement with the vibration as you were without it. In another classic sensory perception experiment, subjects are given prism glasses that alter the visual perception of the position of objects

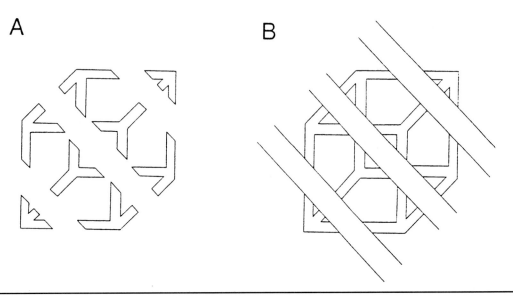

Fig. 6-2. Visualizing the cube in **A** is difficult. In **B**, you perceive a partially occluded object and unconsciously complete the lines so that you visualize a cube. This is an example of the role of visual experience on perception. (From Kanizsa G. Organization of vision. Westport, Conn: Greenwood Publishing Group, 1979.)

in space. When first given the prisms, subjects are unable to reach and grasp an object accurately. Within several trials, they adapt and are very successful with the reaching task.

Perception might be where it all begins, but perception without action isn't going to make your world a better place. You must somehow transform perceptions into a motor act. Even before you have completed formulating your perceptions, your body is ready for action.

Visuomotor reactions

Perceptions dictate how you interact with your environment. Visuomotor coordination is highly dependent on visual perception. Visual perceptions guide motor output. The visual system detects features of objects. These features include its size, shape, texture, orientation to other objects, and the distance and location from your hand and body.[57] Visual perceptions are developed through exposure and experience.[54] For instance, look at Fig. 6-2. What your retinal receptors detect in Fig. 6-2, **A** are a series of lines. But in Fig. 6-2, **B**, based on experience, you use contextual cues to discern the shape of a cube. Unconsciously you complete what you perceive to be the partially occluded lines of a cube. Now, look at Fig. 6-3. This figure might, at first glance, appear to be a random series of ink blobs. But as you continue to look, you will see the outline of a giraffe's head and neck. Do you think you would see the giraffe if you had never seen a picture of one before? Through experience the visual system learns to equate certain visual receptor patterns with object recognition.

In a classic series of experiments that dramatically demonstrated the importance of early experience on pattern recognition, Nobel prize winners Drs. D.H. Hubel and T.N. Wiesel raised newborn animals in environments that lacked light or other aspects of visual inputs (lines, colors, etc.).[42,54,57] Animals raised in this way were forever cortically blind to the visual input of which they were deprived. Retinal receptors

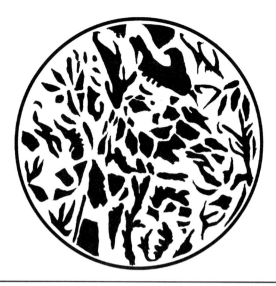

Fig. 6-3. You are probably able to see the outline of a giraffe's head and neck. Visual experience allows you to make figure-ground discriminations. (Design by Jackie Bortoft; reproduced with permission from Bortoft H. Goethe's scientific consciousness. Kent, England: Institute for Cultural Research, 1986.)

responded to the visual cues, but the visual cortex attached no significance to them. Without exposure to visual stimuli during a critical period of development, the ability to perceive was forever altered. Exposure and experience continue to influence perceptions, in a less dramatic fashion, throughout life. With experience you actually learn how to respond to *unseen* properties of objects!

Properties of objects, even those that cannot be directly perceived, influence movement. You learn to associate certain object sizes and textures with particular characteristics. For instance, you know a box of cereal will be lighter than a block of concrete with similar dimensions. Through visual and tactile experience you have gained the ability to perceive differences in object density although this is not something you visually detect directly. Your motor plan for lifting the object will change depending on your perception of the object's density and weight. For instance, during a reaching task, the arm generally accelerates to a target and then decelerates as target acquisition nears. When reaching for fragile objects, such as a light bulb, people spend more time in the deceleration phase to ensure a gentle landing. Visual perception also alters lower extremity reactions. Experiments have shown that people tend to lift their legs higher to clear a fragile obstacle than they do to clear one that they perceive as being more stable.[67]

UE movement trajectories also differ depending on whether vision is involved in the task. Without vision, the initial starting position of the arm appears to bias the arm to move in a certain way.[28] With vision, this bias is eliminated. Reaching trajectories appear to depend on processing visual information about the target location and its intrinsic characteristics (size, texture, etc.), with proprioceptive information of the arm and hand. Later in this chapter we will explore the integrative role of visual and proprioceptive sensory afferent input in more detail. The next section takes us out of the realm of perception and explores the beginnings of the actual mechanics needed to coordinate various body parts to respond to visual input. Head-eye coordination is a good place to start.

■ HEAD-EYE COORDINATION

I have another experiment for you to try. Hold this book a comfortable reading distance away. I now want you to try two different things. First, keep your head still but move the book side-to-side quickly. How well were you able to read while you moved the book? Probably not very well. For the next phase of this experiment, keep the book still but move your head side-to-side. You probably did a bit better with the reading task. Why? The following paragraphs hopefully provide some answers and insights.

Hand-eye coordination is the more typical term applied to the ability to coordinate visual stimuli with accurate arm reaching skills. Hand-eye coordination, however, begins with head-eye coordination. Humans are incapable of detecting visual detail at the periphery of the visual field. An unconscious reflex compensates for this by rotating the eyes so that the object of your desire becomes oriented in the center of your visual field, called the *fovea*. The fovea is where our visual acuity is keenest. It is only about 1 mm in diameter, so for us to see well and to track an incoming fastball traveling at 90 mph, we had better have exquisite control of the muscles that control the eyes. Each eye is controlled by six muscles. These muscles act in concert so that an infinite number of eye positions is possible. *Saccades* is the term used to describe the rapid, staccato-like eye movements that occur during eye tracking or gaze orienting tasks. When the eyes track a moving object, they tend to overshoot the target a bit. Saccades compensate for this by rapidly bringing the eyes back to the target. Saccades are the most rapid movements the human muscular system are capable of producing! As you read this sentence (an eye tracking task), your eyes are performing two to three saccades per second. Even though eye movements are the Olympic sprinters of the human body, they are often not the first to react to a visual stimulus.

When a target is predictable or when target location is away from the midline of the body, the neck and head are the first to move.[5,44] Neck and head muscle contractions stabilize the head and provide a stable base for the higher velocity eye movements. Once the eyes foveate (centralize) on a target, they keep the target in the center of the visual field even as the head continues to move. That is why you were able to read this book while you moved your head side-to-side. You had more difficulty when you held your head stationary and moved the book because you had removed head movement from the tracking task and at times the pages would be in your peripheral visual field.

Saccades are not the only neural mechanism that assists with maintaining visual fixation on an object. *Vestibulo-ocular reflexes* (VORs) allow the eyes to remain fixated on a target even during fast head movements. *Optokinetic reflexes* (OKRs) provide visual tracking assistance during object movement or sustained head movements. *Smooth-pursuit* eye movements are used to keep a moving object centered on the fovea. Smooth-pursuit movements are accomplished by the nervous system's ability to calculate the speed of an object and increase or decrease eye pursuit velocities accordingly.

VORs, OKRs, saccades, and smooth-pursuit eye movements are rather complicated and interact with each other in various ways. The following examples might help in the understanding of these concepts.

Your subject is seated in a chair and instructed to keep the trunk stable and still throughout the experiment. The experiment has three parts. For the first part, the subject is instructed to keep the head stationary while an object is moved horizontally in front of him. For the second part of the experiment, the subject is asked to move the head and the object remains stationary. For the third part, the subject is asked to move the head in the same direction and velocity as the moving object. You, as the experimenter, are to watch the eyes carefully and make a note of eye movement in relation to head movement.

What you note in the first part of the experiment is that with the head held stationary, the subject moves the eyes in the same direction as the moving object (this is referred to as the slow phase of eye tracking). This type of eye tracking task is controlled by the OKR. The eyes tend to overshoot the target a bit and the eyes quickly flick back to the object. This movement is a saccade.

In the second part of the experiment, in which the head moves and the object remains stationary, the eyes move similarly as in the first part of the experiment. The eyes move slowly in the direction opposite the head movement to maintain gaze fixation on the nonmoving object. This movement is controlled by the VOR. Once again, a slight overshoot happens and a rapid saccade occurs in the opposite direction, so that foveation on the object is maintained.

For the third part of the experiment, in which the head moves in the same direction and same velocity as the object moves, eye movement is minimal in relation to head movement. The VOR is suppressed and perfect foveation on the moving object is maintained by the OKR.

All of us were not created equal, unfortunately, with regard to our abilities to track a moving object quickly and accurately or to foveate quickly on a moving object. Some individuals are truly gifted and have superior eye tracking abilities.

As discussed, the VOR coordinates eye and head movements. It is an incredibly fast reflex. From the time the vestibular system detects a change in head position to the time the eyes respond takes less than 10 msec. Highly skilled individuals, such as baseball players, have excellent head-eye coordination. They move their heads more than the rest of us during eye tracking tasks. Their heads cover more of the distance required to focus on an object.[44] The eyes, therefore, do not have to search as wide of an area to locate the target. The benefits of this type of head movement were presented in the explanation of part three of your recently performed experiment.

Not only do elite baseball players have greater excursions with their heads, but they are also more accurate with their head placements. They quickly and accurately move their heads to the target. Experiments have shown that greater head movement results in fewer UE pointing errors.[71] Or, to extrapolate to our current example, greater head movements allow batters to make better contact with a pitched baseball. Most of us are not destined to play Big League baseball. But if it makes you feel any better, your eye tracking skills are superior to other creatures who share our planet.

Once the human eye foveates on a target, it is very good at detecting movement in any direction no matter how subtle. Deer, on the other hand, are almost completely blind to objects at a distance unless movement is involved. That is why, if you are quiet enough and can freeze in place periodically, you can get quite close to deer in the wild. While on the subject of animals, what is it with cats? Have you ever noticed how your housecat constantly moves its head in funny ways? Cat eye muscles have less motility than those of humans and must compensate for this with increased head movements.[36] That cute head tilting behavior you might interpret as intelligent inquisitiveness is, in all likelihood, caused by your cat's desire to get a better look at you. Whether the animal is cat or human, visual acuity depends on the ability to direct and focus the eyes on the object accurately. Head movement is essential to this task.

Accurate tracking of an object requires precise coordination between the head and the eyes. Because this coordination has to be so precise, some have postulated that a single control system drives both head and eye motor circuits. Cells within the superior colliculus, a structure located on the dorsal aspect of the midbrain, coordinate visual, somatic, and auditory information. Individual circuits within the superior colliculus coordinate the head and eyes and saccadic eye movements.[36] Experiments have shown that other areas of the brain are also specialized to detect movement. Certain cells within the visual cortex and lateral geniculate (nucleus within the thalamus concerned with vision) respond only to movement or movements in a certain direction. Other specialized areas exist in the parietotemporal lobes[61] and cerebellar cortex[65] that respond during visual tracking tasks.

Eye contact, a prerequisite for accurate reaching, appears to be achieved by tight coupling between neural circuits that control head and eye muscles. Individual brain stem nuclei might control both head and eye movements during certain tasks. Just as the coupling between head and eye movements has been explored, scientists have wondered whether there is parallel activation of eye and arm movements. Eye and arm movements often occur simultaneously,[44] and it is rare that arm movements don't begin before the termination of head and eye movement to a target. This brings us to the topic of hand-eye coordination.

■ HAND-EYE COORDINATION

Eye contact is the desired goal during visual tracking tasks. Eye contact is also the first phase of eye-hand coordination. As discussed in the previous section, eye contact is accomplished by the cooperation of head and eye muscles. Actual hand contact with the object of your desire requires precise coordination between your eyes and hands. The retinal image must be transformed to internal spatial coordinates in which object location is specified in a body-centered coordinate system, and proprioceptive cues from the moving limb must be superimposed on the same coordinate system so that limb position and object position coincide or are matched.[43] The necessary neural processing that subserves this task remains to be determined.

Eye-hand coordination (often referred to as visuomanual pursuit tracking) requires coordination between various central nervous system (CNS) structures.[46] During visually guided movement the CNS must convert information originating in occipitoparietal visual system brain regions into a pattern of muscle activity that moves the hand to the target.[46] Interestingly, it appears that gaze orientation not only directs placement of the arm during a reach, but also influences the speed of arm movement. Dr. H. Collewijn's group from Denmark instructed subjects to move a stylus as quickly as possible to a moving computer screen target. Even though subjects were instructed to move as quickly as possible during all trials, their arm speed was directly related to the speed of the moving target.[17] The speed by which a target moves across your visual field dictates the speed of your arm's reaction. Purkinje cells of the cerebellum have been implicated in this speed-sensitive, sensory-to-motor transformation.[48,73]

As mentioned previously, because eye and hand movements are so tightly coupled, some have suggested that they might share a common neural drive similar to the one postulated for head-eye coordination. For head and eye control of tracking movements, the common neural drives are the VOR circuitry and other brain stem centers such as those located in the superior colliculus[36,47] and cerebellum.[65]

The organization of hand-eye circuitry, however, is likely to be quite different from that of head-eye circuitry. Dissociating eye and hand movements is easier than dissociating head and eye movements. Rugby players can look in one direction and pass the ball off in quite another. You can watch a movie intently and still be able to reach out and find your popcorn without the aid of vision. In these cases, vision plays a secondary role to kinesthetic senses. The coupled circuits for eye-hand coordination, therefore, need to be more malleable and mutable than head-eye circuitry. Coordination, or more precisely the interaction among various neural processes, once again becomes of paramount importance.

What skill better exemplifies eye-hand coordination than catching a ball? I am sure each of you has direct experience with this motor task, yet I am willing to bet that very few of you have ever considered what factors contribute most to your catching prowess. It appears that several factors are most likely to dictate catching success. The first factor to be considered is the amount of time it takes you to foveate on a moving target. A second factor is the amount of time that elapses between foveation of the target and hand contact with the ball. In general, it appears that the ball (or any incoming projectile) must be seen for at least 240 msec for you to respond accurately to it. Not only must you see the ball for at least 240 msec, but you must make this visual contact no less than 300 msec before contact is to be made with the ball. The duration of visual exposure and the timing relative to contact are the critical variables that determine catching success. Oh yes, one other thing must be considered before you are declared proficient with your catching skills: the ability to move and coordinate your arms and hands in response to visual cues.

Thus far, head-eye coupling and eye-hand coupling have been discussed. These couplings allow you to fixate visually on an object and move in its direction. They have not, as yet, allowed you to actually touch, pick up, or catch the object. For this accomplishment, another closely coupled activity is required: reaching and grasping.

■ REACHING AND GRASPING

Reaching and grasping are yet another tightly choreographed movement sequence. The timing of finger opening and closing must be coordinated with the reach, but it must also be adapted to the size, shape, and texture of the object. Finger movements approximating the size of the object and force generations appropriate for the estimated weight of the object begin during reaching. Reaching is an anticipatory reaction involving visuomotor transformations. Reaching and grasping represent excellent examples of the parallel processing of visual input. At almost the same time as you reach for an object, the hand starts to mimic the shape of the object. It does this without any tactile cueing. Somehow the intrinsic properties of the object (size, shape, texture) that are detected visually are conveyed to the hand musculature. The arm responds to visual cues about the location and orientation of the object. The hand appears to respond to object size and perceived weight.

Many questions exist regarding the coordination of reaching and grasping. How do we choose which muscles to activate to cover the distance required to obtain an object? How do we know when to open the hand to grasp a glass or catch a ball? How do we judge how hard to contract certain muscles to pick up a rock or a fragile eggshell? Are these conscious acts or are generator circuits, once initiated, acting autonomously? These difficult questions won't be answered definitively in this book or in anyone's laboratory in the near future. An incredible amount of work is being done in this area to identify the anatomical locations and guiding physiological principles of UE reach and grasp coordination.

Reaching typically involves a triphasic muscle activity pattern and an accompanying triphasic acceleration-deceleration pattern. The triphasic muscle pattern consists of an agonist contraction to initiate the movement, an antagonist contraction to decelerate the movement, and a final bursting of the agonist to move and reach the target. These patterns occur with or without visual feedback and appear to reflect a UE motor program.

Researchers have proposed that, similar to circuits that exist for lower extremity locomotion, specialized circuits exist in the brain stem and spinal cord that are dedicated to reaching. Different portions of the cerebral cortex are involved in various aspects of reaching, but the primary motor cortex appears to be involved in most aspects of reaching tasks. Reaching movements might originate in the motor cortex, but a spinal circuit involving propriospinal neurons appears to generate the synergy necessary for the movement.[27] The circuit could theoretically be completed by connectivity known to exist between cervical spinal cord propriospinal neurons to the reticular nucleus of the brain stem, which then projects to the cerebellum. The cerebellum is involved in visual tracking[48,73] and it projects back to the motor cortex via the thalamus.

Beyond doubt, the primary motor cortex is involved in reaching tasks. Interestingly, however, different areas of this cortical area are active during different aspects of a reaching task. Scanning techniques indicate that activity within a specified region (field) of the primary motor cortex and premotor cortex is related to the efferent control of muscle contraction. Two other fields have been identified. One is involved in postural preparatory movements needed for reaching, and the other is active only after the learning of a particular task that involves reaching.[49] Furthermore, visual cues related to intrinsic properties appear to travel a different neural route than cues related to distance and direction.[47] Evidence also suggests that the nervous system encodes hand direction separately from other aspects of hand function such as force production.[34] These findings represent excellent examples of parallel processing within the human nervous system.

Identifying the brain structures involved in reaching still does not tell us how the human nervous system coordinates grasping and reaching. What strategies does the nervous system use to control these coupled movements? What sensory modalities do we rely on for these movements after perturbations to UE movement or during unexpected load changes? Researchers from around the world are constantly developing wonderfully novel approaches to these questions.

Dr. Paul Cordo and his group from Portland, Ore., have unraveled one neuroscientific mystery of hand and arm coordination: the frisbee toss. As every college student and Ultimate Frisbee player knows, the key to a good frisbee toss is in the wrist snap. The hand and fingers need to open at precisely the right instant to obtain maximum spin and distance (Fig. 6-4). In an elegant set of laboratory experiments, Dr. Cordo's group has shown that the timing of hand opening depends on arm velocity and joint angular change at the elbow[11] (Fig. 6-4). They have shown that proprioception is used by the nervous system to assist in the control of multijoint movements occurring at the arm and hand. Additionally, their findings indicate that muscle spindles are an important source of this proprioceptive input.[12]

Dr. Cordo's work identifies some of the sensory modalities that contribute to arm and hand coordination. But how does the arm and hand know how fast and how far to move to achieve its purpose?

One idea that has emerged is that accurate reaching and grasping are accomplished by the nervous system's internal creation of a coordinate system. A coordinate system is created as follows. Afferent stimuli, such as vision, provide the nervous system with a knowledge of final target position. Initial hand position (proprioceptive input) provides the nervous system with an awareness of the distance and amplitude the arm and hand must move to cover the distance to the target. In this way, multiple movement strategies can be internally generated to move to the target accurately. Your internal representation of the object, and your relation to it, allow one joint or muscle to alter its trajectory or force production based on what another body segment is doing. Target acquisition is the parameter that is the driving force. Some investigators believe more proximal body parts such as the shoulders dictate the more distal movements of the hand,[44] whereas others believe hand position drives more proximal movements.[33] Some evidence indicates that distance and direction use two different cues. For the control of distance parameters during reaching, the shoulder might be the primary reference point in the coordinate system, and for directional control, visual cues appear to be the most important.[1]

If reaching circuitry is similar to other movement-related neural circuits, then the control parameters probably change depending on the task. In all probability a multiplicity of reference points change not only with the task but also with an individual's preferred movement pattern, sensory context, and instructional set.[1] The concept of an internal coordinate system provides a testable hypothesis of how the CNS might control multiple degrees of freedom during complex, multijointed movements such as reaching.

Drs. Claude Ghez and James Gordon, from Columbia and Long Island Universities, respectively, have conducted experiments that have yielded unique insight into the sensory modalities that potentially contribute to our internal coordinate system.[35] Patients with large fiber peripheral neuropathies are essentially without peripheral sensation. They have lost tactile sensation and position sense and are without stretch reflexes. Obviously, without vision they make many errors during target acquisition tasks because they receive no feedback from the moving limb. What is intriguing is that Drs. Ghez and Gordon have discovered that these patients also experience deficits in the *planning* of reaching movements. As previously presented, proprioceptive information contributes to the execution of coordinated movements. Drs. Ghez and Gordon propose that proprioceptive information helps to form and update internal representations of limb properties. Without this constant updating, the coordinate system used to guide movement becomes dysfunctional and accurate reaching is no longer possible. One modality—proprioception—with possibly two very different functions!

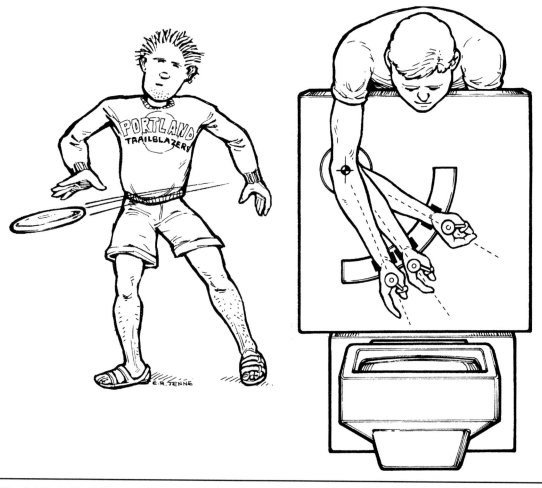

Fig. 6-4. Left, The frisbee toss might have been the inspiration for a creative experiment in motor control. **Right,** A diagram of the actual experimental set-up. (Redrawn from Cordo P, Carlton L, Bevan L, Carlton M, Kerr GK. J Neurophysiol 1994;71:1849.)

■ THE ROLE OF SENSORY INFORMATION IN THE GUIDANCE OF UPPER EXTREMITY MOVEMENT

Multijoint control

UE control can be divided into four main components:

1. Descending motor commands,
2. Intake of sensory information,
3. Internal coding of descending and sensory information, and
4. The generation of movement.

Inherent to, but not explicitly included, in these four components is the role of sensory input on descending motor commands. Sensory input is involved in reflex functions, but it is also involved in modulating or even directing descending supraspinal input. Refer back to Chapters 2 and 3 for a review of some of the potential mechanisms, such as presynaptic inhibition, that are involved.

The role of feed-forward and feedback sensory systems in UE control is considerable. A wide array of sensory inputs has the potential to contribute to the control of UE movement. Encoding of visual information that contributes to UE control requires the convergence of different types of visually related afferent input. This input includes retinal signals, information about eye position, and information about the position of the head, arm, and hand in relation to the body.[71] Proprioceptive inputs from a multitude of muscle, skin, and joint receptors make an equally significant and diffuse contribution. The relative contributions of vision and proprioception are the focus of the next discussion.

Vision and proprioception

Obviously, UE movement is possible either in the absence of vision or in the absence of proprioceptive input. Visually challenged individuals can still coordinate arm and hand movements. Individuals with sensory neuropathies are still capable of generating voluntary movement. Closer examination, however, reveals that either situation results in some problems, especially in multijoint control during complex tasks. Central motor programs acting without sensory input might be sufficient to control simple, learned movements, but sensory feedback is needed for dexterous movements, to recover from a perturbation, and for the initial stages of motor learning.[26] The degree to which we normally rely on vision and proprioception for these movements is where the debate begins. Findings thus far indicate that reliance on a specific type of sensory input is task specific.

Most common, everyday arm movements are controlled visually. A critical value exists, however, when movement becomes too fast for visual guidance. During fast movements, vision plays less of a role and proprioceptive feedback becomes more important. It takes approximately 190 to 260 msec for visual feedback to influence the accuracy of a UE movement.[50] For proprioceptive input, the latency is considerably shorter. A UE stretch reflex has a response latency of less than 20 msec. To respond voluntarily to a stretched muscle takes less than 100 msec. For quick UE movements, the sensory cues for the control of the movement come from the moving limb and not the eyes. The longer it takes to perform a movement, the more the eyes are used.

This does not mean that proprioceptive information is not used during slow movements or that vision is not used during fast ones. For instance, muscle spindle activity is just as active during visually guided tasks as it is during a nonvisual task.[76] It also does not indicate that vision and muscle spindles don't act in concert. A unique and creative experiment demonstrates the symbiotic relationship between vision and proprioception in the control of movement.[17]

Subjects were asked to point to an ever-changing series of blinking lights. Eye gaze to the light stimulus always preceded the finger tap (e.g., a light came on, the subject oriented his or her gaze to the light, and then pointed to the light. The next light came on, and so forth). Initially some eye gaze errors occurred (overshoots or misdirections), but these errors were minimized in a short period. Subjects quickly learned the task. Subjects were then asked to look but *not* point and tap with their hands. In the absence of arm movements, subjects took longer to gaze at each light stimulus, had more gaze orienting errors, and took longer to learn the task. These results provide evidence that UE proprioception contributes to the learning and accuracy of eye tracking tasks. In addition, multisensorial input increases accuracy, speed, and motor learning abilities.

Speed and accuracy

Fitt's Law states that as the speed of limb movements increase, accuracy diminishes (see Fig. 6-1). This makes intuitive sense, and a number of studies have demonstrated this concept. Not surprisingly, movements that rely solely on proprioceptive input are prone to have an increased number of errors. In contrast, visual guidance results in more accurate performance during reaching tasks. The problem with total reliance on vision is that it slows you down. Motor responses to visual input have considerably longer latencies than responses to proprioceptive input.

A downhill mogul run on your favorite ski slope serves as an excellent example of the cooperative yet divergent responsibilities of visual and proprioceptive sensory feedback. In this case we aren't talking solely about UE control. When you are skiing down difficult terrain, you do not want to be looking at the tips of your skis. You want to direct your gaze downhill to plan your descent strategy. You must rely on your quick-responding lower extremity proprioceptors to correct for the ever-changing terrain and snow conditions underfoot. Visual input primarily contributes to motor planning and perhaps postural set, whereas proprioceptive input corrects for spontaneous disruptions to your equilibrium.

Movements involved with skiing, of course, involve more than one extremity. Most functional movements, in fact, are not isolated to a single joint but rather involve the control of multiple joints and muscles. The control of limb accuracy and coordination of multijoint movements are the subjects of considerable debate. At the heart of this debate is the Equilibrium-Point Hypothesis.

The Equilibrium-Point Hypothesis

Dr. Anatol Feldman, a Russian physicist and neuroscientist, first proposed the Equilibrium-Point Hypothesis in 1965. The hypothesis states that multijoint movements are accomplished via springlike muscle properties, peripheral reflexes, and feedback loops without the need for complex brain computations or involvement.[19-21]

Data from some experiments with human reaching movements are consistent with this theory.[53,79] No doubt that muscle compliance and the springlike properties of muscles contribute to motor control. The hotly contested issue is whether the peripheral neuromuscular system can generate accurate movements without ongoing supraspinal input. Inherent to the Equilibrium Point Hypothesis is the concept that the body (brain) can only control what it senses.

This premise has some significant contradictions. First, after deafferentation (destruction of sensory input), some movements are still well controlled. Also, during fast, ballistic-type movements, afferent feedback is too delayed to contribute to the task. Furthermore, highly trained movements have little or no reliance on sensory input. Finally, control of one variable might rely on the sensing of quite another (i.e., the swing phase of gait might be triggered by unweighting of a limb, hip extension, or increased extensor muscle output).[62]

Other experimental work challenges the Equilibrium Point Hypothesis. Drs. Gomi and Kawato of Kyoto University in Japan provided evidence that equilibrium point calculations did not predict actual arm trajectories.[30] They suggest that the brain develops an internal model of the desired movement based on visual information. In this way the brain computes final joint angles and muscle lengths needed to reach the object. This implies that learning has a tremendous role to play in the acquisition of accurate reaching and that reflexes are a secondary player. These data fit nicely with results from young children that show their accuracy in reaching and grasping is not as accurate as that of a learned adult.[18,22]

The disputes pertaining to the control of multijoint movement will continue well beyond my lifetime. This difficult and complex area of study has generated some of the most creative motor control experiments to date. Another area of interest involves the relationship between proactive postural responses during tasks that involve UE movement.

■ POSTURAL CONTRIBUTIONS TO VOLUNTARY UPPER EXTREMITY MOVEMENT

Postural stabilization appears to be a prerequisite for accurate UE movements. Any type of UE movement will displace the body's center of gravity (Fig. 6-5). Any change in the center of gravity results in a loss of equilibrium, unless an opposing movement counteracts the destabilizing UE movement. Every high

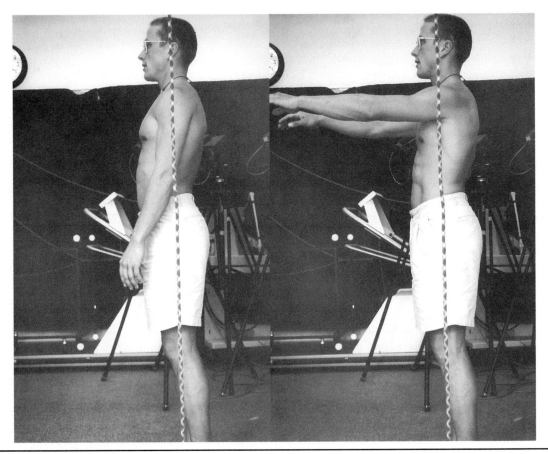

Fig. 6-6. As the arms come forward, the body needs to lean backward a bit to maintain the center of gravity over the feet. Note the head (ear) position relative to the plumb line.

school physics student knows that for every action there is a reaction. This is the best analogy I can think of when it comes to explaining the relationship between voluntary arm movements and postural adjustments. If arm movement destabilizes the body's center of gravity, another body part must contract or move to prevent the potential loss of equilibrium. The intriguing aspect of the association of postural reactions and voluntary movements is the temporal sequence of events.

Losing one's equilibrium is a condition to be avoided if possible. The nervous system appears to be able to anticipate the loss of equilibrium that results from voluntary UE movement. Rather than reacting to the loss of equilibrium, the nervous system takes a proactive role. Many postural reactions to voluntary UE movements actually precede UE movement. You might think that as you initiate the thought process to pick up a glass of water, you naturally send a neural message to the prime movers of the arm. Before any message activating the arm, however, messages activate postural muscles (neck, back, and leg) so that subsequent arm movements don't knock you off balance. It is as if the postural reactions needed to counteract any resultant change in the center of gravity elicited by UE movement are part of the UE motor program. Experimental evidence does indeed suggest that postural adjustments to UE movements are pre-programmed.[6,25] These studies indicated that postural muscle activity always preceded arm movements and that the postural activations were predictable and task specific. As might be predicted, postural responses were also modified by the body's initial position.[13]

The fact that postural sets change depending on initial body position and task is not a matter of any small significance. The latency and sequence of postural muscle activations that precede UE movements appear to be designed to be the most mechanically and energy-efficient means to compensate for any type of a destabilizing influence. For instance, most postural reactions to arm movements or small perturbations involve activation of distal musculature before more proximal activations.[63] Activation of smaller, distal muscles is more energy efficient than activation of larger, proximal muscles. Somehow the human nervous system appears to be able to modulate its activity based on biophysical and biomechanical principles. No peripheral receptors detect center of gravity changes or limb accelerations, yet certainly a knowledge of these conditions helps to control multijoint movements. Piecing together this puzzle is not easy, but let's briefly look at the postural responses of standing subjects during a UE reaching task to see if any ideas pertaining to the coordination of postural control and UE movement emerge. Several laboratories have examined postural reactions during UE reaching. Some of the postural changes that precede UE reaching movements from a standing position include activation of the legs and trunk,[66] contralateral arm,[58] and ipsilateral leg.[74] Interestingly, these postural adjustments that precede UE reaching movements share some of the same characteristics as postural responses that result from perturbations (loss of balance).[13] It is, therefore, possible that some of the same neural circuits might be used to control postural stability regardless whether the responses are elicited as part of a UE synergy or as a response to loss of equilibrium.[13] Furthermore, one can speculate that the neural circuitry involved might include spinal cord propriospinal pathways.[60,70] Activation of these pathways could result in a stereotyped motor response even if triggered by different descending supraspinal input (i.e., motor commands from the sensorimotor cortex or after input from vestibular nuclei). In this way dissimilar input could yield the same motor output. The common denominator for both situations is the preservation of equilibrium.

Remember that propriospinal pathways are divergent and ascend and descend throughout the spinal cord. They can activate a wide array of neurons or functional neural groupings (e.g., motor neurons innervating the paraspinals). In this way different muscles could act synergistically in response to a particular descending or sensory afferent input. Perhaps propriospinal pathways will prove to be the key to understanding the multijoint control needed to coordinate postural and UE movements. Or, perhaps not. Perhaps postural reactions to perturbations and postural reactions that precede voluntary movement are controlled by totally independent processes.[24]

Body position and task specificity are not the only determinants to the coupling of postural reactions and UE movement. Instructional set, experience, anxiety, and learning can all influence postural reactions.[3,8,9,24,40,41] Something as simple as holding a glass of water totally changes postural reactions to perturbations of a standing subject even though every other aspect of initial body position is the same. Subjects' responses also change with exposure to a task or postural perturbation. People become increasingly more efficient with their movements and learn to anticipate after repeated exposures to the same perturbation—unless the subject being tested has had damage to the cerebellum. Subjects with cerebellar damage do not seem capable of adapting postural responses based on experience or learning.[40] The adaptability of the coupling between postural responses and UE movements does not appear consistent with a more hard-wired propriospinal neural network concept. Rather, findings that cognitive factors and situational context alter reactions are more consistent with the concept of an internal representation of a voluntary movement that preprograms postural adjustments according to a goal. This would involve feedforward mechanisms and include the basal ganglia and cerebellum.[6,24,25,59]

These issues, like so many in the neural control of movement, have not been resolved. Insights into the relationships between postural reactions and voluntary movement and between automatic reactions and voluntary movement will be important for clinicians involved in eliciting and optimizing movement from their patients. For instance, a certain instructional set of directions may be more effective than another, or a certain starting position may be more favorable than another for the initiation of movement.

Results thus far indicate four main characteristics regarding postural adaptations to voluntary movement:

1. Postural reactions are anticipatory and attempt to minimize body displacement during voluntary movement
2. Postural reactions are adaptable to conditions and context,
3. Postural reactions are influenced by the individual's intent and emotional state, and
4. Postural reactions can be modified by learning and experience.

■ BIMANUAL COORDINATION: DOES THE RIGHT HAND REALLY KNOW WHAT THE LEFT HAND IS DOING?

Can you pat your head and rub your belly simultaneously? Chances are good that this task initially feels a bit awkward, but given a little practice, you probably do pretty well. Now for your next test. Place your hands on top of a table, palms down. With your dominant hand, begin alternately tapping with your index and middle fingers. Do this as fast as possible. Now begin the same alternate tapping with the other hand. Without being told to do so, it is extremely likely that your tapping is bilaterally synchronized. In other words, both index fingers tapped the table at the same time while you lifted the middle fingers, and vice versa. Experiment with how fast you can perform this alternate tapping.

For the next phase of this exercise, try asynchronous tapping. The taps should still alternate between the index and middle fingers of each hand, but now the right index finger and left middle finger should tap the table at the same time (Fig. 6-6). All of a sudden this isn't so easy. What happened? You aren't taxing the muscles any differently. Postural stability has not changed. The only thing that has really changed has been the intended sequence of activations. The tendency for the CNS to want to synchronize both extremities is a neural demon with which musicians and other athletes must wrestle on a daily basis to succeed. Your ability to coordinate movements occurring solely on one side of the body differs from coordinating both sides of the body. Getting both sides of the body to move at different velocities or rhythms is difficult. Force generation also suffers during bimanual tasks.[29,64]

The following paragraphs focus on the differences in neural control between unimanual and bimanual tasks. I'll let the cat out of the bag a little early: it appears that unimanual and bimanual UE control might be controlled by different parts of the brain.

Examining the neural connectivity of the brain can often provide keys to function. In the case of bimanual coordination, it can also be more than a bit misleading. A premise established years ago was that bimanual tasks are controlled as if they represented a single task[4] and thus are controlled simultaneously by similar brain regions or regions that are richly interconnected via callosal projections (projections that connect the two cerebral hemispheres). Neuroanatomical investigations, however, have shown that the two primary hand areas of each hemisphere share very sparse callosal projections.[45] It is tempting to use this as an argument in favor of each hand being independently controlled. Other strategies of connectivity, however, would allow one cerebral hemisphere to control both UEs.

Cortical neurons project to brain stem nuclei and spinal cord propriospinal neurons. These brain stem nuclei and propriospinal neurons have bilateral connections within the spinal cord. One cortical area, therefore, by nature of its projections to the brain stem and spinal cord, could control both halves of the body. Other findings also provide evidence for bilateral control that originates from a single cortical

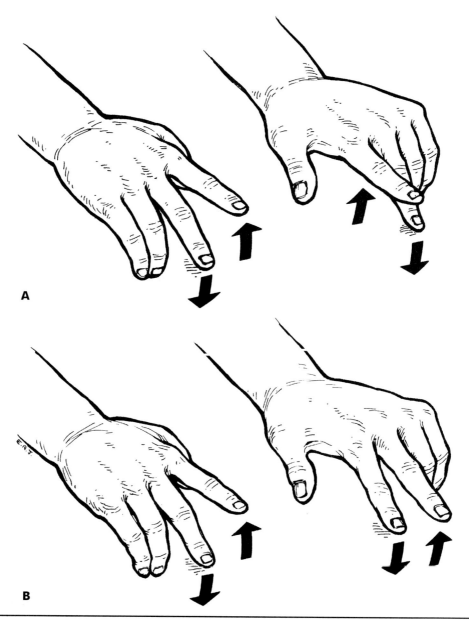

Fig. 6-5. A, Synchronous finger tapping and **B,** asynchronous finger tapping. Synchronous finger tapping is easier; at faster tapping speeds, asynchronous tapping gets increasingly more difficult to maintain.

source. Isolated areas appear to exist within the primary hand motor area that are active only during bimanual tasks.[2] Unlike the primary motor cortex, association areas of the sensorimotor cortex have dense bilateral connections to each other.[52] Also, the precedent exists for one cortical area controlling bilateral motor activities. Drs. Liu and Chambers showed that the motor cortical area of one cerebral hemisphere controls trunk and proximal muscles bilaterally.[56]

An obvious but important point to bear in mind with these studies, however, is that this type of connectivity work is typically done with monkeys and other nonhumans. We have previously discussed the problems inherent to drawing direct correlates to human neural organization and behavior from studies in nonhuman animals. So, let's examine behavioral studies in humans to determine whether any correlates or similarities to data from nonhuman animal work exist.

This might be a case where science is busy trying to catch up to intuition and common sense. The opening paragraphs of this section provided anecdotal and experiential data demonstrating that synchronized UE movements are easier to coordinate than asynchronous ones. One of the hallmarks of motor learning is the ability to break out of innate patterns of synchronized connectivity. The ability to fractionate movement quickly and efficiently is a good indicator of the acquisition of a motor skill.

The learning of a motor task typically involves processing sensory input and generating an appropriate motor response to this input. This is true regardless whether the task involves unimanual or bimanual movements. Adult humans are able to transfer sensory information, such as the weight of objects, obtained from one limb to control the movement of the other limb.[32] Other investigators have found, however, that disrupting sensory input from one limb does not negatively impact the motor skills of the other.[7] So what sensory modalities or movement parameters control bimanual activities? An interesting series of studies by Dr. John Scholz from The University of Delaware shed some light on this issue. Dr. Scholz showed that humans preferred to move fingers synchronously but were also capable of asynchronous activations, with one exception: as the frequency (speed) of movement increased, they increasingly failed to maintain the asynchronous pattern.[72] This finding implies that bimanual asynchronous tasks might depend on sensory feedback to higher brain centers to a larger degree than other movements.[78] Fast movements occur at speeds that exceed the sensory systems' ability to feedback changes or perturbations to the movement pattern. Fast movements, therefore, revert back to a more hard-wired, subcortical synchrony. Asynchronous bimanual tasks, because they appear to rely on sensory processing by higher brain centers, require more concentration and are slower. Synchronous bimanual tasks might have less cortical dependency than unimanual tasks.[44]

Do the above findings indicate that therapists might be more successful in eliciting movement in their patients with head injury or stroke if synchronous bilateral exercises are used? The differences in the neural control of various tasks and the potential clinical implications make for interesting conjectures and testable hypotheses. Human brain scanning techniques and functional testing of patient populations after various treatment interventions should help to illuminate these issues in the not-too-distant future. Increasingly, imaging techniques during functional movements in humans indicate that different areas of the brain serve very specialized functions (see Chapter 4 for presently available data in this area).

■ CHILDRENS' DEVELOPMENT OF UPPER EXTREMITY CONTROL

Considering the multiple levels at which the nervous system needs to coordinate activity for reaching and grasping, it should come as no surprise that UE control does not come easily. Although some interlimb coordination is inherent and present at birth,[18,38,75] UE control involves a rather extended learning process. Ask the parents of a "tendency to drop and break everything" teenager, and they will swear the process takes forever. Actually, the majority of maturational processes needed for UE sensory system integration takes about 5 to 7 years.[23] These processes, however, begin quite early.

Take time out of your busy life sometime and watch an infant. Try to do it with an unbiased and unemotional eye. When the infant is in the supine position, you will notice a lot of activity. The arms and legs appear to be in constant motion. The more awake and engaged the child, the more activity. You might

TABLE 6-1 Selected hand and upper extremity developmental milestones

Motor behavior	Age at onset	Integration
Traction response	28 wk	2-5 mo
Palmar grasp	Birth to 2 mo	4-6 mo
Instinctive grasp	4 to 11 mo	Persists
Bilateral hand play (>50% of time)	4 to 5 mo	Persists
Thumb-finger grasp	8 to 9 mo	Persists
Pincer grasp	8 to 9 mo	Persists
Page turning and block stacking	12 to 15 mo	Persists
Imitates vertical crayon stroke	16 to 18 mo	Persists

interpret these movements as purposeless flailings or spontaneous reflex activity. Nothing could be further from the truth. In reality, the infant is establishing a relationship between herself and her environment. The next time the relatives and neighbors are oohing and aahing over the antics of some infant, just lay the following informational tidbit on them: "Actually, her motor output is simply being compared with the resultant afferent feedback of her movements to develop an internal body reference scheme." Chances are you won't have to worry about buying a gift for the next baby shower—you won't be invited.

As unsentimental as it might seem, it appears to be the truth. Babies tend to move the arms to bring the hands within their visual field.[75] The reaching and grasping motions of a 4- to 5- month-old infant are not purposeless, but are an attempt to judge how long the arm is in relation to the distance from the desired object.[75] The baby needs to learn body dimensions and needs to be able to interpret visual cues. The rapid growth of human infants further compounds their problem. The child needs to adapt and recalibrate his or her internal coordinates constantly based on new body dimensions. That is why a visually challenged child or one with a disorder that limits visual or motor exploration might be at risk for developing future sensorimotor difficulties.[55,75]

Clinicians who work with children are very adept at identifying certain milestones of UE development (Table 6-1; Fig. 6-7). If a milestone is not achieved by a certain age, intervention might be indicated. Increasingly, neuroscientists are discovering that nervous system maturation and connectivity depend on activity.[9,24,51,77]

Clinicians are equally adept at identifying difficulties in movement quality or movement retardation. In discussions among themselves, clinicians talk about a child's lack of movement or a UE or lower extremity movement that doesn't appear "typical." Even though experienced clinicians develop an intuitive feel in these areas and recognize a deficit when they see it, until recently correlations between paucity or quality of infant movement and potential developmental difficulties have not been made. Some work is now being done in this area that might help to validate and quantify the clinicians' observations.[10,68]

Movement and exploration are the keys to infant development. Reaching and grasping, as discussed previously, are not separated from other motor functions. They rely on the development of other motor skills such as anticipatory postural reactions.

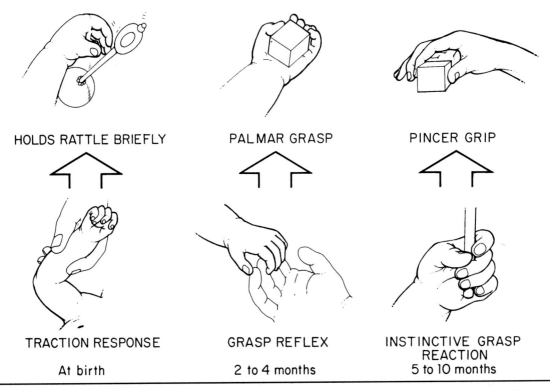

HOLDS RATTLE BRIEFLY · PALMAR GRASP · PINCER GRIP

TRACTION RESPONSE · GRASP REFLEX · INSTINCTIVE GRASP REACTION

At birth · 2 to 4 months · 5 to 10 months

Fig. 6-7. Some hand developmental milestones. (From Twitchell TE. In: Growth and development: an anthology. Washington: American Physical Therapy Association, 1975.)

It is no accident that the reaching and grasping that begins at approximately 4 to 5 months of age coincide with the development of neck righting. As infants develop postural control, they establish a more stable base of support from which to extend their extremities. If the base is unstable, accuracy of distal arm and hand movements suffers. An infant who has not yet developed adequate neck strength or control has difficulty with reaching. If the neck is supported, for instance by a parent's hands, the infant has much better success.

It is important for infants to experience success with their reaching. The act of reaching encourages the development of postural control. Moving the arms contributes to an unstable base of support. The infant must compensate for this instability with postural control strategies. Initially postural adaptations are reactive in nature,[37-39,63] but with experience and time postural reactions become anticipatory and precede voluntary movement. Through reaching, the infant acquires object manipulation skills. Object manipulation contributes to bimanual coordination and developing internalized representations between object texture, size, and weight. These skills relate unequivocally to a child's ability to grasp an object appropriately.

We generally reach out for something to grasp it. Once we grasp an object, we tend to lift it. The relationship between grip force and load force (the amount of force we exert to lift an object) is a linear one. The heavier the object, the harder you have to grip it and the more force you have to exert to lift it. Adults are very good at estimating size and weight of an object by using visual cues.

Adults, as they reach out for a familiar object, open their hands to an appropriate width while the arm is still reaching toward the object. Once they reach the object, they grip it with just enough force so that it doesn't drop out of the hand during the lifting phase (Fig. 6-8, **A**). These movements cannot be solely dependent on tactile input because they begin before contact with the object is ever made. Adults are also very good at adapting grip and load forces to unexpected weights. Children are not as accomplished with any of these tasks.

Children do not relate grip forces with object texture or size. Finger posturing during visual grasping does not develop until approximately 20 weeks of age.[44] By 1 to 2 years old, children have some ability to adjust grip force to object texture, but their abilities are less than perfect. Children less than 2 years old tend to use a higher grip force than is necessary (Fig. 6-8, **B**). This tendency has been termed a "high safety margin."[22] Once they grasp an object, they tend not to lift it immediately. Rather, they push down on the object and then lift. The relationship between grip force and load force is not linear. Instead, they tend to lift by means of trial and error. As might be expected for any learning situation, a lot of variability exists among children and from trial to trial of the same child. Beyond the age of 2 years, the grip/load force synergy becomes much more adultlike.[22] And by 3 years of age the child can use visual cues to estimate weight. By 6 to 8 years their responses approximate those of an adult. Children with damage to the sensorimotor cortex are delayed in these skills.[15,16]

At 2 years of age, the child acquires an additional milestone for yet another UE synergy: using the two hands together for a common goal. *Bimanual coordination*, the ability to use both hands to achieve a common purpose, follows a fairly predictable developmental sequence. A 2- or 3-month-old infant, when lying on his or her back, reaches for objects with both hands.[10,18] This early bimanual reaching perhaps indicates a rudimentary neural network capable of controlling multijoint movements bilaterally in an infant. At 6 months the infant is actually showing some coordinated actions of the two hands, although at this age the child prefers to use a single arm to reach for an object.[69] By 9 months the two hands are acting in unison to accomplish a goal. The movements, however, have poor temporal organization and tend to be synchronous.[18] Between the ages of 9 and 12 months, the movements become less synchronous and more sequential. This is a prelude to having the two hands perform two different functions to accomplish the same task; for instance, using one hand for a prop while the other reaches for an object, or a later skill, having one hand pick up a box lid while the other reaches for the object inside. From 1 to 2 years of age the child increases mastery of these bimanual skills and becomes quite proficient. A good portion of "the terrible twos" can be attributed to newly found motor skills, not only in locomotion but also bimanual manipulative skills. Maturational changes needed for bimanual movements include postural control, distal hand control, increased opportunities for object manipulation, and maturation of interhemispheric and spinal cord connectivity.[18]

Upper extremity coordination develops secondary to nervous system maturation and feedback from ongoing motor activity (learning).[18,38] UE motor development appears to begin with basic synergistic patterns present at birth. These patterns, via experience and learning, become modified and modulated into a plethora of new programs. Activity and exploration dictate our ultimate movement repertoire. *Epigenetic factors* (environmental factors or learning that act on a genome to express morphology or function) play a key role in the UE development of children. It might look like play to you and me, but that kid is putting in long hours of hard work, literally learning how he or she fits into this world.

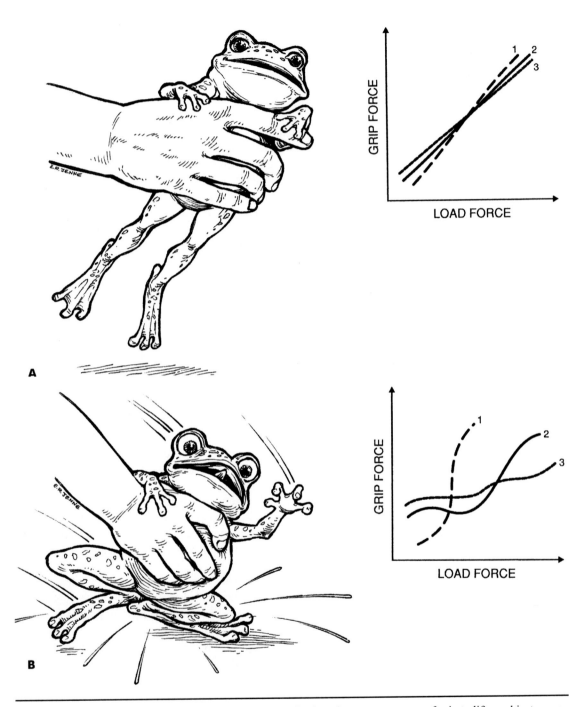

Fig. 6-8. A, An adult, with a mature grip/load synergy, applies just the correct amount of grip to lift an object appropriately and not squeeze too hard or too lightly. Graph insert shows consistent linear relationship between grip and load forces during three lifting trials. **B,** A child does not yet have a mature grip/load synergy and tends to squeeze objects with excess force and also pushes the object downward before lifting. Graph insert shows lack of a linear relationship between grip and load forces and also the greater degree of variability among lifting trials.

SUGGESTED READINGS

Abrams RA, Pratt J. Rapid aimed limb movements: differential effects of practice on component submovements. J Motor Behav 1993;25:288-98.

Albright TD. My most true mind thus makes mine eye untrue. Trends Neurosci 1995;18:331-3.

Badke MB, Di Fabio RP. Effects of postural bias during support surface displacements and rapid arm movements. Phys Ther 1985;65:1490-5.

Bennett KMB, Lemon RN. Corticomotoneuronal contribution to the fractionation of muscle activity during precision grip in the monkey. J Neurophysiol 1996;75:1826-42.

Bizzi E. Intermediate representations in the formation of arm trajectories. Curr Opin Neurobiol 1993;3:925-31.

Blouin J. On-line versus off-line control of rapid aiming movements. J Motor Behav 1993;25:275-9.

Carson RG, Goodman D, Chua R. Asymmetries in the regulation of visually guided aiming. J Motor Behav 1993;25:21-32.

Cordo P, Bevan L, Gurfinkel V, Carlton L, Carlton M, Kerr G. Proprioceptive coordination of discrete movement sequences: mechanism and generality. J Pharm Pharmacol 1995;73:305-15.

Decety J, Kawashima R, Gulyas B, Roland PE. Preparation for reaching: a PET study of the participating structures in the human brain. Neuroreport 1992;3:761-4.

Donkelaar P, Lee RG, Gellman RS. Control strategies in directing the hand to moving targets. Exp Brain Res 1992;91:151-61.

Eden GF, VanMeter JW, Rumsey JM, Masiog JM, Woods RP, Zeffiro TA. Abnormal processing of visual motion in dyslexia revealed by functional brain imaging. Nature 1996;382:66-9.

Fetz EE. Cortical mechanisms controlling limb movement. Curr Opin Neurobiol 1993;3:932-9.

Flament D, Fortier PA, Fetz EE. Response patterns and post-spike effects of peripheral afferents in dorsal root ganglia of behaving monkeys. J Neurophysiol 1992;67:875-89.

Forssberg H, Hirschfeld H. Postural adjustments in sitting humans following external perturbations: muscle activity and kinematics. Exp Brain Res 1994;97:515-27.

Gahery Y, Massion J. Co-ordination between posture and movement. Trends Neurosci 1981;378:199-202.

Gentilucci M, Jeannerod M, Tadary B, Decety J. Dissociating visual and kinesthetic coordinates during pointing movements. Exp Brain Res 1994;102:359-66.

Georgopoulos AP. Current issues in directional motor control. Trends Neurosci 1995;18:506-10.

Ghez C, Gordon J, Ghilardi MF. Impairments of reaching movements in patients without proprioception. II. Effects of visual information on accuracy. J Neurophysiol 1995;73:361-72.

Ghez C, Gordon J, Ghilardi MF. Programming of extent and direction in human reaching movements. Biomed Res 1993;14:1-5.

Ghez C, Gordon J, Ghilardi MF, Christakos CN, Cooper SE. Roles of proprioceptive input in the programming of arm trajectories. In: Cold Spring Harbor Symposia on Quantitative Biology. Cold Spring Harbor Laboratory Press, 1990:837-47.

Ghez C, Hening W, Gordon J. Organization of voluntary movement. Curr Opin Neurobiol 1991;1:664-71.

Gordon J, Ghilardi MF, Ghez C. In reaching, the task is to move the hand to a target. Behav Brain Res 1992;15:337-8.

Gottlieb GL. The generation of the efferent command and the importance of joint compliance in fast elbow. Exp Brain Res 1994;97:545-50.

Gottlieb GL, Latash ML, Corcos DM, Liubinskas TJ, Agarwal GC. Organizing principles for single joint movements. V. agonist-antagonist interactions. J Neurophysiol 1992;67:1417-27.

Haas G, Diener CH, Bacher M, Dichgans J. Development of postural control in children: short-, medium-, and long latency EMG responses of leg muscles after perturbation of stance. Exp Brain Res 1986;64:127-32.

Hashimoto M, Ohtsuka K. Transcranial magnetic stimulation over the posterior cerebellum during visually guided saccades in man [abstract]. Brain 1995;118:1185-93.

Henn V. Neuronal control of eye movements. In: Berthoz A, ed. Multisensory control of movement. Oxford: Oxford University Press, 1993:7-26.

Hogan N, Winters JM. Principles underlying movement organization: upper limb. In: Winters JM, Woo SL-Y, eds. Multiple muscle systems: biomechanics and movement organization. New York: Springer-Verlag, 1990:182-94.

Jeannerod M, Arbib MA, Rizzolatti G, Sakata H. Grasping objects: the cortical mechanisms of visuomotor transformation. Trends Neurosci 1995;18:314-20.

Lacquaniti F, Carrozzo M, Borghese N. Feedback and feedforward mechanisms for the control of multijointed limbs. In: Berthoz A, ed. Multisensory control of movement. Oxford: Oxford University Press, 1993:341-62.

Lacquaniti F, Carrozzo M, Borghese N. The role of vision in tuning anticipatory motor responses of the limbs. In: Berthoz A, ed. Multisensory control of movement. Oxford: Oxford University Press, 1993:379-93.

Lee TD, Swinnen SP, Verschueren S. Relative phase alterations during bimanual skill acquisition. J Motor Behav 1995;27:263-74.

Levin MF, Feldman AG, Milner TE, Lamarre Y. Reciprocal and coactivation commands for fast wrist movements. Exp Brain Res 1992;89:669-77.

Loeb GE. Past the equilibrium point. Behav Brain Sci 1992;15:774.

Martin JH, Ghez C. Differential impairments in reaching and grasping produced by local inactivation within the forelimb representation of the motor cortex in the cat. Exp Brain Res 1993;94:429-43.

Pennisi E. Tilting against a major theory of movement control. Science 1996;272:32-3.

Prochazka A. Comparison of natural and artificial control of movement. IEEE Trans Rehab Eng 1993;1:7-17.

Redding GM. Adaptive coordination and alignment of eye and hand. J Motor Behav 1993;25:75-88.

Roucoux A, Crommelinck M. Orienting gaze: a brief survey. In: Berthoz A, ed. Multisensory control of movement. Oxford: Oxford University Press, 1993:130-49.

Schmied A, Ivarsson C, Fetz EE. Short-term synchronization of motor units in human extensor digitorum communis muscle: relation to contractile properties and voluntary control. Exp Brain Res 1993;97:159-72.

Sidaway B, Sekiya H, Fairweather M. Movement variability as a function of accuracy demand in programmed serial aiming responses. J Motor Behav 1995;27:67-75.

Smeets JBJ, Erkelens CJ, Denier Van Der Gon JJ. Perturbations of fast goal-directed arm movements: different behavior of early and late EMG responses. J Motor Behav 1995;27:77-88.

Theeuwen M, Miller LE, Gielen CCAM. Are the orientations of the head and arm related during pointing movements? J Motor Behav 1993;25:242-50.

Theeuwen M, Miller LE, Gielen CCAM. Is the orientation of head and arm coupled during pointing movements? J Motor Behav 1993;25:242-50.

van Ingen Schenau GJ, Boots PJ, deGroot G, Snackers RJ, van Woensel WW. The constrained control of force and position in multi-joint movements. Neuroscience 1992;46:197-207.

Vandonkelaar P, Fisher C, Lee RG. Adaptive modification of oculomotor pursuit influences manual tracking responses. Neuroreport 1994;5:2233-6.

Viviani P, Stucchi N, Laissard G. Issues in perceptuo-motor coordination. In: Berthoz A, ed. Multisensory control of movement. Oxford: Oxford University Press, 1993:394-423.

Wierzbicka MM, Wiegner AW. Effects of weak antagonist on fast elbow flexion movements in man. Exp Brain Res 1992;91:509-19.

REFERENCES

1. Abeele SV, Crommelinck M, Roucoux A. Frames of reference used in goal-directed arm movement. In: Berthoz A, ed. Multisensory control of movement. Oxford: Oxford University Press, 1993:63-78.

2. Aizawa H, Mushiake H, Inase M, Tanji J. An output zone of the monkey primary motor cortex specialized for bilateral hand movement. Exp Brain Res 1990;82:219-21.

3. Allum JHJ, Honegger F. Synergies and strategies underlying normal and vestibulary deficient control of balance: implication for neuroprosthetic control. Prog Brain Res 1993;97:331-58.

4. Bernstein N. The coordination and regulation of movements. Oxford: Pergamon Press, 1967.

5. Bizzi E, Polit A, Morasso P. Mechanisms underlying achievement of final head position. J Neurophysiol 1976;39:435-44.

6. Bouisset S, Zattara M. A sequence of postural movements precedes voluntary movement. Neurosci Lett 1981;22:263-70.

7. Bullen AR, Brunt D. Effects of tendon vibration on unimanual and bimanual movement accuracy. Exp Neurol 1986;93:311-9.

8. Burleigh A, Horak F. Influence of instruction, prediction, and afferent sensory information on the postural organization of step initiation. J Neurophysiol 1996;75:1619-28.

9. Burleigh AL, Horak FB, Malouin F. Modification of postural responses and step initiation: evidence for goal-directed postural interactions. J Neurophysiol 1994;72:2892-902.

10. Corbetta D, Thelen E. A method for identifying the initiation of reaching movements in natural prehension. J Motor Behav 1995;27:285-93.

11. Cordo P, Carlton L, Bevan L, Carlton M, Kerr GK. Proprioceptive coordination of movement sequences: role of velocity and position information. J Neurophysiol 1994;71:1848-61.

12. Cordo P, Gurfinkel VS, Bevan L, Kerr GK. Proprioceptive consequences of tendon vibration during movement. J Neurophysiol 1995;74:1675-88.

13. Cordo PJ, Nashner LM. Properties of postural adjustments associated with rapid arm movements. J Neurophysiol 1982;47:287-302.

14. Elbert T, Pantev C, Wienbruch C, Rockstroh B, Taub E. Increased cortical representation of the fingers of the left hand in string players. Science 1995;270: 305-7.

15. Eliasson A, Gordon AM, Forssberg H. Impaired anticipatory control of isometric forces during grasping by children with cerebral palsy. Dev Med Child Neurol 1992;34:216-25.

16. Eliasson AC, Gordon AM, Forssberg H. Tactile control of isometric fingertip forces during grasping in children with cerebral palsy. Dev Med Child Neurol 1995;37:72-84.

17. Epelboim U, Steinman RM, Kowler E, et al. The function of visual search and memory in sequential looking tasks. Vision Res 1995;35:3401-22.

18. Fagard J. Manual strategies and interlimb coordination during reaching, grasping, and manipulating throughout the first year of life. In: Interlimb coordination: neural,

dynamical, and cognitive constraints. New York: Academic Press, 1994:439-60.

19. Feldman AG. Control of the length of the muscle. Biofizika 1974;19:749-53.

20. Feldman AG. Superposition of motor programs. I. Rhythmic forearm movements in man. Neuroscience 1980;5:81-90.

21. Feldman AG. Superposition of motor programs. II. Rapid forearm flexion in man. Neuroscience 1980;5:91-5.

22. Forssberg H, Eliasson AC, Kinoshita H, Westling G, Johansson RS. Development of human precision grip. IV. Tactile adaptation of isometric finger forces to the frictional condition. Exp Brain Res 1995;104:323-30.

23. Forssberg H, Nashner LM. Ontogenetic development of postural control in man: adaptation to altered support and visual conditions during stance. Neuroscience 1982;2:545-52.

24. Frank JS, Earl M. Coordination of posture and movement. Phys Ther 1990;70:855-63.

25. Friedli WG, Cohen L, Hallett M, Stanhope S, Simon SR. Postural adjustments associated with rapid voluntary arm movements. II. Biomechanical analysis. J Neurol Neurosurg Psychiatry 1988;51:232-43.

26. Gandevia SC, Burke D. Does the nervous system depend on kinesthetic information to control natural limb movements? Behav Brain Sci 1992;15:614-32.

27. Georgopoulos AP, Grillner S. Visuomotor coordination in reaching and locomotion. Science 1989;245:1209-10.

28. Ghilardi MF, Gordon J, Ghez C. Learning a visuomotor transformation in a local area of work space produces directional biases in other areas. J Neurophysiol 1995;73:2535-9.

29. Glencross DJ, Piek JP, Barrett NC. The coordination of bimanual synchronous and alternating tapping sequences. J Motor Behav 1995;27:3-15.

30. Gomi H, Kawato M. Equilibrium-point control hypothesis examined by measured arm stiffness during multijoint movement. Science 1996;272:117-9.

31. Goodwin GM, McCloskey DI, Matthews PBC. The contribution of muscle afferents to kinaesthesia shown by vibration induced illusions of movement and by effects of paralysing joint afferents. Brain 1972;95:705-48.

32. Gordon AM, Forssberg H, Iwasaki N. Formation and lateralization of internal representations underlying motor commands during precision grip. Neuropsychologia 1994;32:555-67.

33. Gordon J, Ghilardi MF, Cooper SE, Ghez C. Accuracy of planar reaching movements. II. Systematic extent errors resulting from inertial anisotropy. Exp Brain Res 1994;99:112-30.

34. Gordon J, Ghilardi MF, Ghez C. Accuracy of planar reaching movements I. Independence of direction and extent variability. Exp Brain Res 1994;99:97-111.

35. Gordon J, Ghilardi MF, Ghez C. Impairments of reaching movements in patients without proprioception. I. Spatial errors. J Neurophysiol 1995;73:347-60.

36. Guitton D. Control of eye-head coordination during orienting gaze shifts. Trends Neurosci 1993;16:214-8.

37. Hirschfeld H, Forssberg H. Development of anticipatory postural adjustments during locomotion in children. J Neurophysiol 1992;68:542-50.

38. Hirschfeld H, Forssberg H. Epigenetic development of postural responses for sitting during infancy. Exp Brain Res 1994;97:528-40.

39. Hirschfeld H, Forssberg H. Phase-dependent modulations of anticipatory postural activity during human locomotion. J Neurophysiol 1991;66:12-9.

40. Horak FB, Diener HC. Cerebellar control of postural scaling and central set in stance. J Neurophysiol 1994;72:479-93.

41. Horak FB, Diener HC, Nashner LM. Influence of central set on human postural responses. J Neurophysiol 1989;62:841-53.

42. Hubel D, Wiesel T. Receptive fields, binocular interaction and functional architecture in the cat's visual cortex. J Physiol (Lond) 1962;160:106-54.

43. Jeannerod M. A neurophysiological model for the directional coding of reaching movements. In: Paillard J, ed. Brain and space. Oxford: Oxford University Press, 1991:49-69.

44. Jeannerod M. The neural and behavioural organization of goal-directed movements. Oxford: Oxford Science Publications, 1990.

45. Jones EG. Connectivity of the primate sensory-motor cortex. In: Jones EG, Peters A, eds. Cerebral cortex. New York: Plenum Press, 1986:113-83.

46. Kalaska JF, Crammond DJ. Cerebral cortical mechanisms of reaching movements. Science 1992;255:1517-23.

47. Kandel ER, Schwartz JH, Jessell TM. Principles of neural science, 3rd ed. Norwalk: Appleton & Lange, 1991.

48. Kawano K, Shidara M. Information representation by Purkinje cells in the cerebellum during ocular following responses. Neurosci Res 1994;21:13-7.

49. Kawashima R, Roland PE, O'Sullivan BT. Fields in human motor areas involved in preparation for reaching, actual reaching, and visuomotor learning: a positron emission tomography study. J Neurosci 1994;14:3462-74.

50. Keele SW, Posner MI. Processing of visual feedback in rapid movements. J Exp Psychol 1968;77:155-8.

51. Kocsis JD. Competition in the synaptic marketplace: activity is important. Neuroscientist 1995;1:185-7.

52. Kunzle H. Cortico-cortical efferents of primary motor and somatosensory regions of the cerebral cortex in Macaca fascicularis. Neuroscience 1978;3:25-39.

53. Latash ML. Control of human movement. Champaign: Human Kinetics, 1993.

54. Le Vay S, Wiesel TN, Hubel DH. The development of ocular dominance columns in normal and visually deprived monkeys. J Comp Neurol 1980;191:1-51.

55. Leonard CT. Motor behavior and neural changes following perinatal and adult-onset brain damage: implica-

tions for therapeutic interventions. Phys Ther 1994;74:753-67.

56. Liu CN, Chambers WW. An experimental study of the cortico-spinal system in the monkey (Macaca mulatta). The spinal pathway and pre-terminal distribution of degenerating fibers following discrete lesions of the pre- and postcentral gyri and bulbar pyramid. J Comp Neurol 1964;123:257-84.

57. Livingstone M, Hubel D. Segregation of form, color, movement, and depth: anatomy, physiology, and perception. Science 1988;240:740.

58. Marsden CD, Merton PA, Morton HB. Anticipatory postural responses in the human subject. J Physiol (Lond) 1977;275:47-8.

59. Massion J. Postural changes accompanying voluntary movements. Normal and pathological aspects. Human Neurobiol 1984;2:261-7.

60. Mazevet D, Pierrot-Deseilligny E. Pattern of descending excitation of presumed propriospinal neurones at the onset of voluntary movement in humans. Acta Physiol Scand 1994;150:27-38.

61. McCarthy G, Spicer M, Adrignolo A, Luby M, Gore J, Allison T. Brain activation associated with visual motion studied by functional magnetic resonance imaging in humans. Human Brain Mapping 1995;2:234-43.

62. McCloskey DI, Prochazka A. The role of sensory information in the guidance of voluntary movement: reflections on symposium held at the Twenty-Second Annual Meeting of the Society of Neuroscience. Somatosens Mot Res 1994;11:69-76.

63. Nashner LM, Forssberg H. Phase-dependent organization of postural adjustments associated with arm movements while walking. J Neurophysiol 1986;55:1382-94.

64. Oda S, Moritani T. Maximal isometric force and neural activity during bilateral and unilateral elbow flexion in humans. Eur J Appl Physiol 1994;69:240-3.

65. Ohtsuka K, Noda H. Discharge properties of Purkinje cells in the oculomotor vermis during visually guided saccades in the macaque monkey. J Neurophysiol 1995;74:1828-40.

66. Pal'tsev YI, El'ner AM. Preparatory and compensatory period during voluntary movement in patients with involvement of the brain of different localization. Biofizika 1967;12:142-7.

67. Patla AE, Rietdyk S, Martin C, Prentice S. Locomotor patterns of the leading and the trailing limbs as solid and fragile obstacles are stepped over: some insights into the role of vision during locomotion. J Motor Behav 1996;28:35-47.

68. Prechtl HFR. Qualitative changes of spontaneous movements in preterm infants are a marker of neurological dysfunction. Early Hum Dev 1990;23:151-9.

69. Rochat P. Hand-mouth coordination in the newborn: morphology, determinants, and early development of a basic act. In: Savelsbergh GJP, ed. The development of coordination in infancy. Amsterdam: Elsevier, 1992.

70. Roll JP, Roll R. From eye to foot: a proprioceptive chain involved in postural control. In: Amblard B, Berthoz A, Clarac F, eds. Posture and gait: development, adaptation and modulation. Amsterdam: Elsevier, 1988:155-64.

71. Rossetti Y, Tadary B, Prablanc C. Optimal contributions of head and eye positions to spatial accuracy in man tested by visually directed pointing. Exp Brain Res 1994;97:487-96.

72. Scholz JP, Kelso JAS. A quantitative approach to understanding the formation and change of coordinated movement patterns. J Motor Behav 1989;21:122-44.

73. Shidara M, Kawano K, Gomi H, Kawato M. Inverse-dynamics model eye movement control by Purkinje cells in the cerebellum. Nature 1993;365:50-2.

74. Traub MM, Rothwell JC, Marsden CD. Anticipatory postural reflexes in Parkinson's disease and other akinetic-rigid syndromes and in cerebellar ataxia. Brain 1980;103:393-412.

75. van der meer ALH, van der Weel FR, Lee DN. The functional significance of arm movements in neonates. Science 1995;267:693-5.

76. Wessberg J, Vallbo AB. Human muscle spindle afferent activity in relation to visual control in precision finger movements. J Physiol (Lond) 1995;482:225-33.

77. Westerga J, Gramsbergen A. The effect of early movement restriction: an EMG study in the rat. Behav Brain Res 1993;59:205-9.

78. Wiesendanger M, Wicki U, Rouiller E. Are there unifying structures in the brain responsible for interlimb coordination? In: Swinnen S, Hever H, Massion J, Caesar P, eds. Interlimb coordination: neural, dynamical, and cognitive constraints. New York: Academic Press, 1994:179-207.

79. Won J, Hogan N. Stability properties of human reaching movements. Exp Brain Res 1995;107:125-36.

The Neuroscience of Motor Learning

An Introduction to Motor Learning Concepts
Neural Structures Involved in Motor Learning
The Physiology of Motor Learning
Changes Within the Nervous System Induced by Training
Developmental Plasticity and Adult Motor Learning
Factors That Influence and Enhance Motor Learning
Motor Learning After Brain Damage

Motor learning is not a term that represents a singular entity. Motor learning involves perception and transferring perceptions into actions and skilled behaviors.[49] Motor learning also involves sensory processing, motor control, motor skill acquisition, the ability to perform the skill during various conditions, and retention/memory of the acquired skill. Performance of a skill is different from learning, and learning is different from memory. Performance of a skill typically refers to motor control issues: the execution of the task. Motor learning is modification of the behavior by experience. Memory is the retention of these modifications. Designing experiments that assess each of these processes separately is an ongoing challenge for researchers.

■ AN INTRODUCTION TO MOTOR LEARNING CONCEPTS
Definitions
Various types of motor learning are recognized: adaptive, conditioned-associative, nonassociative, and skill learning. *Adaptation* refers to an individual's ability to modify a motor output in response to a changing sensory input. This can be via conscious effort or, in many cases, is carried out automatically and without conscious effort via reflex pathways in the spinal cord and brain stem. Modification of the vestibulo-ocular reflex (VOR) is a good example of adaptive learning. The VOR integrates eye and head movements to maintain visual fixation on an object. Eye movements are related to head movements. The magnitude and direction of eye movements depend on resting head position, speed of head movement, and relation of the eyes to the object.[58] The ability of the VOR to respond rapidly to these varying conditions reflects adaptive learning. *Conditioned-associative responses* are a type of learning that can be considered adaptive and automatic. Pavlov's dogs learned to associate the ringing of a bell to being fed and were thus conditioned to salivate to the ringing of a bell.

Conditioned responses can also be *nonassociative.* Nonassociative learning involves habituation or sensitization to repetitive stimuli. Suppression of a response to a stimulus is referred to as *habituation* and accentuation of a response to a stimulus (usually associated with pain) is referred to as *sensitization.* Habituation and sensitization appear to involve different neural mechanisms. In fact, all the types of learning presented thus far involve a wide array of shared and dissimilar mechanisms. And, they all contribute to the type of motor learning that will be the main focus of this chapter; motor skill learning. *Motor skill learning* is the formation of new or novel movement sequences to gain speed, precision, accuracy, and efficiency in a task.[35] It is the most complex of the types of motor learning and in all likelihood involves, to various degrees, some of the same mechanisms associated with the other types of learning. However, additional mechanisms and neural structures are called into play whenever you seek to acquire and retain a new skill.

Evidence suggests that acquiring a motor skill (learning) and retaining that skill (memory) are two different processes involving different neural mechanisms.[77] The enhanced motor performance that accompanies practice does not necessarily represent motor learning or transfer to memory. Researchers have developed transfer tests that distinguish between performance enhancement and motor learning. With practice you might be able to enhance a motor skill, such as tapping your fingers in a certain rhythm or sequence, but if you cannot use this new sequence in the context of a new skill or at a future date, you have not retained or learned the skill. To add further to the complexity, motor skill learning appears to occur in phases, with each phase being associated with a different neural process.

Motor skill learning can be divided into three phases:[40]

1. The early-cognitive phase,
2. The intermediate phase, and
3. The late-autonomous phase.

At this point, take time to reflect on a motor skill you have acquired recently. Think about the phases you went through to master the skill. Initially, it took quite a bit of concentration for you to perform the task. No one gets on a snowboard, surfboard, or windsurfer the first time and experiences the exhilaration of speed and weightlessness. The beginner typically talks himself through the skills necessary to maintain an upright posture. You either recall what your instructor told you or what you read in a book. This represents the cognitive phase of learning. This phase is similar to what psychologists refer to as declarative learning. *Declarative learning* deals with concepts and facts that usually can be expressed and communicated consciously. Declarative learning is distinct from procedural learning. *Procedural learning*, of which motor skill acquisition is a part, refers to learned behaviors or habits that are performed automatically without excessive mental concentration. Various authors and texts use different terms to distinguish between these two types of learning (Table 7-1).

Brain scanning techniques have indicated that during the early-cognitive phase of motor skill acquisition, the language centers of the brain (located primarily in the frontal, temporal, and parietal lobes) are active.[71,121] These are the same areas that are active during declarative learning.[80] Cortical area 2, a somatosensory area, is also active during the early stages of learning, but it is not as active once a movement sequence is learned.[4] Area 2 relays sensory information to motor areas of the brain.

The intermediate phase of motor learning reflects a trial-and-error period. During this time you attempt different strategies and compare your results. "What happens if I edge my board a little more?" "What happens if I weight my back foot a bit more?" Based on your success or failure, you either adopt or reject the strategy. During this phase of learning, the motor and sensorimotor association areas of the brain appear to be selectively stimulated.[55,121]

Once you have progressed through the rites of passage known as the cognitive and intermediate phases, you enter "the zone," "the sweet spot," or, to put it more scientifically, the late-autonomous phase. This is the hallmark of motor skill mastery. Within this realm you are no longer burdened with excessive ver-

TABLE 7-1 Different terms used to indicate two types of memory

Declarative	Procedural
Fact memory	Skill memory
Memory	Habit
Explicit	Implicit
Knowing that	Knowing how
Cognitive mediation	Semantic
Conscious recollection	Skills
Elaboration	Integration
Autobiographical memory	Perceptual memory
Representational memory	Dispositional memory
Vertical association	Horizontal association
Locale	Taxon
Episodic	Semantic
Working	Reference

From Squire LR. Memory and brain. New York: Oxford University Press, 1987.

bal processing and mental concentration. You no longer need to try various strategies; you and your body know what works. Now, the more you practice, the more fluid you become. Now it doesn't matter what the snow, surf, or wind conditions might be. You are able to adapt, compensate, and react without undue conscious effort. Your associative brain areas are left to contemplate other matters, because now brain activity that accompanies performance of a learned movement skill is shifted elsewhere, such as the basal ganglia.[71,121]

Theories of motor learning

This chapter deals with the neuroscience of motor learning. It will be helpful for you to put this basic science information in context with previously established theories of motor learning. Most of these theories have been derived from behavioral research. The theories are many and reflect overlap as well as divergence. They include Adam's Closed Loop Model, Schmidt's Schema Model, Anderson's Act Model, Mackay's Node Structure, Dynamic Systems, and Newell's Theory. These theories are succinctly reviewed in "Motor Control: Theory and Practice Applications" by Shumway-Cook and Woollacott,[122], "Handbook of Research On Sport Psychology" by Singer, Murphey, and Tennant,[123] and "Motor Control and Learning" by Schmidt.[120] I encourage you to refer to these references and attempt to synthesize these theories with the basic science data to be presented subsequently in this chapter.

Behavioral theories provide a framework for the development of testable questions regarding the mechanisms that contribute to motor learning. As data continue to be collected, some of the theories will need to be modified or dropped entirely in favor of others that best fit the data. Continuing to develop theories of motor learning is important. Testable theories provide scientists with a broad framework within which to develop specific experiments. Testable theories also have the potential to provide educators, therapists, and trainers with a set of generalized concepts that can be applied to their specific needs.

Plasticity

Whoever first coined the term *plastic* with regard to brain function must have been a linguist. Engineers and polymer chemists have very precise definitions for the term, but forget these for a moment and think of the adjectives you associate with the word. My cerebral thesaurus conjures up "pliable," "moldable," and "malleable." When I think of the physical characteristics of plastic, I imagine a substance that is vulnerable to changes in the environment. If it is cold, plastic becomes brittle; if it is warm, I can mold it. Older plastic seemingly undergoes some chemical metamorphosis such that it is less malleable than when new. These characteristics, with some obvious modifications, can be applied to the "plastic" changes that occur within the nervous system during learning.

The nervous system is not a static structure. Rather, it is continuously being reshaped according to environmental needs and demands. Plasticity is present throughout life, but never equals that which is available to the younger animal. Plasticity is somewhat of a generic term and is used to encompass the many and multifarious mechanisms associated with learning, development, and recovery from damage to the nervous system. Subsequent sections of this chapter discuss plasticity as it relates to these events. As you will read, the neural mechanisms you use to learn to snowboard might not be so different from those you used to learn how to walk. Furthermore, the processes involved in recovery from brain damage might also share some of these same mechanisms. Each type of learning has some unique characteristics. As neuroscientists learn more about the nuances associated with different types of neural plasticity, there is hope that the mechanisms involved can be enhanced.

As is typical of this type of wishful thinking, it is much easier said than done. As you have already read, motor learning is not a singular entity and does not occur within a single region of the nervous system. So, one of the first daunting tasks facing neuroscientists is the identification of structures within the nervous system that are involved with the various types of motor learning. Each structure or pathway might use its own unique molecular mechanism to accomplish its specified task. Subsequent sections of this chapter introduce some of the neural structures and the physiology involved in motor skill learning.

■ NEURAL STRUCTURES INVOLVED IN MOTOR LEARNING

Traditionally, experiments that attempted to identify neural structures associated with motor learning used neurophysiological recordings of cell activity while a nonhuman animal performed a motor task. These types of experiments remain crucial to our understanding of brain function. In recent years, however, we have seen an explosion of human brain imaging studies. Imaging techniques (reviewed in Chapter 4) permit scientists to identify the areas of the brain that are active in fully conscious humans while they perform a variety of tasks. Imaging techniques do not record neural activity, but rather changes in blood flow or metabolism of brain regions.

The generalizations to follow make use of results obtained by neurophysiological and scanning methods. The neurophysiological methods are far more precise than scanning methods and provide a better understanding of the underlying mechanisms that produce the changes in cerebral activations. These techniques are limited, however, because they cannot be used with humans and because they examine single cell function and not overall brain activity.

Scanning techniques are limited in both spatial and temporal resolution (i.e., neighboring structures cannot always be quantitatively differentiated in their level of activation, and scans have a temporal delay from performance of the task to visualization of the scan). Despite these limitations, brain imaging techniques provide a window by which we can observe the human brain at work.

There is no singular area within the brain that controls all aspects of learning. For instance, clearly the areas of the brain that are involved with the procedural learning of some motor tasks are distinctly different from those engaged during declarative learning. As introduced earlier, the actual execution or performance of a motor task and the various phases of motor learning involve different structures. Also, remember that humans are not a very homogeneous group. Individuals learn at different rates and use different strategies to perform a skill. Group analysis of scans or other techniques might possibly obscure important individual differences.[119] This is perhaps a contributing factor to the disparities that exist in the literature pertaining to motor learning. With these caveats in mind, what follows are brief, generalized summaries of what has been hypothesized to be aspects of motor learning attributed to a given neural structure.

Declarative vs. procedural memory

Declarative (semantic) memory involves the acquisition of conceptual and factual knowledge. Procedural memory allows us to learn new motor skills and acquire habits.[115] Procedural memory can be further subdivided into adaptive responses, conditioned responses, and skilled movements.[35] Declarative and procedural memory appear to be separate and parallel learning systems.[78]

The hippocampus, a part of the archicortex deeply embedded within the medial temporal lobe, has long been known to be involved with declarative memory. Bilateral damage to the hippocampus results in a loss in the ability to store new memories. However, this damage does not appear to impair the ability to recall old memories.[129] The hippocampus, therefore, is involved with information storage, but it is not the storage site for memory. Memory storage probably occurs at various sites within the brain.[66] In contrast to the impairments in declarative memory processes that occur after hippocampal damage, motor learning does not seem to be affected.[89] Data from positron emission tomographic studies show that areas of the brain that are activated by declarative memory do not change activation levels during procedural learning.[121] Areas of the brain that are typically activated during declarative memory skills include the hippocampus, medial temporal cortex, mediodorsal thalamus, and mammillary bodies (all of which are part of the limbic system). Procedural learning and task performance typically involve the sensorimotor cortex, supplementary motor cortex, premotor cortex, cerebellum, various parietal regions, prefrontal cortex, and basal ganglia. As discussed in Chapter 4, however, motor tasks that involve spatial memory involve the hippocampus and posterior parietal regions. The distinctions between the two types of learning are not always clear, and neither are the patterns of cortical activations.

The role of afferent information

Many motor learning theories emphasize the role of sensory information in the acquisition of motor skills (e.g., Adams' Closed Loop Theory, Schmidt's Schema Theory). Many rehabilitation techniques make use of the sensory system to initiate and guide movement. It makes sense. We learn by trial and error. Without sensory feedback, how would we know whether our motor output achieved the desired goal? The brain apparently makes use of the sensory information generated by our movements, as indicated by the increase in neural activity within the sensory areas of the brain during the initial learning of a motor skill.[121]

Lesioning the dorsal roots of animals (thereby eliminating all peripheral sensory input of the lesioned extremity) results in impairments in the ability to learn new movements.[14] Well-trained movements that were learned before the lesioning, however, are retained. Individuals with dense peripheral neuropathies are capable of learning, but the time course is protracted and they substitute other sensory systems (e.g., vision) to compensate for the loss of proprioception and other sensations.[47,53,111] Drs. Rothwell and Marsden, from Great Britain, report an interesting and revealing anecdotal story about one of their experimental subjects with a large fiber peripheral neuropathy.[111] This subject had driven an old, standard-shift car for many years, and continued to do so successfully even as his neuropathy progressed to the degree that he lost all proprioception and deep tendon reflexes. He was unable, however, to learn to drive a new vehicle. Unfortunately, he was unable to accommodate to the subtle changes in motor output necessary to drive an unfamiliar vehicle. This story provides a graphic example of the ability to carry out previously learned motor programs independent of sensory feedback. It also illustrates the problems inherent in trying to learn new motor skills, no matter how closely related they are to previously learned ones. Afferent input appears to regulate and adapt movement.[98]

Given these findings, you would expect that peripheral receptor activity and afferent sensory feedback might change during the acquisition of a motor skill. Drs. Prochazka and Hulliger, from Edmonton and

Calgary, Canada, respectively, have shown that gamma motor neuron activity depends on the type of motor task being performed.[101] Other investigators, however, have reported that muscle spindle activity does not change with the various stages of learning involved in adapting a motor response to an imposed movement.[130] Furthermore, other researchers have shown that the learning of fast, sequential hand movements can occur independently of somatosensory feedback.[121]

These apparently disparate findings might not be as contradictory as they appear at first glance. Methodologies must be examined closely when comparing studies. The role of afferent input might change based on the type of learning taking place and the sensory modality involved (e.g., visually guided movements vs. nonvisually guided movements, or fast vs. slow movements). Perhaps the way the nervous system makes use of sensory information might also change depending on a particular stage of the learning process. The fact that activity within parietal cortical areas decreases with learning[121] provides some indirect evidence for this idea. Possible also, is that afferent discharge doesn't change during motor learning, but the integration of the convergent, multifarious sensory input within the central nervous system (CNS) does. It is also possible that the CNS might place greater emphasis on certain sensory signals during different stages of learning even if the actual output of the peripheral receptor does not change.

Spinal cord adaptability associated with motor learning

Learning is not all in your head. Strong evidence indicates that changes occurring within the spinal cord contribute to our success or failures as athletes, musicians, and craftsmen. Perhaps I slightly overstate the point, because the work identifying changes in the spinal cord associated with motor learning has only involved rats and monkeys. Nonetheless, the case is a strong one, and indirect evidence already exists that the same processes occur in humans.[140]

Dr. Jonathan Wolpaw and his group from Albany, N.Y., have spent innumerable hours training rats and monkeys, via operant conditioning, to upregulate or downregulate their H-reflexes. The H-reflex reflects the summation of excitatory and inhibitory influences on motor neurons. It has been referred to as the electrical analog of the spinal stretch reflex. An increase in H-reflexes is synonymous with relative excitability (depolarization) of the motor neuron pool, and a decrease in H-reflexes reflects inhibition (hyperpolarization) of the pool. Monkeys, rats, and humans demonstrate the ability to upregulate or downregulate these reflexes.[27,140,141] With nonhuman animals, Dr. Wolpaw has demonstrated physiological and morphological changes in the involved spinal cord circuitry that are associated with the learning of this regulation.[24,25,39] The spinal cord motor neurons of the animals that had learned to downregulate their reflexes had a shift away from action potential threshold, so that an increase in excitatory input was needed for these neurons to reach threshold.[24] The physiological picture was not as clear for the upregulated animals,[25] but a morphological analysis of the motor neurons of these animals revealed fewer and smaller inhibitory synaptic terminals.[39] These results clearly demonstrate that plastic changes in the spinal cord accompany conditioned learning. Interestingly, and confoundingly, up- and downregulation of spinal reflexes do not appear to involve similar mechanisms.[25] Whether similar plastic changes occur in the human and accompany other forms of procedural learning remains to be determined. For instance, skilled learning (unlike the conditioned responses of Wolpaw's monkeys) involves a conscious effort on our part. Skilled learning is typically associated with higher brain functions—which brings us to the next phase of our discussion, plastic changes occurring within the cerebral cortex associated with learning.

The cerebral cortex

It is logical to assume that the cerebral cortex has something to do with motor learning. In fact, the consensus is growing that the cerebral cortex is the primary location of declarative and procedural memory.[87] Because we are discussing motor behaviors, what better place to begin our investigations than the motor cortex?

Neurons within the primary motor cortex (MI) fire before and during movement.[2,3,100] Therefore, they appear to be involved with the preparation and execution of movement. Neural activation patterns within the MI encode force and direction.[45,46] The MI is involved in spatial transformations (i.e., matching and transferring sensory perceptions to motor acts), trajectory control, and the modulation of brain stem and spinal cord activity.[125] Refer to Chapter 4 for additional information regarding the functioning of the motor cortex. The function that most concerns us now is its possible role in motor learning and memory.

Certain physiological mechanisms have been identified as being involved with learning:[35]

1. activity-dependent synaptic plasticity,
2. long-term potentiation,
3. changes in the excitability of the postsynaptic neuron, and
4. growth of new connections.

These mechanisms are discussed later in this chapter. What is important for the present discussion is that neurons within the MI exhibit these properties.

Brain scanning studies have indicated plastic changes in the activation of the MI during the learning of a motor skill.[55,71,75,121] During early stages of learning, widespread activation of the MI becomes more focused. Activity within the cerebellum and prefrontal cortex, both of which project to the MI, also decreases during early learning. It is possible, therefore, that the decrease in MI activation might reflect a decrease in the inputs to the MI during this phase of learning.[71] During later stages of learning, a larger area of the MI becomes active. This later increase in activation can last for months and is consistent with a long-term, experience-dependent reorganization of the MI. Some have argued that these later changes in MI activation patterns reflect circuitry devoted to memory and not to performance execution.[75] MI connectivity provides some clues as to how it might contribute toward transferring a motor skill into a motor memory.

The MI is organized into vertical and horizontal circuits. Inputs coming from outside the MI (e.g., thalamus and other cortical areas such as frontal, parietal, and premotor areas) form vertical pathways. Vertical columns are composed of vertical pathways. These columns are interconnected by horizontal projections. Horizontal projections travel throughout the MI and form extensive connections. Many of these projections connect synergistic muscle groups.[35,62] The majority of these horizontal projections originate in layer V of the cortex. This is the site of pyramidal cells that also form the bulk of MI projections to the brain stem, spinal cord, and other cortical areas. Based on connectivity alone, one can visualize how this type of organization can contribute to a motor memory and execution of this memory.

Visualize yourself learning a new motor skill. As you gain proficiency in the skill, you will most likely use synergists in a very controlled way. You will also begin to activate muscles proactively to stabilize your posture before you activate the primary movers. You might embellish the movement a bit to add drama and flair to your performance. All of these activities require additional neural circuitry. Through practice, long-term changes occur within the organization of this circuitry such that all it takes is activation of one part of the circuit to begin the cascade of activity that manifests as graceful, effortless movement.

Electrophysiological studies provide support for changes in the organization of movement control during the acquisition of a motor skill.[95] These changes include but are not limited to the MI. Some researchers have proposed that a type of cortical engram of movement develops for motor memory.[87] A *cortical engram* is a widely distributed group of neurons comprising multiple smaller functional groupings. Each engram overlaps with the others and can influence other engrams. Memory develops over time and is represented not by the activity of single cells or single circuits, but rather by cell assemblies. These assemblies are plastic and are modified by experience. *Cell assemblies* consist of cells that tend to fire synchronously during a movement. The various parts of the assembly are linked. The linkages are strengthened, via physiological mechanisms, through repetition.[87]

The MI has a role to play in transferring the engram's message into an executable motor act. It contributes to the learning of new movement sequences that influence our attainment of precision, speed, accuracy, and efficiency.[35] Also, cells within the MI activate differently during a memorized task vs. a nonmemorized task.[125] But, what of the other areas of the cerebral cortex? What might they contribute to motor learning, and how do they interact with MI circuitry? Engrams or cell assemblies are not limited to the MI.

The sensorimotor cortices are intimately involved with receiving sensory information and transferring its perceptions to other cortical areas including the premotor and motor cortices. The primary somatosensory area (SI) is extremely plastic, demonstrating considerable reorganization after amputations, deafferentations,[76,85,86] and sensory stimulation.[87,132] These plastic changes will be discussed later in this chapter in the section dealing with changes induced by training. Researchers generally agree that parietal (sensory) areas are active during the learning of a new complex motor task.[71,121] These same studies are a bit more contradictory with regard to the role of sensory areas during fast, automatic movement. The apparent discrepancies might be related to performance of a task rather than to a difference in the role of parietal areas in learning. Studies that indicate decreased activations in parietal areas with automatic movements might not have taken into account the fact that fast movements are less reliant on sensory feedback for their control, and hence would have less of a requirement for activation of cortical sensory areas. With regard to the learning of complex, sensory-dependent movements, the parietal areas of the brain appear to work in conjunction with the thalamus and motor areas of the brain in a process referred to as conditioned (associative) long-term potentiation. *Long-term potentiation* (LTP) is a physiological mechanism whereby afferent input induces long-term changes in the excitability of the pathway involving the stimulated axons and their postsynaptic cells. (Refer to Chapter 3 for a review of LTP. LTP is also discussed in the section of this chapter devoted to the physiology of motor learning.) Conditioned LTP is a change in the excitability of a pathway that depends on repetitive input from more than one afferent system.[35]

One of the mechanisms by which sensory areas of the brain contribute to motor learning might involve conditioned LTP. The MI receives projections from the somatosensory cortex and from the ventrolateral nucleus of the thalamus. Projections from the thalamus cannot cause LTP in the MI. Together with input from the sensory cortex, however, thalamic input can cause LTP in MI circuitry. Interestingly, after repeated and concomitant stimulations to the sensory cortex and the thalamus, input from the thalamus alone can induce LTP in the MI.[4] Removal of area 2 (sensory cortex) before learning a motor skill results in the failure of thalamic stimulation to induce LTP in the MI and in deficits in motor learning.[4] This provides further evidence that sensory areas in the brain are necessary for motor learning and is consistent with the mechanism involving conditioned LTP.

Learning that depends on sensory feedback might be dependent on input from the sensory cortex and from the thalamus (to meet the requirements of conditioned LTP). Once learning takes place, no sensory feedback is necessary (e.g., playing the piano), and so activity in the parietal areas lessens and only input from the thalamus is necessary to activate appropriate circuitry in the MI.[4] This concept is consistent with brain scanning data that have shown decreases in activation of parietal areas and increased activation in deeper cortical structures (including the thalamus) during later stages of learning. Procedural learning also appears to involve other cortical areas in addition to the sensorimotor cortex.

The premotor (PM) and supplementary motor (SMA) areas also appear to contribute to motor learning. They both receive large inputs from somatosensory areas. The PM appears to be involved with the learning of new movement sequences. It is especially important to movements that are guided by external sensory cues.[71] The PM might function very similarly to the MI during the learning of a visuospatial task.[125] The SMA is preferentially activated during the performance of a prelearned sequence. This is typically a movement that is less reliant on external sensory cues.

Prefrontal (PF) areas are active during the initial phases of learning and much less so during automatic movements. Regardless of whether the movement involves the right or left extremities, the right hemisphere demonstrates more activation than the left hemisphere.[71] Perhaps this is because learning a new task usually involves spatial processing, a function attributed to right PF lobe activity.

Similar to the PF areas, the anterior cingulate gyrus is active during new learning but not during automatic movements. In fact, it tends to be active whenever the PF areas are active.[71] The PF areas and the cingulate gyrus share rich interconnectivity and appear to be important for directed attention and motivational aspects of motor learning.[119] The cingulate gyrus also has input to the forelimb area of the MI.[119]

The cerebellum

Earlier in this book I referred to the cerebellum as enigmatic. Nowhere is this characteristic more apparent than during discussions of the cerebellum's possible role in motor learning. The cerebellum is intimately involved with the control of movement. It has also been hypothesized that the cerebellum influences and modulates sensory input to various parts of the CNS.[18,42] The cerebellum is involved in the temporal sequencing of movement and the coordination of complex, multijoint movements. Most of the studies that have attempted to define the cerebellum's role in motor learning have stressed its role in reflex adaptation. Adaptation of the VOR has been shown to involve cerebellar pathways.[68,71] The controversy begins regarding its possible role in classical conditioning. Some studies have clearly implicated the cerebellum as a storage site for conditioned responses,[68,107] whereas others have challenged this view.[15,16] The debate really gets heated when discussing the cerebellum's potential contribution to the learning of voluntary skilled movements.

Dr. W. Thomas Thach, who has done much to define the cerebellum's role in motor control, provides a good review of the differing viewpoints.[127] Those who contend that the cerebellum plays a role in the adaptation and acquisition of movement point to experiments that have shown a correlation between cerebellar cell activity and learning, the role of the cerebellum in detecting errors in performance, and the impairments in adaptive learning experienced by patients with cerebellar damage.

Those who question a direct role for the cerebellum in skilled motor learning emphasize that learning is distributed throughout the nervous system, depends on the task and strategy used, and is not localized to the cerebellum. These investigators point to experiments that have shown that some types of motor learning that have been attributed to the cerebellum can be accomplished by brain stem structures in the absence of cerebellar input. Data have also not indicated that the cerebellum is necessary for memory storage. Furthermore, studies of patients with lesions do not add much insight into actual learning because results are so clouded by impairments in performance.

I think the following two quotes are representative of the present state of an understanding/agreement regarding cerebellar contributions to motor learning:

> "Purkinje cells...[have] behaved in a manner consistent with the Marr-Albus theory* of motor learning."[127] (*The Marr-Albus theory contends that previous patterns of movement and the acquisition of new ones is a cerebellar function)

> "It is concluded that there is no convincing evidence, at this time, to support the view that a long-term modification of Purkinje cell activity is either the basis of motor learning or an authentic mechanism of cerebellar function."[83]

I encourage you to read the related references listed at the end of this chapter and form your own opinion. It does appear that the cerebellum is involved in adaptive learning, but that this type of learning is not restricted to the cerebellum. In fact, if agreement exists anywhere in the cerebellar/motor learning literature, it is that the learning of complex, voluntary skilled motor behaviors involves multiple sites within the nervous system. The relative contribution of the cerebellum to this process remains to be determined.

The basal ganglia and striatal pathways

The basal ganglia and their associated pathways are intimately involved with motor control. Similar to the cerebellum, the basal ganglia receive afferent projections from the sensorimotor cortex. Unlike the cerebellum, however, the input from the cortex to the basal ganglia is not limited to sensorimotor areas. The basal ganglia receive input from all areas of the cerebral cortex.[32] There is a massive convergence of cortical afferents to a portion of the basal ganglia referred to as the *neostriatum* (caudate and putamen).[23,32] Unlike the cerebellum, whose efferent projections indirectly project back to the premotor and motor cortices, basal ganglia projections are more widespread and include associational motor areas. The basal ganglia, more than the cerebellum, appear to be involved in higher-order, cognitive aspects of motor control.[32]

The substantia nigra also has major inputs to the neostriatum.[78] Individuals with Parkinson's disease, a disorder primarily involving cells of the substantia nigra, exhibit deficits in procedural but not declarative learning.[55,78] These clinical findings, together with the known connectivity of the basal ganglia, clearly indicate involvement of the basal ganglia in motor learning.

The neostriatum is essential for motor learning and habit formation. The neostriatum is important not only for motor learning, but also for nonmotor tasks that require the formation of associations and tendencies.[112] Researchers have hypothesized that the putamen is involved in the transfer of a skill into memory and the performance of a prelearned movement.[71] As discussed previously in Chapter 2, the basal ganglia appear to be involved in the motivational aspects of learning a new task. Basal ganglia circuits and corticostriatal pathways appear to process information in parallel.[1] Whether certain aspects of motor learning or procedural memory storage are exclusive domains of the basal ganglia is unknown at this point.

Changes in structural activations associated with different motor learning phases

By now you have gained an appreciation for the fact that the various aspects of procedural learning—adaptive, conditioned, and skilled—involve different brain regions and different mechanisms. Involved regions also differ depending on the type of motor task being performed. Different regions also appear to be preferentially activated during early vs. later phases of learning a new motor skill (Fig. 7-1).

The areas of the brain that show the most activation during the actual performance of a motor skill involving eye-hand coordination are the sensorimotor cortex, the SMA, the PM, the associational parietal areas, and the anterior lobe of the cerebellum.[55,121]

During early acquisition of the skill, activation levels increase and then decrease in the parietal areas, thalamic nuclei, and the pars triangularis region of the inferior frontal cortex (part of Broca's speech area).[55,121] During early phases of motor learning, we appear to be reliant on the processing of sensory information and the sensory feedback that results from our motor performance. It also appears that we talk to ourselves during this phase of motor learning, as indicated by the activation of speech areas within the brain.

Motor skill acquisition can be said to have occurred when the task is carried out with increased accuracy, smoothness, and speed. During this phase the skill becomes automatic. The individual no longer has to devote a concentrated effort for successful completion of the task. This is reflected by changes in activation patterns during this phase of learning. The MI remains active during automatic skilled movements, but cortical association areas decrease in activity.[4,121] During this phase, cells within the putamen and globus pallidus (basal ganglia nuclei) increase their activity.[121] One of the more significant challenges for researchers in this area is designing experiments that manage to separate out areas of the nervous system that are involved in the actual performance of a task vs. those that are used during learning of that task. For instance, if an area of the brain shows increased activity after an experimental subject has learned a fast sequential finger sequence (such as is involved in keyboard use), is this related to learning of the task? Or, is the increased activity related to the fact that the individual is now moving his fingers with increased velocity, less muscle cocontraction, more synergist muscle activation, and increased accuracy? In fact, the

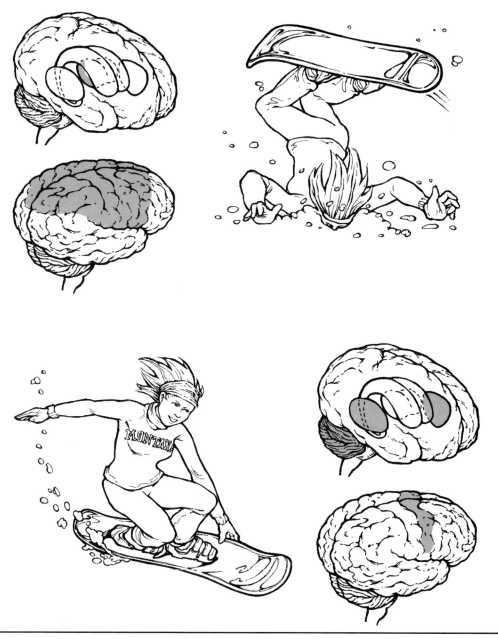

Fig. 7-1. Brain areas reported to be active during the early and late learning phases of a complex, multijoint movement. Early learning involves the primary sensorimotor cortex, sensorimotor association areas, supplementary motor cortex, premotor cortex, parietal areas, prefrontal areas, pars triangularis, and selected thalamic nuclei. During the performance of a learned skill, cortical activation decreases. The primary motor area continues to be active along with the cerebellum and striatum.

recognition of these technical problems has led to a considerable debate regarding how the brain learns a new motor skill.

This debate centers around the interpretation of the data presented in the preceding paragraphs. Brain mapping is an inexact science and data can be quantified and analyzed in various ways. What exactly does it mean when one brain area increases its activity during the learning of a task? Was the area involved in the performance of the task and subsequently increased its relative role once the task was learned? Or, was it uninvolved in the acquisition of the task and became involved only when procedural memory occurred?

Some researchers contend that the same circuits are used to perform and learn a movement.[1,15,55] Those who adhere to this viewpoint hypothesize that learning takes place by reinforcement of synaptic connectivity involved in the performance of the skill. The reinforcement and strengthening of synaptic contacts occurs through repetition of the skill.

Other experimental evidence and alternative interpretations indicate that performance and learning do not necessarily involve the same neural circuitry. Adherents to this viewpoint place emphasis on the widely varying activation patterns that accompany the various phases of motor learning. Initial learning involves limiting brain activation to those areas most intimately involved with the skill.[129] Later, additional cells and circuits from various structures are recruited into the network.[75,129] The relative roles of the different structures change with the different phases of motor learning.

Parallel processing and multiple representations of memory

Increasingly, motor programming theories of motor learning that are based on neural connectivity are being displaced by theories that emphasize physiology and process. Most motor programming theories take a connectionist view on things. For example, afferent information is conveyed to higher brain centers such as the cerebellum, where this information is used to correct ongoing movement. The cerebral cortex has the blueprint of the plan, which it has shared with the cerebellum. The cerebellum compares the plan with the afferent information and initiates the necessary corrections. As we repeat the behavior, association areas of the cortex and the cerebellum aren't needed as much, so the execution of the more automatic movement is transferred to other brain centers such as the basal ganglia. There, somehow, and in a specific location yet to be determined, these repeated motor acts are committed to memory.

Neurophysiological data have not been consistent with motor programming theories.[1] The literature indicates that procedural memory is not something that occurs in a specific location. The various types of motor learning and the various motor learning phases involve different neural structures to varying degrees. Almost certainly the system has overlap, with the relative contribution of each depending on the sensory modality involved, the task, or even the context of the task. Motor learning incorporates neural networks interconnected in such a way as to allow for parallel processing of information. Information is not stored in discrete locations, but rather in the gestalt of patterned activity. That is why multimodal imaging techniques (see Chapter 4) hold such great promise for opening up a window of understanding to processes of human memory. The patterns of neural activity are not fixed, but are incredibly variable. As you have read previously, cortical maps change depending on activity. But this is not all. Any given connection can vary in strength. Structural connectivity doesn't necessarily dictate the formation of procedural learning memories, but the physiology of that connectivity endows the nervous system with increased plasticity and variability. Physiological mechanisms associated with motor learning are the next topics to be considered.

■ THE PHYSIOLOGY OF MOTOR LEARNING
Synapse modification

Learning is a form of synaptic plasticity. Changes in synaptic efficacy are the physiological substrate for memory storage.[109] Memory mechanisms do not necessarily depend on structural changes, but rather on the strength of preexisting connections.[73] Adaptive and conditioned procedural learning does not depend

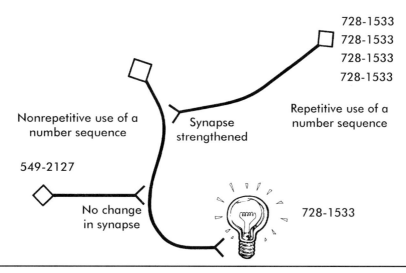

Fig. 7-2. Hypothetical example of the contribution of LTP to declarative memory. Repetitive stimuli of a neural pathway during the memorization of a series of numbers will strengthen the synapse, thus enhancing transmission along this pathway and making future recall of the number series easier.

on neurons specializing in memory. Rather, learning occurs as a result of synaptic changes in the neurons that were part of the sensorimotor pathway.[73] These changes either enhance or depress neural transmission. Short-term changes involve changes in neural transmission, whereas long-term changes involve changes in gene expression. The actual number of synapses changes over time and fluctuates based on the amount of activity within the pathway. The basic message here is that synapses are dynamic and subject to various influences that will strengthen or weaken their synaptic transmission. Some synapses are more susceptible to change than others. The synapses between sensory and motor neurons appear to be exceptionally vulnerable to activity-dependent ebbs and flows in strength.[67] The changes in the efficacy of synaptic neural transmission appear to be one of the primary ways the nervous system encodes memories.[103,109,126] Some of the mechanisms that contribute to synaptic plasticity have been discussed in Chapter 3 and will be reviewed again here in the context of motor learning.

Long-term potentiation and depression
LTP was first discovered in the hippocampus (for an interesting story on its discovery, see reference 7). LTP has now been found to exist in the cerebellum, motor cortex, and other CNS regions.[67] LTP induces enhanced neural transmission between the stimulated axon and its postsynaptic cell that can last for hours or weeks. It is a highly selective process. Regardless of how many synapses a neuron receives, only the synapse that is highly active, secondary to increased stimulation, will exhibit LTP and thus enhanced activity (Figs. 7-2 and 7-3). This contributes to selective memory, or why a particular input will have more of an affect on a target neuron than another typically less active one (spouses and significant others, please take note: there truly appear to be physiological reasons why some things are remembered and others are not).

LTP has two interesting properties. One is cooperativity and the other is associativity. Strong presynaptic stimulation may not always be sufficient to induce LTP. In some cases presynaptic stimulation must

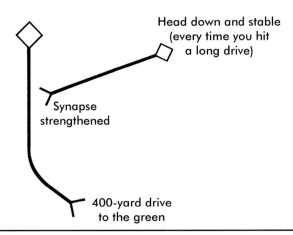

Fig. 7-3. Hypothetical example of the contribution of LTP to procedural memory of a golf swing. Motor sequences or postures that are habitually associated with successful performance of a skill are strengthened over time and become part of the movement engram.

be paired with depolarization of the postsynaptic neuron from other sources.[7] This type of pairing is termed *cooperativity. Associativity* is a selective LTP property by which a weak stimulus, if it is consistently paired with a strong stimulus, becomes potentiated and thus strengthens its synapse over time (Fig. 7-4).

These concepts are perhaps of some relevance to rehabilitation specialists. For example, let us assume that hip extension contributes to the initiation of hip flexion and the swing phase of gait.[56,57] Your patient is unable to generate sufficient hip extension during overground locomotion to accomplish this functional task. You now pair hip extension with a cutaneous stimulation to the sole of the foot (which you already know can enhance hip flexion).[41] The cutaneous stimulation is the strong input and over time, via associativity (or cooperativity if the cutaneous input is sufficient to depolarize the desired neurons), synapses transmitting hip extension information input become strengthened, such that less input is now needed to initiate the swing phase (Fig. 7-4). It is a huge leap of faith to take studies of LTP, primarily done in a petri dish, and apply them to an intact human. However, it is a start, and the basic biological mechanisms provide a good theoretical framework and testable clinical questions.

Long-term depression (LTD), as you might surmise by the name, has the opposite effect as LTP. LTD is a mechanism that can selectively weaken synapses. Unopposed LTP has been linked to seizures and epilepsy, in which even small sensory stimulations can cause massive depolarizations.[103] LTD can depress excitatory postsynaptic potentials and erase the effects of LTP. LTD does not represent a single mechanism. For instance, the mechanisms subserving LTD in the hippocampus appear to be considerably different from those in the cerebellum.[68,103]

LTP and LTD depend on molecular mechanisms that depend on ionic interactions (e.g., calcium, magnesium), protein activations (e.g., kinase C), and specific postsynaptic receptors (e.g., *N*- methyl-D-aspartate [NMDA]). For instance, associative LTP involves the release of the neurotransmitter glutamate. Glutamate binds to a postsynaptic receptor (e.g., NMDA). The NMDA receptor is especially important for learning. For the NMDA receptor channel to open, it must not only bind glutamate, but the postsynaptic cell must also be depolarized. The depolarization is accomplished by afferent input. The depolar-

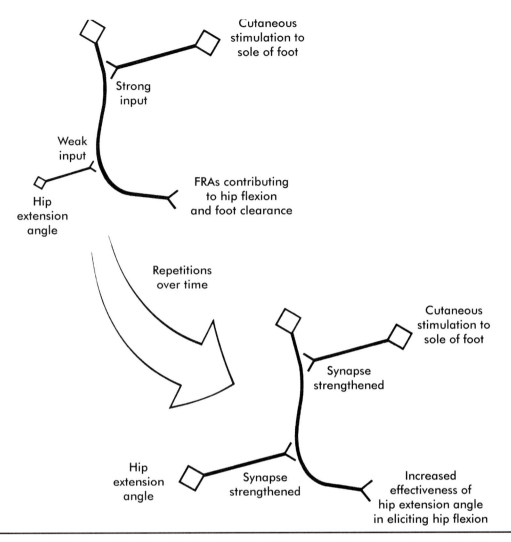

Fig. 7-4. Hypothetical example of the role of associativity of LTP. A strong input (e.g., cutaneous stimulation of the foot) might always elicit the desired movement (e.g., activation of flexor reflex afferents [FRAs] for hip flexion). A weaker input (e.g., hip extension) might not be sufficient to elicit the desired movement, but if it is consistently paired with the stronger input, its synapse will, via associativity, be strengthened over time.

ization removes magnesium from the receptor and allows the influx of calcium, which initiates activation of protein kinases and the enhancement of synaptic transmission. This is, needless to say, quite the cascade of events. Knowing that a multitude of steps is involved in modulating just one synapse, perhaps you won't feel so guilty about your forgetfulness. It is no minor miracle that we remember anything at all. Refer to a neuroscience textbook for more information on these molecular processes.

LTP and LTD represent neural mechanisms that can cause long-term changes in the transmission characteristics of a synapse. Despite the fact that they cause relatively long-term changes, the changes are not permanent. They represent molecular mechanisms that are transient and thus cannot subserve long-term memory. To form a permanent memory, other mechanisms must be involved.

Long-term memory: genes and proteins

Long-term memory apparently requires the synthesis of new proteins. The proteins are used to form new synapses. One of the triggers for the synthesis of new proteins appears to be activity within the pathway and LTP. Long-term memory is associated with the formation of new synapses.[7]

The number and type of proteins synthesized regulate the growth and remodeling of synapses.[112] The synthesis of new proteins involves genetic transcription in the cell body. One of the quandaries currently challenging researchers is how long-term memory can maintain synaptic specificity if proteins are created in the cell body and then transported to all of its synapses. One neuron might contact thousands of other neurons, yet changes in synaptic size and strength associated with long-term memory might occur in only a select few synapses.[112,126] How this occurs is yet another neuroscientific mystery. The two main theories currently being pursued are: (1) that gene expression and protein synthesis preferentially affect certain axons, and (2) that changes in the postsynaptic neuron dictate the effectiveness of the newly synthesized protein.[112,126]

■ CHANGES WITHIN THE NERVOUS SYSTEM INDUCED BY TRAINING

Locations of plastic changes

The nervous system exhibits many plastic changes that are associated with activity and learning. The plasticity associated with motor learning begins with the muscle and neuromuscular junction, extends throughout the involved neural pathways in the spinal cord and brain stem, and includes higher brain centers such as the cerebellum, basal ganglia, and cerebral cortex.

Plasticity begins with muscle. Evidence indicates that muscle motor unit recruitment changes during the learning of a motor task. For instance, variability in the recruitment of motor units decreases concomitant with motor learning.[91] Furthermore, there are significant increases in the frequency of motor unit firing after extended practice of tasks requiring fast movements.[90,91] Morphological and physiological changes occurring within the spinal cord that are associated with motor learning[24,25,39] have been discussed previously. LTP, a process important for learning, exists in the cerebellum.[69,103] Exercise during critical periods of development affects growth and development of Purkinje cells located within the cerebellum.[105] Brain scanning experiments indicate dramatic changes in brain metabolic activity associated with motor learning and memory.[55,71,75,121] These plastic changes occur rapidly, even within performance from one movement trial to the next. These plastic changes in metabolic activity, however, typically involve transient, short-term changes. They probably reflect processes such as LTP and changes in the input/output characteristics of the areas under study. Previously, I indicated that the repository for memory is probably located in the cerebral cortex and that long-term memory involves structural changes such as the addition of synapses. Thus, it would be of interest to know whether training and practice have an impact on long-term changes in cortical organization.

Experience-dependent changes

During perinatal development, activity has a dramatic effect on neural transmission and certain aspects of cerebral cortex organization.[21,36,61,81,93] But your interests might be in developing the perfect tennis serve, mastering the keyboard, teaching gymnastics, or rehabilitating patients. For these activities, we need to examine the evidence for adult cortical plasticity.

Evidence collected to date suggests that some degree of cortical plasticity remains throughout life. This plasticity is not of the same degree as during critical periods of ontogenetic development, but, similar to the plasticity associated with development, it shows activity/experience dependency. Adult cortical plasticity has been demonstrated in several areas, including sensory and motor cortices.

Within the sensory cortex, each neuron has a specific receptive field. The receptive field corresponds to an area of the body to which stimulation will cause activation of this neuron. In the adult, the size and representation of these receptive fields can show plastic changes. Amputation of a digit will cause the cortical receptive field of the missing digit to change. These neurons will now respond to stimulation of the neighboring intact digits.[86] Furthermore, if an animal is trained to use a digit repetitively, the cortical representation of this digit will expand.[87] If an animal is forced to use two digits together for every activity or if simultaneous, synchronous stimulation is applied to the two digits, their representation within the SI becomes integrated. Interestingly, the thalamus does not appear to undergo similar reorganization during these experimental paradigms.[132] Either not all CNS structures have plastic capabilities, or their mechanisms differ.

The adult MI also shows a plasticity that depends on activity. The MI has considerable interconnectivity between the representations of muscles that tend to behave synergistically. Synergist muscles or movement combinations that were frequently activated together increase their area of representation within the MI.[96] Therefore, similar to the sensory cortex,[132] specific activity or synchronous activity among different cell populations can induce changes in MI organization.

These studies, and others of a similar nature, have now been expanded, and evidence suggests that the same processes occur in the human. For instance, evidence suggests that the human motor cortex reorganizes after a partial upper extremity amputation.[29] Other brain regions show differences in activation and organization after damage to the cerebral cortex and its projections.[28,133] These changes in cortical representation are not without functional significance. An increase in the size of sensory areas within the brain has been correlated with increased sensory discriminatory capabilities.[86,143] Not all increases in cortical representations, however, lead to increased discriminatory abilities.[22] Monkeys trained to use the hands repetitively in a specified manner for 20 weeks experienced a dedifferentiation of the normally segregated areas of hand representation in the sensory cortex (area 3b). The normally separated representations between the different digits of the hand were replaced by overlapping receptive fields of adjacent digits.

Data suggest that considerable variability exists in brain activation patterns associated with the learning of a motor task.[119] This might reflect differences in individual capabilities and differences in the way individuals' brains are organized. In turn, these individual differences might reflect differences in accumulated experiences. Studies in nonhuman animals indicate that animals raised in enriched environments have a thicker cerebral cortex and increased dendritic branching.[17,34] These studies are not limited to nonhuman species. A correlation exists between the complexity of dendritic systems in the human brain and the type of work in which the individual participated during his or her lifetime.[117] For instance, individuals involved in occupations that demanded hand dexterity had increased dendritic branching within primary motor areas; those who depended on talking and communication skills had increased cortical area devoted to speech areas. The auditory association cortex of musicians with perfect pitch is larger than that of less-gifted musicians.[118] Perhaps genetics rather than activity can account for this, but activity appears to play at least a part. For example, one study found the cortical somatosensory hand area of string players to be enlarged.[37] The earlier the individual began to play, the larger the cortical area devoted to finger dexterity. These findings suggest that use of the extremity contributed to the cortical enlargement.

Mechanisms contributing to plasticity

The mechanisms that contribute to adult cortical plasticity associated with training are poorly understood. Rewiring and axonal growth to the extent that occurs during development is unlikely. More likely is that synapses that are normally present but physiologically silent, either due to presynaptic inhibition or other neural mechanisms, become strengthened when an adjacent area is damaged or when demands on its circuitry are increased. Changes in synaptic strength and cortical representations during learning appear to follow Hebbian mechanisms (i.e., if one neuron continuously activates another, over time the strength of that synapse will be enhanced). The Law of Effect, first developed by E.L. Thorndike in the early 1900s, is also potentially applicable here. This concept proposes that responses that are followed by a reward tend to be repeated, and those that are not tend not to be repeated.[128]

Several times I have alluded to the fact that the plastic changes available to the adult differ somewhat from those observed during development. The differences and similarities associated with plastic changes that occur during development vs. those associated with the mature, fully developed nervous system are the focus of the next section.

■ DEVELOPMENTAL PLASTICITY AND ADULT MOTOR LEARNING
Processes of plasticity during development
From conception onward through the first or second year of life, the human nervous system is a tsunami wave of development and change. The processes guiding these changes are many and involve such things as cell migration and differentiation, axonal growth, dendritic arbor formation, neurotransmitter synthesis, glial-neural interactions, and synaptogenesis. Regressive events such as cell death and retraction of projections are an equally vital part of development. Some of these processes are genetic, some depend on tropic (guide axons toward a target) and trophic (support cell survival) molecules. Some developmental processes depend on activity. These activity-dependent processes involve neural organization from the neuromuscular junction[104] to the cerebral cortex.[36] The activity can range from spontaneous electrical activity in utero to postnatal sensory and motor experiences. Competition for synaptic sites is one of the determinants of final connectivity. This Darwinian characteristic was discussed in Chapter 3.

Differences between developmental and adult plasticity
The global and dramatic plastic changes in projections and connectivity that occur during development do not recur again in the human brain. The growth and retraction of adult axons is very restricted. Cell death and dendritic arborization continue throughout life, but not to the extent that they occur during development. In fact, once a critical period of development has been passed, plastic changes become limited. However, adults are capable of learning, and this learning must reflect plastic changes within the nervous system. Plasticity that is associated with development is heavily reliant on structural changes (cell migration, axon growth, synapse formation, and regressive events). The plastic changes available to the adult brain are generally considered not to be secondary to major structural change but are largely attributable to changes in synaptic strength. Some similarities do exist, however, between development and adult plasticity.

Shared mechanisms between development and adult learning
Repetitive stimulation and activity within a neural pathway are important during development and during the processes associated with adult learning. How many of the activity-dependent mechanisms involved with adult learning are the same as activity-dependent mechanisms used during critical periods of development remains to be determined.[30,73]

Competition at the synaptic site appears to be an important determinant in both situations. In the developing nervous system, the precise pattern of neural connectivity (reflecting pruning of excess synaptic connections and formation and retention of new ones) depends on competition.[79] One process that enhances competitive survival is synaptic activity. A synapse that is used is preferred over one receiving less activity.[30] In the adult, a similar process occurs. A highly used synapse will undergo LTP and thus strengthen its synaptic connection. Note that during development, enhanced synaptic activity contributes to the survival of that connection. In the adult, an established synapse is likely to survive regardless of its level of activity. It is the strength of the synapse that changes with activity.

LTP is one mechanism by which an active synapse in a mature animal is strengthened. In the developing animal, this same process appears to contribute to the process of cell survival and fine-tuning of synaptic connections.[74] Long-term changes such as synapse formation depend on the synthesis of new proteins. The modulation of synapses in the adult and synapse formation in the developing animal might rely on the same associations between LTP and transcription activation of protein synthesis. Signalling molecules, whose release is initiated by LTP, are retrogradely transported back to the cell body. These molecules initiate protein synthesis needed for long-term synaptic change.[74] Are the same molecules used during development as during the process of learning in the adult? This remains unknown, but there are many similarities between the molecular mechanisms subserving development and adult learning.

The adult brain retains some plasticity, albeit not to the degree of the developing animal. The plasticity depends on activity and can be altered by training and experience. The following section briefly presents some factors that influence adult motor learning and, by association, plastic changes within the CNS.

■ FACTORS THAT INFLUENCE AND ENHANCE MOTOR LEARNING

Motor learning is accompanied by plastic changes. These plastic changes are activity dependent. Repetitive stimulation enhances transmission within a neural pathway. Repetition and activity dependency are constantly repeated themes in the neuroscience of motor learning literature. One might be tempted to take the basic science literature, apply it to human performance, and assume that the adage of "practice makes perfect" has a biological basis and is an adequate principle on which to base our training and rehabilitation efforts. In certain aspects this is true. Practice and repetition enhance motor skill acquisition. Two parameters are most influential in determining the speed and proficiency of motor skill acquisition: (1) the number and strength of reinforcing variables, and (2) the amount of repetition. Nonetheless, an evolving body of knowledge indicates that the conditions under which we practice, the type and amount of feedback we receive from our coaches and therapists, how we group our practice sessions, and the type of sensory feedback we receive during practice all influence our acquisition and retention of motor skills. Yes, practice does make perfect, but researchers have found that there are ways to optimize practice sessions.

Acquisition and retention

Skill *acquisition* (execution and learning) and *retention* (memory) do not represent the same neural processes. Retention of a skill does not necessarily follow its acquisition. How we practice a motor skill influences our abilities to acquire and retain that skill. Practice sessions have inherent variables. These variables include how much verbal feedback we receive and the conditions under which we practice (e.g., a quiet room vs. a noise-filled stadium). Also, is it more advantageous to repeat the same skill over and over again during a single practice session, or should we practice different skills within a session? Factors such as mental concentration and fatigue also need to be considered.

Separate factors appear to contribute to the fast acquisition of a skill and its retention. If your goal is to acquire a skill as quickly as possible (e.g., you have 2 days to teach a patient to transfer from bed to chair independently), you will want to plan your practice sessions a certain way. If you want to ensure that your patient will retain these skills for a lifetime, your practice sessions should be organized somewhat differently. Of course, the goal is usually both to acquire and to retain a skill.

Read the following sections with the behavioral differences of acquisition and retention in mind. Also do two additional things: (1) think about practical applications for the motor learning concepts that are presented, and (2) relate the behavioral findings on motor learning with possible underlying neural mechanisms.

Grouping of practice sessions

A classic example illustrating the differences between acquisition and retention of a motor skill involves the grouping of practice sessions. When you attempt to learn a new skill, you can either devote entire practice sessions to its attainment, or you can practice a number of different skills during a particular session. Repetitively practicing a skill over and over again within a practice session is referred to as *blocked practice.* Mixing skills during practice is known as *random practice.*

Controlled studies have examined the effects of blocked vs. random practice on the acquisition and retention of motor skills. As you might have suspected, these studies indicate that blocked practice sessions resulted in faster acquisition and better initial performance of a complex motor skill.[120] Transfer tests (designed to assess retention of a learned skill) revealed, however, that random practice sessions resulted in better retention of the skill. Thus, blocked practice sessions result in better acquisition and random practice sessions result in better retention.

The neuroscientific bases of these findings are unknown. It is logical to assume that blocked practice sessions, if they involve more trials of a particular skill during a practice session, will result in more repetitive use of the involved pathways and thus more associated changes such as LTP. But, why would retention suffer under these circumstances?

Blocked practice sessions bear some semblance to stimulus-response classical conditioning. Conceivably, the learning associated with classical conditioning is more vulnerable to extinction over time than other types of procedural learning that involve increased associative relationships. Perhaps randomizing practice results in the new skill being integrated into other more established movement engrams in which enhanced neural transmission is already present. Randomization might also result in the learned behavior being represented in a number of different pathways rather than a more singular circuit. Representation of the skill among numerous pathways perhaps results in the skill being less susceptible to changes associated with inactivity of a single pathway, such as might occur between practice sessions. You should realize that these are conjectural ideas that have not yet been tested directly. Innumerable other equally plausible explanations abound. Graduate students in motor control and learning should have no fear that this area of study will fail to yield even more questions in the future.

Sensory feedback: specificity in training and practice settings

The acquisition of most complex motor skills relies on sensory feedback. Fast movements are the exception and can be accurately performed independent of sensory feedback. However, most movement does not occur solely within this strict temporal confine. Movement, therefore, requires a constant sensory awareness of our changing environment, the relation of body parts to each other and the environment, and the resultant sensory feedback of our movements. The importance of sensory cuing and feedback for the acquisition of a new motor skill has been discussed previously in this chapter.

The Specificity of Learning Hypothesis states that a skill should be learned under the conditions in which it is to be performed. This hypothesis really encompasses two quite different concepts. The first concept involves sensory feedback during motor learning, and the other involves the setting in which practice occurs.

We learn a motor skill by matching ongoing and resultant sensory feedback during movement with the achievement of the movement goal. If our goal is to perform a perfect tennis serve, we practice the serve until we achieve the proper "feel" of the movement. In other words, through trial and error, we determine the optimal height to toss the ball, the proper amount of back extension, and the correct timing for contacting the ball. Good tennis players know when they've made a good serve without ever having to look at their opponent's side of the net; they know, via sensory feedback, when they have met the necessary movement criteria for successful completion of the task. This is where sport-specificity of training comes into play. Studies have shown that practicing movement patterns that are close to, but not exactly, those required for the desired skill might be detrimental to performance of that skill. For instance, a skilled volleyball player making the transition to tennis may encounter difficulties. The volleyball spike serve and tennis serve are initiated in a similar way. They differ, however, in important but perhaps subtle aspects of forearm pronation and wrist movement.

The neurological reasons for the difficulties faced in mastering two similar movement patterns are not entirely clear, but educated speculation is possible. If the brain establishes engrams of movement patterns and these engrams are initiated in response to a particular sensory signal, then the beginning of a movement sets in motion a cascade of events that are essentially preprogrammed. Because the movement is preprogrammed, you will have to exert extraordinary concentration to change the program midstream to adapt the movement to a new task. Concentration involves the cerebral cortex. Every time you use this organ, you slow down (nothing personal—this is scientific fact). Slowing down the movement will affect every other aspect of the movement pattern and a less-than-optimal performance is the likely result.

It would also be a detriment if the tennis serve were practiced all day using a heavier ball or a racket strung to a different tension. This is because the serve will now have been learned under different sensory conditions than those involved during competitive play.

Two additional examples provide further evidence for the importance of practicing skills under the same sensory influences as those expected during performance. The first involves competition anxiety. Nervousness robs athletes and musicians of their skills. You might be a backyard hero, but put you in front of a crowd in a stressful situation and you fall apart. Some of this coliseum fright can be attributable to the fact that nervousness impacts sensory and motor set. If you are tense, you will tend to cocontract your muscles. As you now attempt to hit that foul shot or make that difficult gymnastic move on the uneven bars, you are no longer performing the task under the same sensory conditions in which you practiced.

A second example is the motor performance of individuals with spasticity. Spasticity is a motor disorder that often accompanies damage to upper motor neurons and their pathways. It often results, among other things, in accentuated muscle tone. Some procedures, such as inhibitive casting, drug management, and surgical lesioning of sensory fibers (dorsal root rhizotomies), can help alleviate the condition. However, studies have shown that if an individual learned a skill in the presence of spasticity, alleviating the spasticity will result in detriments of the learned skill.[48] The individual needs to relearn the skills under the new sensory complement (i.e., in the absence of spasticity).

The Specificity of Learning Hypothesis also states that transfer of motor learning is optimized by practicing in the same setting as that expected during performance. Now the issue gets a little cloudy. You have already read that variable practice results in better retention than blocked practice. These findings might be interpreted as being somewhat contradictory to the Specificity of Learning Hypothesis. Perhaps not, however. If later performance of a motor skill will take place under various conditions, practice conditions that are varied would appear to be the most appropriate mode of practice.[136] Varying practice conditions appears to increase problem solving skills and enables individuals to develop numerous strategies by which to solve a particular motor problem.[136,137] So, if you are an athlete, vary your practice setting if possible (e.g., don't practice your foul shots at the same end of the gym every day). If you are a therapist, vary the conditions under which you have your patient practice.

Augmented feedback: knowledge of results

Not all sensory feedback is endogenously created. Therapists, coaches, and trainers are forever attempting to optimize performance by providing physical and verbal input. This type of feedback is referred to as *augmented feedback*.

Therapists are typically called upon to assist their patients with their movements. The temptation is to guide them physically toward the desired goal. Research has shown, however, that a high frequency of physical guidance results in the poorest retention of the motor skill.[138] The reasons for this include the fact that the sensory complement used during an active movement differs considerably from that used during a passive movement. Passive movements are not likely to contribute to the learning of a complex motor skill.

Knowledge of results refers to verbal feedback that provides postresponse information about the movement or errors in the movement. You might be tempted to think that the more verbal feedback, the better; controlled studies suggest otherwise. With regard to motor skill retention, reducing the amount of verbal correction given to an individual appears to be beneficial to the individual's ability to retain that skill.[137,139] Furthermore, randomizing the feedback and giving feedback only when performance falls outside specified guidelines also appear to have beneficial effects on motor learning.[136,139]

Once again, the neural basis of such findings is poorly understood. Perhaps constantly providing verbal feedback prevents an individual from internalizing his own corrective strategies or establishing a reliance on his own abilities for error correction.[120] Or, perhaps frequent knowledge of results creates more variability in corrective responses or actually results in maladaptive responses.[139] When individuals are faced with a conflict between endogenous sensory feedback and knowledge of results from an outside source, they tend to rely more on the outside source than their own innate abilities. This tendency, however, can be reversed if an individual has had sufficient practice in using sensory feedback to correct movement.[19] Once a subject has learned to rely on intrinsic sensory feedback, he or she will ignore erroneous knowledge of results being provided by an outside source. These results provide additional support for the importance of permitting individuals to internalize learning processes.

Component vs. whole task practice

When learning a complex movement, is practicing the entire required sequence as a whole more advantageous, or should you break down the movement into component parts? Although the literature is contradictory, breaking down a movement into its component parts appears to be the better strategy. This is especially true for complex movements. Breaking down a movement into component parts is referred to as *part-task training*. The caveat to part-task training is that it should be a natural part of the whole movement.[120] For instance, practicing a component part slowly might not carry over to the whole movement if a fast response of the component part is required.[120,136] The best examples of the benefits of part-task training involve sports such as figure skating, gymnastics, and diving. Can you imagine trying to learn an entire routine without first mastering the component parts?

This aspect of motor learning is very similar to findings with verbal processing skills. The beginning and end of a verbal phrase are remembered easier than words within the middle of the phrase. This is also true of motor skill retention. Although somewhat task dependent, skills involved at the beginning and the end of a movement sequence tend to be retained better than those occurring in the middle of a movement. Breaking down a movement into component parts gives you more beginnings and endings. Perhaps this contributes to better retention.

Fatigue and motor learning

How appropriate that I would begin the writing of this section at this particular moment. I have just returned from an afternoon of backcountry telemark skiing in the mountains of Montana. Because my legs aren't exactly pistons of power and my turns through the steep and deep aren't exactly effortless, I am exhausted. My heart continues an attempt to pound an escape out of my chest and my legs are trembling. My hands, poised above the keyboard, are also slightly tremulous. As I type, I notice that my speed is a bit less thatn beofre I left and I am making a few more errors. There is no doubt in my mind, or within the literature, that fatigue affects motor performance. It also appears to affect motor learning.

Controlled studies have shown that practicing a motor skill while in a state of heavy aerobic physical fatigue is detrimental to both motor performance and learning.[26] Bear in mind that the test/retest variables were assessed in a nonfatigued state. In other words, subjects were tested on a motor skill, exercised to fatigue before the practice sessions, and then, after complete recovery, retested on the same motor skill. Subjects who learned the task under the fatigued condition did not perform as well as subjects who learned the task in a nonfatigued state.

Many sensory and central changes are associated with muscle fatigue.[11,12] The effects of fatigue range from changes in muscle activation characteristics,[92] to changes in sensory afferent information being sent to the nervous system,[43,44,82] to changes in the central drive to alpha motor neurons.[10,142]

Questions regarding the effects of muscle fatigue are of obvious importance to industry, the military, athletes, the space program, and rehabilitation specialists. Many questions remain regarding the limits of fatigue, differences in central effects of aerobic vs. muscular fatigue, parameters of performance and central change that are most affected, and, of course, what can be done to reduce the changes imposed by fatigue.

Mental imagery

Jean Claude Kiley, one of the most accomplished skiers of all time, was well known for mentally rehearsing his run down a slalom course before a competition. He is said to have been so skilled in mental imagery that his times during mental rehearsal were unerringly close to his actual performance time. In related studies, a Swedish researcher, Johnny Nilsson, tested elite skiers and recreational skiers to assess their abilities to memorize and mentally rehearse a slalom course. He found that elite skiers were much more accurate with mental rehearsal than recreational skiers (personal communication).

In 1984 the United States Army Research Institute funded The National Academy of Sciences to conduct a review of the literature pertaining to mental imagery and mental practice.[38] Several studies have reported a beneficial effect, whereas others have questioned its efficacy. A meta-analysis (a statistical procedure that allows grouping of the results from numerous studies) revealed a beneficial effect of mental practice. Mental practice was most effective in facilitating learning in tasks requiring accuracy (e.g., marksmanship, shooting fouls) or motor performance (e.g., dribbling a ball, driving a car). Mental practice did not appear to improve strength, endurance, speed, or balance.

Mental practice, however, was effective in improving accuracy and motor performance only if two other parameters were met. First, to benefit from mental imagery, the individual must have already had a certain amount of proficiency in the skill. Second, mental practice alone did not seem to have much of an effect. Its beneficial effects were apparent only when mental practice was paired with actual physical performance of the skill.

Many of the same neural circuits are activated during mental imagery as during actual performance of a motor skill.[54,70,124] Reflex amplitudes of the limbs that are imagined to move actually increase.[70] In some cases, electromyographic activity during mental rehearsal simulates that of actual performance.[120] This activity is at a very low level, so no actual movement occurs. Some cerebral cortex activation patterns during mental rehearsal of a motor skill are similar to areas activated during actual performance.[33,124] Some notable differences exist, however, between mental imagery and physical performance.

The cerebellum demonstrates a strong activation during mental imagery of motor tasks.[113] The cerebellar areas that are activated, however, are regionally distinct from areas that are activated during actual movement.[54] The SMA appears to be especially active during mental imagery, but similar to the cerebellum, the area of activation is separate from the area activated during actual movement.[54] Other cortical areas that are active during mental imagery of a motor skill involving the hand include the inferior frontal cortex (area 44), middle frontal cortex, caudal inferior parietal cortex, and premotor cortex.[54] These areas share a close association with language processing.

Music and motor learning

Athletes have always used music to enhance performance. Athletes report getting "psyched up" after listening to their country's national anthem or a favorite piece of music. Much of this performance enhancement can be attributed to increased arousal. Studies have shown an increase in arousal and endurance after listening to music.[8] Is there a relationship, however, between music and motor learning that is independent of its arousal effects?

Much of the work that has examined the effects of music on performance has examined spatial task performance. Classical music, typically Mozart sonatas, has been the music of choice during these experimental explorations. In fact, the relationship between music and motor performance is sometimes referred to as "the Mozart effect." Although some studies report no Mozart effect,[94] others have reported enhanced spatial performance after subjects listened to a Mozart sonata.[106,108] Enhanced performance while listening to Mozart has been correlated with changes in electroencephalographic activity.[108] While these studies did not assess motor learning directly, spatial awareness and reasoning skills are an inherent aspect of motor learning.

Why Mozart sonatas, and what is the possible relationship between a sonata and movement skill? Surely it is just coincidence that sonata-form is also referred to as "first-movement form." A sonata is typified as having a beginning (usually repeated), a middle, and an end. The different themes are connected by appropriate transitions: "...the energy of a work [sonata], its motoric principle, come largely from the sequence—the repetition of patterns..."[110] All motor skills have a beginning, a middle, and an end. Part-task motor learning literature indicates that, similar to verbal memorization skills, beginnings and endings of a movement sequence are remembered more easily than middles. Furthermore, transitions are often the most problematic. Perhaps the temporal similarity between a sonata and movement skill acquisition underlies the Mozart effect. Or, perhaps listening to a sonata concomitant with learning a motor skill involves more parts of the brain devoted to temporal sequencing. Or, maybe listening to music forms associations that ease future recall of motor patterns. Researchers really don't know yet. Plenty of clues are out there and much work remains to be done. Therapists have already discovered that music can enhance verbal communication and temporal aspects of gait of patients with stroke.[102,116]

Nicotine, glutamate and other pharmacological interventions

The year is 2075. The scene is the victorious locker room of the Bejing Dragons, who have just won the World Field Hockey title, a sport that long ago displaced The World Cup and The Super Bowl as the number one most popular sporting event. The room is filled with smoke, and not just from the media. The athletes are smoking up a storm. Their jerseys are emblazoned with the logos from various tobacco companies. The television commercials for this special event were dominated by advertisements for smoking. What has happened to cause such an extreme shift away from the late twentieth century, when no serious athlete would even think about smoking? Smokers were shunned members of society forced to partake of their habit only in special reserved smoking sections in the deserts of Nevada. Some say the turnaround began in the 1990s, when researchers ranging from Houston to California found that nicotine enhanced memory formation.[9]

Nicotine's enhancement of memory appears to have a sound biological basis. We have long known that the brain has receptors for nicotine. What they were doing there, other than contributing to the addictive qualities of tobacco, was unknown. Researchers have now found that interaction between nicotine and their receptors enhances the entry of calcium into the presynaptic terminal during an action potential. The more calcium that enters the terminal, the more neurotransmitter is released. Increasing the amount of available neurotransmitter increases the likelihood that the postsynaptic neuron will become activated. Over time this synapse will be strengthened—a mechanism that contributes to LTP, learning, and memory. Other drugs, perhaps less harmful to the body than the carcinogens associated with tobacco, are also known to enhance memory.

The neurotransmitter, glutamate, and the postsynaptic receptors, NMDA and mGlu, have a strong connection with learning. Injection of drugs that block NMDA and mGlu receptors can impair learning and the acquisition of motor memories.[103] Glutamate agonists given after training enhance memory formation.[109] Perhaps of considerable importance, corticostriatal projections (which are hypothesized to be essential for the transfer of a learned motor skill to memory) use glutamate.[23] mGlu receptors, via second messenger mechanisms, appear to be one of the methods that repetitive short-term neural activations use to initiate long-lasting intracellular changes.[109] These long-term changes, in turn, might be the signal to initiate genetic transcription and protein synthesis, which are necessary for memory formation.

Other drugs ranging from caffeine to cocaine have an affect on learning and motor skill acquisition. The rehabilitation of patients with neurological disorders increasingly encompasses innumerable drug protocols. Many of these, such as dantrolene or baclofen, are used to decrease spasticity. Other drugs, however, apparently have a more direct effect on motor learning and the ability to enhance coordinated patterns of muscle contraction. Amphetamine, when paired with physical therapy procedures, enhances the speed and extent of motor skill recovery.[131] Other drugs that are precursors or agonists of different neurotransmitters appear to enhance orderly muscle contraction.[5,6] In all cases, the pairing of the drug with functional training appears to provide the most beneficial effect.

■ MOTOR LEARNING AFTER BRAIN DAMAGE

"...we may need to revise our notions of localization of function to account for recovery, or perhaps to question the assumption that recovery represents the return of the same motor mechanisms that were lost because of a lesion, rather than an adaptation of residual mechanisms."[50]

Michael Goldberger (1935-1992)

The progress in understanding the mechanisms involved in motor learning is impressive. Nonetheless, many issues remain unresolved regarding the acquisition and retention of motor skills. Included among these unresolved issues are the effects of brain damage on motor learning. We cannot assume that the principles underlying motor learning in individuals without disability apply equally to individuals with damage to various brain structures. Various brain structures contribute to different aspects of motor learning, and different stages of motor learning involve different neural pathways. Therefore, it is highly likely that damage to various areas of the brain will result in deficits of various aspects of motor learning. Of equal importance is determining the processes that contribute to recovery after brain damage.

Theories of motor recovery
Michael Goldberger, a neuroscientist extraordinaire and one of my all-time heroes, devoted much of his career to understanding the mechanisms mediating recovery after damage to the CNS. Two of his early reviews on this subject[50,52] remain relevant and important reading today. In these reports he outlines theoretical possibilities for recovery that still serve as a framework for current investigations. Mass action (equipotentiality), vicarious function, functional reorganization, and substitution are theories upon which many testable questions and experiments have been based.

Mass action theory, also referred to as *equipotentiality*, asserts that various parts of the nervous system can mediate the same motor function. This suggests that a function that is lost secondary to damage to a specific region of the nervous system can be mediated by a surviving structure or pathway. The finding that certain aspects of vestibulo-ocular adaptation can be mediated by the cerebellum or by brain stem pathways is consistent with mass action theory.[58]

Vicarious function theory contends that undamaged CNS regions have latent capabilities that can respond to or control actions originally mediated by the damaged areas. This might involve synapses that originally had a very weak input into a system, but after damage to the stronger input their activity becomes manifest. Many examples of this type of neural organization[20,62,88,99] and its unmasking after injury[28,63,133] can be found.

Functional reorganization theory suggests that a neural system can alter its function depending on need and secondary to damage to related areas. Studies demonstrating somatosensory cortex plasticity that depends on activity and plastic changes that accompany various types of damage provide clear evidence of this concept.[28,29,86,96,97,132]

The *theory of substitution* proposes that a motor behavior can be performed by a different mechanism than that which originally controlled the behavior. In other words, the end is achieved by different means. Three types of substitution exist. Sensory substitution after CNS damage refers to a movement that is similar to the original, but the sensory cue that triggers the movement is different. Functional substitution states that the lost and recovered movement do not differ, but the underlying mechanisms subserving the movement are different. Behavioral substitution proposes that the strategy used for the recovery of a movement is different from the original. Considerable clinical and experimental[13,28,31,51,52,63] evidence exists for the theory of substitution.

Motor learning deficits associated with specific brain regions
Refer to Chapters 2 and 4 for a discussion of sensory and motor functions associated with various regions of the brain and nervous system. Chapter 4 also discusses the effects of damage to specific areas of the cerebral cortex. The following section discusses the effects of damage as it specifically relates to motor learning. Remember, there does not appear to be a single location for motor memory and retrieval, and many of the factors that impact motor learning are not related to a structure, but rather to physiological mechanisms that modulate synaptic transmission.

The cerebellum. The cerebellum is apparently not involved in some motor learning tasks.[119] Clearly, however, lesions to the cerebellum result in motor performance impairments and motor learning deficits. The cerebellum is involved in the temporal aspects of movement and is involved in combining simple movements into complex synergies. It might also play a role in sensory processing.[18,42] Synapses within the cerebellum exhibit LTP and LTD, mechanisms associated with learning. Lesions to the cerebellum result in loss of task-specific reflex adaptations[59] and conditioned responses.[80] Lesions also result in impairments in the ability to make use of prior knowledge for reflex adaptation.[65]

Basal ganglia and striatal pathways. Lesions to the basal ganglia result in poor habit formation, impaired stimulus-response reactions, and a decrease in the acquisition of motor tasks involving visual pursuit movements. Individuals with Parkinson's disease can visually track an object, but they cannot initiate these pursuit movements from memory.[59] They also have difficulty generating sequential movements.[121] This is perhaps related to the fact that individuals with Parkinson's disease do not activate the SMA (which is involved in internally generated sequential movements and motor planning) during motor tasks.[55] These individuals have deficits in procedural learning,[55] yet do not have significant impairments in declarative memory.[78]

Apparently, the entire corticostriato-cerebellar loop must be intact for a motor skill to be assimilated.[55] The specific functions associated with this loop have yet to be determined.

Supplementary and premotor cortical areas. Damage to either of these regions of the brain results in deficits in motor memory, although of a somewhat different nature. Damage to the SMA results in a loss of the ability to initiate memorized movement sequences. PM lesions also result in impairments in learned sequential movements, but the movements most affected are those initiated by sensory cuing. Individuals with damage to the PM experience a decreased ability to respond to sensory cuing, especially visual signals.[59]

Parietal cortex. Perhaps no other areas within the cerebral cortex have larger roles to play in motor learning than parietal areas. Lesions to various aspects of the parietal cortex result in dramatic impairments in learned motor behaviors.[59] *Apraxia* (the loss of ability to perform familiar movements in the absence of motor or sensory impairment), loss of motor memory, and difficulties in storage and retrieval of motor skills can result. The conceptualization of motor behavior appears to share circuitry with neural circuits involved with language comprehension.

Effects of training and rehabilitation

As more and more individuals are surviving strokes and other CNS disorders, one of the greatest challenges facing researchers and clinicians today is the development of treatment interventions that will have a beneficial effect on motor control and motor learning. Previously in this chapter I discussed various factors that enhance motor learning. The studies relied on for this information involved subjects without disability. Researchers are now making determinations as to whether these same principles can be applied to individuals with disabilities. Dr. Carolee Winstein and her group from The University of Southern California are among those conducting research in this area. This laboratory and others are exploring the relationships between specific training techniques, associated plastic changes within the CNS, and related functional outcomes.

In some cases, techniques that have been used to enhance motor learning of individuals without disabilities have also been shown to be effective with patient populations. Augmented feedback during training of motor skills for individuals without disability is effective for immediate acquisition of the skill, but reliance on this type of feedback appears to be detrimental to retention. A study of patients with adult-onset stroke reports that these individuals responded similarly: augmented feedback improved immediate performance but decreased retention.[84] Studies have also reported that random practice was more effective than blocked practice for motor skill retention in survivors of stroke.[60] Again, this is similar to findings in individuals without disability.

Encouragingly, researchers are finding that plastic changes associated with learning are not limited to individuals without disability. Electroencephalographic studies have shown that mental rehearsal of a motor task activates similar brain regions in individuals who have had a stroke as is involved in individuals without disability.[134,135] Evidence exists for limited plastic reorganization of the cerebral cortex after a stroke.[28,72,97,114] Positron emission tomographic scans have provided evidence that the undamaged cortex increases its activity and perhaps reorganizes so that it contributes to the control of movement of the involved extremity after a stroke.[28] And perhaps the most promising findings are that rehabilitation procedures can affect the reorganization of undamaged cortical pathways after brain injury.[97] My guess is that the field of rehabilitation medicine is about to embark on an exciting journey. As scientists continue to determine how the brain responds to injury and how training affects these responses, therapies will be developed that target specific impairments and disabilities. No longer will a single rehabilitation procedure or single drug be used to treat stroke or other movement and motor learning disorders. Procedures will be developed that are specific to the location of the pathologic area. Motor learning disabilities secondary to parietal lesions or premotor areas will likely be treated differently than disabilities caused by damage to other cortical regions.

SUGGESTED READINGS

Abbe J, Winstein CJ. Functional contributions of rapid automatic sensory-based adjustments to motor output. In: Jeannerod M, ed. Attention and performance XIII. Hillsdale: Lawrence Erlbaum, 1990:627-52.

Adolphe B. The mind's ear. St Louis: MMB Music, 1996.

Alkon DL. Memory storage and neural systems. Sci Am 1989;261:42-50.

Allen G, Buxton RB, Wong EC, Courchesne E. Attentional activation of the cerebellum independent of motor involvement. Science 1997;275:1940-3.

Astington JW. The child's discovery of the mind. Cambridge: Harvard University Press, 1993.

Bach-y-Rita P. Receptor plasticity and volume transmission in the brain: emerging concepts with relevance to neurologic rehabilitation. J Neuro Rehab 1990;4:121-8.

Bizzi E, Mussa-Ivaldi FA, Giszter S. Computations underlying the execution of movement: a biological perspective. Science 1991;253:287-91.

Brown TH, Chapman PF, Kairiss EW, Keenan CL. Long-term synaptic potentiation. In: Kelner KL, Koshland DE, eds. Molecules to models: advances in neuroscience. Washington, DC: American Association for the Advancement of Science, 1989:196-204.

Burleigh A, Horak F. Influence of instruction, prediction, and afferent sensory information on the postural organization of step initiation. J Neurophysiol 1996;75:1619-28.

Calvin WH. The cerebral symphony. New York: Bantam Books, 1990.

Churchland PM. The engine of reason, the seat of the soul. Cambridge, Mass: Massachusetts Institute of Technology Press, 1997.

Corcos DM, Gottlieb GL, Jaric S, Cromwell RL, Agarwal GC. Organizing principles underlying motor skill acquisition. In: Winters JM, Woo SLY, eds. Principle muscle systems: biomechanics and movement organization. New York: Springer-Verlag, 1990:251-67.

Cordo PJ, Nashner LM. Properties of postural adjustments associated with rapid arm movements. J Neurophysiol 1982;47:287-302.

De Luca CJ, Erim Z. Common drive of motor units in regulation of muscle force. Trends Neurosci 1994;17:299-305.

Earl EM, Frank JS. The influence of task demands on the coordination of posture and movement. In: Woollacott M, Horak F, eds. Posture and gait: control mechanism, vol 1. Portland: University of Oregon Books, 1992:135-9.

Ebner TJ, Flament D, Shanbhag SJ. The cerebellum's role in voluntary motor learning: clinical, electrophysiological, and imaging studies. In: Bloedel JR, Ebner TJ, Wise SP, eds. The acquisition of motor behavior in vertebrates. Cambridge, Mass: Massachusetts Institute of Technology Press, 1996:235-60.

Eliasson A, Gordon AM, Forssberg H. Impaired anticipatory control of isometric forces during grasping by children with cerebral palsy. Dev Med Child Neurol 1992;34:216-25.

Frank JS. Spinal motor preparation in humans. Electroencephalogr Clin Neurophysiol 1986;63:361-70.

Funakoshi H, Belluardo N, Arenas E, et al. Muscle-derived neurotrophin-4 as an activity-dependent trophic signal for adult motor neurons. Science 1995;268:1495-9.

Germain L, Lamarre Y. Neuronal activity in the motor and premotor cortices before and after learning associations between auditory stimuli and motor responses. Brain Res 1993;611:175-9.

Goldberger ME. The role sprouting might play during the recovery of motor function. In: Flohr H, Precht W, eds. Lesion-induced neuronal plasticity in sensorimotor systems. Heidelberg: Springer-Verlag, 1981:130-9.

Goldberger ME, Murray M. Patterns of sprouting and implications for recovery of function. Adv Neurol 1988;47:361-85.

Goldberger ME, Murray M. Recovery of function and anatomical plasticity after damage to the adult and neonatal spinal cord. In: Cotman CW, ed. Synaptic plasticity. New York: Guilford Press, 1985:77-110.

Gordon AM, Forssberg H, Iwasaki N. Formation and lateralization of internal representations underlying motor commands during precision grip. Neuropsychologia 1994;32:555-67.

Halsband U, Ito N, Tanji J, Freund HJ. The role of premotor cortex and the supplementary motor area in the temporal control of movement in man. Brain 1993;116:243-66.

Hammond G, Choo C. Changes in spinal reflex excitability in a countermanded timed response task. J Motor Behav 1994;26:187-95.

Higgins S. Motor skill acquisition. Phys Ther 1991;71:123-39.

Hinshaw KE. The effects of mental practice on motor skill performance: critical evaluation and meta-analysis. Imagination Cognition and Personality 1991;11:3-35.

Hutton RS, Atwater SW. Acute and chronic adaptations of muscle proprioceptors in response to increased use. Sports Med 1992;14:406-21.

Jeannerod M, Decety J. Mental motor imagery: a window into the representational stages of action. Curr Opin Neurobiol 1995;5:727-32.

Jenkins WM, Merzenich MM. Reorganization of neocortical representations after brain injury: a neurophysiological model of the bases of recovery from stroke [abstract]. Prog Brain Res 1987;71:249-66.

Kasai T, Komiyama T. Soleus H-reflex depression induced by ballistic voluntary arm movement in human [abstract]. Brain Res 1996;714:125-34.

Keele SW, Cohen A, Ivry R. Motor programs: concepts and issues. In: Jeannerod M, ed. Attention and performance XIII: motor representation and control. Hillsdale: Lawrence Erlbaum, 1990:77-110.

Latash ML, Anson JG. What are "normal movements" in atypical populations? [abstract] Behav Brain Sci 1996;19:55-106.

Lee TD, Swanson LR, Hall AL. What is repeated in a repetition? Effects of practice conditions on motor skill acquisition. Phys Ther 1991;71:150-6.

Lisberger SG. The neural basis of learning of simple motor skills. In: Kelner KL, Koshland DE, eds. Molecules to models: advances in neuroscience. Washington, DC: American Association for the Advancement of Science, 1989:205-18.

Maki BE, Whitelaw RS. Influence of experience, expectation and arousal on posture control strategy and performance. In: Woollacott M, Horak F, eds. Posture and gait: control mechanisms, vol 1. Portland: University of Oregon Books, 1992:123-6.

Marks R, Quinney HA. Effect of fatiguing maximal isokinetic quadriceps contractions on ability to estimate knee-position. Percept Mot Skills 1993;77:1195-202.

Mcintyre J, Mussaivaldi FA, Bizzi, E. The control of stable postures in the multijoint arm [abstract]. Exp Brain Res 1996;110:248-64.

Muller K, Homberg V. Development of speed of repetitive movements in children is determined be structural changes in corticospinal efferents. Neurosci Lett 1992;144:57-60.

Nielsen J, Petersen N, Deuschl G, Ballegaard M. Task-related changes in the effect of magnetic brain stimulation on spinal neurones in man. J Physiol (Lond) 1993;471:223-43.

Oda S, Moritani T. Maximal isometric force and neural activity during bilateral and unilateral elbow flexion in humans. Eur J Appl Physiol 1994;69:240-3.

Pascual-Leone A, Grafman J, Hallett M. Modulation of cortical motor output maps during development of implicit and explicit knowledge. Science 1994;263:1287-8.

Prochazka A, Hulliger M. Muscle afferent function and its significance for motor control mechanisms during voluntary movements in cat, monkey, and man. In: Desmedt JE, ed. Motor control mechansims in health and disease. New York: Raven Press, 1983:93-132.

Rogers MW. Influence of task dynamics on the organization of interlimb responses accompanying standing human leg flexion movements. Brain Res 1992;579:353-6.

Rumelhart DE, Norman DA. Simulating a skilled typist: a study of skilled cognitive-motor performance. Cogn Sci 1982;6:1-36.

Sanes DH, Takacs C. Activity-dependent refinement of inhibitory connections. Eur J Neurosci 1993;5:570-4.

Sanes JN, Dimitrov B, Hallett M. Motor learning in patients with cerebellar dysfunction. Brain 1990;113:103-20.

Sanes JN, Mauritz K, Evarts EV, Dalakas MC. Motor deficits in patients with large-fiber sensory neuropathy. Proc Natl Acad Sci USA 1984;81:979-82.

Schallert T, Jones TA. Exuberant neuronal growth after brain damage in adult rats: the essential role of behavioral experience. J Neural Transplant Plast 1993;4:193-8.

Stein DG, Brailowsky S, Will B. Brain repair. New York: Oxford University Press, 1995.

Stelmach GE. Motor learning: toward understanding acquired representations. In: Bloedel JR, Ebner TJ, Wise SP, eds. The acquisition of motor behavior in vertebrates. Cambridge, Mass: Massachusetts Institute of Technology Press, 1996:391-408.

Taub E, Miller NE, Novack TA, et al. Technique to improve chronic motor deficit after stroke. Arch Phys Med Rehabil 1993;74:347-54.

Thach WT, Goodkin HP, Keating JG. The cerebellum and the adaptive coordination of movement. Ann Rev Neurosci 1992;15:403-42.

Thompson RF. The neurobiology of learning and memory. In: Kelner KL, Koshland DE, eds. Molecules to models: advances in neuroscience. Washington, DC: American Society for the Advancement of Science, 1989:219-34.

VanSant AF. Life-span development in functional tasks. Phys Ther 1990;70:788-98.

Von T, Deitz JC, McLaughlin J, DeButts S, Richardson M. The effects of chronic otitis media on motor performance in 5- and 6-year-old children. Am J Occup Ther 1988;42:421-6.

Walters ET, Alizadeh H, Castro GA. Similar neuronal alterations induced by axonal injury and learning in aplasia. Science 1991;253:797-9.

Ward SE. Order effects on selected perceptual motor tests. Am J Occup Ther 1973;27:321-5.

Wickens J, Hyland B, Anson G. Cortical cell assemblies: a possible mechanism for motor programs. J Motor Behav 1994;26:66-82.

Winstein CJ, Abbe J, Petashnick D. Influences of object weight and instruction on grip force adjustments. Exp Brain Res 1991;87:465-9.

Winstein CJ, Gardner ER, McNeal DR, Barto PS, Nicholson DE. Standing balance training: effect on balance and locomotion in hemiparetic adults. Arch Phys Med Rehabil 1989;70:755-62.

Winstein CJ, Grafton ST, Pohl PS. Motor task difficulty and brain activity: investigation of goal-directed reciprocal aiming using positron emission tomography. J Neurophysiol 1997;77:1581-94.

Winstein CJ, Knecht HG. Movement science and its relevance to physical therapy. Phys Ther 1990;70:759-62.

Wise SP. Evolution of neuronal activity during conditional motor learning. In: Bloedel JR, Ebner TJ, Wise SP, eds. The acquisition of motor behavior in vertebrates. Cambridge, Mass: Massachusetts Institute of Technology Press, 1996:261-86.

Wolpaw JR, Maniccia DM, Elia T. Operant conditioning of primate H-reflex: phases of development. Neurosci Lett 1994;170:203-7.

Yeh SR, Fricke RA, Edwards DH. The effect of social experience on serotonergic modulation of the escape circuit of crayfish. Science 1996;271:366-9.

Zajac FE. Muscle coordination of movement: a perspective. J Biomech 1993;26:109-24.

REFERENCES

1. Alexander GE, DeLong MR, Crutcher MD. Do cortical and basal ganglionic motor areas use "motor programs" to control movement? Behav Brain Sci 1992;15:656-65.

2. Armstrong DM. The supraspinal control of mammalian locomotion. J Physiol (Lond) 1988;405:1-37.

3. Armstrong DM, Drew T. Discharges of pyramidal tract and other motor cortical neurones during locomotion in the cat. J Physiol (Lond) 1984;346:471-95.

4. Asanuma H. Neuronal mechanisms subserving the acquisition of new skilled movements in mammals. In: Bloedel JR, Ebner TJ, Wise SP, eds. The acquisition of motor behavior in vertebrates. Cambridge, Mass: Massachusetts Institute of Technology Press, 1996:387-90.

5. Barbeau H, Chau C, Rossignol S. Noradrenergic agonists and locomotor training affect locomotor recovery after cord transection in adult cats. Brain Res Bull 1993;30:387-93.

6. Barbeau H, Fung J. New experimental approaches in the treatment of spastic gait disorders. In: Forssberg H, Hirschfeld H, eds. Movement disorders in children. Switzerland: Karger, 1992:234-47.

7. Bear MF, Connors BW, Paradiso MA. Neuroscience: exploring the brain. Baltimore: Williams & Wilkins, 1996.

8. Becker N, Brett S, Chambliss C, et al. Mellow and frenetic antecedent music during athletic performance of children, adults, and seniors. Percept Mot Skills 1994;79:1043-6.

9. Begley S. Memories are made of ... nicotine? New clues to how it affects the brain. Newsweek Nov 4 1996;68.

10. Bigland-Ritchie B, Johansson R, Lippold OCJ, Smith S, Woods JJ. Changes in motoneurone firing rates during sustained maximal voluntary contractions. J Physiol (Lond) 1983;340:335-46.

11. Bigland-Ritchie B, Jones DA, Hosking GP, Edwards RHT. Central and peripheral fatigue in sustained maximum voluntary contractions of human quadriceps muscle. Clin Molec Med 1978;54:609-14.

12. Bigland-Ritchie B, Woods JJ. Changes in muscle contractile properties and neural control during human muscular fatigue. Muscle Nerve 1984;7:691-9.

13. Bishop B, Craik RL. Neural plasticity [abstract]. Neural Plast 1982;62:1-52.

14. Bizzi E, Abend W. Posture control of trajectory formation in single and multi-joint arm movements. In: Desmedt RE, ed. Motor control mechanisms in health and disease. New York: Raven Press, 1983:31-45.

15. Bloedel JR, Bracha V, Kelly TM, Wu J. Substrates for motor learning, does the cerebellum do it all? Ann NY Acad Sci 1991;627:305-18.

16. Bloedel JR, Bracha V, Shimansky Y, Milak MS. The role of the cerebellum in the acquisition of complex volitional forelimb movements. In: Bloedel JR, Ebner TJ, Wise SP, eds. The acquisition of motor behavior in vertebrates. Cambridge, Mass: Massachusetts Institute of Technology Press, 1996:319-42.

17. Bower AJ. Plasticity in the adult and neonatal central nervous system. J Neurosurg 1990;4:253-64.

18. Bower JM. The cerebellum as a sensory acquisition controller. Human Brain Mapping 1995;2:255-6.

19. Buekers MJ, Magill RA, Sneyers KM. Resolving a conflict between sensory feedback and knowledge of results, while learning a motor skill. J Motor Behav 1994;26:27-35.

20. Burke D, Gracies JM, Mazevet D, Meunier S, Pierrot-Deseilligny E. Convergence of descending and various peripheral inputs onto common propriospinal-like neurones in man. J Physiol (Lond) 1992;449:655-71.

21. Burleigh AL, Horak FB, Malouin F. Modification of postural responses and step initiation: evidence for goal-directed postural interactions. J Neurophysiol 1994;72:2892-2902.

22. Byl NN, Merzenich MM, Cheung S, Bedenbaugh P, Nagarajan SS, Jenkins WM. A primate model for studying focal dystonia and repetitive strain injury: effects on the primary somatosensory cortex. Phys Ther 1997;77:269-84.

23. Calabresi P, Pisani A, Mercuri NB, Bernardi G. The corticostriatal projection: from synaptic plasticity to dysfunctions of the basal ganglia. Trends Neurosci 1996;19:19-24.

24. Carp JS, Wolpaw JR. Motoneuron plasticity underlying operantly conditioned decrease in primate H-reflex. J Neurophysiol 1995;72:431-42.

25. Carp JS, Wolpaw JR. Motoneuron properties after operantly conditioned increase in primate H-reflex. J Neurophysiol 1995;73:1365-73.

26. Carron AV. Motor performance and learning under physical fatigue. Med Sci Sport Exerc 1972;4:101-6.

27. Chen XY, Wolpaw JR. Operant conditioning of H-reflex in freely moving rats [abstract]. J Neurophysiol 1995;73:411-5.

28. Chollet F, DiPiero V, Wise RJS, Brooks DJ, Dolan RJ, Frackowiak RSJ. The functional anatomy of motor recovery after stroke in humans: a study with positron emission tomography. Ann Neurol 1991;29:63-71.

29. Cohen LG, Bandinelli S, Findley TW, Mattett M. Motor reorganization after upper limb amputation in man. Brain 1991;114:615-27.

30. Colman H, Nabekura J, Lichtman JW. Alterations in synaptic strength preceding axon withdrawal. Science 1997;275:356-61.

31. Corcos DM. Strategies underlying the control of disordered movement. Phys Ther 1991;71:25-38.

32. Cote L, Crutcher MD. The basal ganglia. In: Kandel ER, Schwartz JH, Jessell TM, eds. Principles of neural science, 3rd ed. Norwalk, Conn: Appleton & Lange, 1991.

33. Decety J. Do imagined and executed actions share the same neural substrate. Brain Res Cogn Brain Res 1996;3:87-93.

34. Diamond MC, Johnson RE, Protti AM, Ott C, Kajisa L. Plasticity in the 904 day old male rat cerebral cortex. Exp Neurol 1985;87:309-17.

35. Donoghue JP, Hess G, Sanes JN. Substrates and mechanisms for learning in motor cortex. In: Bloedel JR, Ebner TJ, Wise SP, eds. The acquisition of motor behavior in vertebrates. Cambridge, Mass: Massachusetts Institute of Technology Press, 1996:363-86.

36. Easter SS, Purves D, Rakic P, Spitzer NC. The changing view of neural specificity. Science 1985;230:507-11.

37. Elbert T, Pantev C, Wienbruch C, Rockstroh B, Taub E. Increased cortical representation of the fingers of the left hand in string players. Science 1995;270:305-7.

38. Feltz DL, Landers DM, Becker BJ. A revised meta-analysis of the mental practice literature on motor skill learning. National Academy Press, 1984.

39. Fengchen KC, Wolpaw JR. Operant conditioning of H-reflex changes synaptic terminals on primate motoneurons [abstract]. Proc Natl Acad Sci USA 1996;93:9206-11.

40. Fitts PM. Perceptual-motor skill learning. In: Melton AW, ed. Categories of human learning. New York: Academic Press, 1964:243-85.

41. Fung J, Barbeau H. Effects of conditioning cutaneomuscular stimulation on the soleus H-reflex in normal and spastic paretic subjects during walking and standing. J Neurophysiol 1994;72:2090-104.

42. Gao JH, Parsons LM, Bower JM, Xiong JL, Li J, Fox PT. Cerebellum implicated in sensory acquisition and discrimination rather than motor control. Science 1996;272:545-7.

43. Garland SJ, Garner SH, McComas AJ. Reduced voluntary electromyographic activity after fatiguing stimulation of human muscle. J Physiol (Lond) 1988;401:547-56.

44. Garland SJ, McComas AJ. Reflex inhibition of human soleus muscle during fatigue. J Physiol (Lond) 1990;429:17-27.

45. Georgopoulos AP, Ashe J, Smyrnis N, Taira M. Motor cortex and the coding of force. Science 1992;256:1692-5.

46. Georgopoulos AP, Schwartz AB, Kettner RE. Neuronal population coding of movement direction. Science 1986;233:1416-9.

47. Ghez C, Gordon J, Ghilardi MF. Impairments of reaching movements in patients without proprioception. II. Effects of visual information on accuracy. J Neurophysiol 1995;73:361-72.

48. Giuliani CA. Dorsal Rhizotomy for children with cerebral palsy: support for concepts of motor control. Phys Ther 1991;71:248-59.

49. Glencross D. Human skill: ideas, concepts, and models. In: Singer RN, Murphey M, Tennant LK, eds. Handbook of research on sport psychology. New York: MacMillan Publishing Co, 1993:242-56.

50. Goldberger ME. Motor recovery after lesions. Trends Neurosci 1980;3:288-91.

51. Goldberger ME. Partial and complete deeafferentation of cat hindlimb: the contribution of behavioral substitution to recovery of motor function. Exp Brain Res 1988;73:343-53.

52. Goldberger ME. Recovery of movement after central nervous system lesions in monkeys. In: Stein D, Rosen J, Butters N, eds. Plasticity and recovery of function in the central nervous system. New York: Academic Press, 1974:265-337.

53. Gordon J, Ghilardi MF, Ghez C. Impairments of reaching movements in patients without proprioception. I. Spatial errors. J Neurophysiol 1995;73:347-60.

54. Grafton ST, Arbib MA, Fadiga L, Rizzolatti G. Localization of grasp representations in humans by positron emission tomography. 2. Observation compared with imagination. Exp Brain Res 1996;112:103-11.

55. Grafton ST, Mazziotta JC, Presty S, Friston KJ, Frackowiak RSJ, Phelps ME. Functional anatomy of

human procedural learning determined with regional cerebral blood flow and PET. J Neurosci 1992;12:2542-8.

56. Grillner S. Control of locomotion in bipeds, tetrapods, and fish. In: Brooks VB, ed. Handbook of physiology, vol 2. The nervous system. II. Motor control. Bethesda: American Physiological Society, 19811:179-236.

57. Grillner S, Rossignol S. On the initiation of the swing phase of locomotion in chronic spinal cats. Brain Res 1978;146:269-77.

58. Hallett M, Pascual-Leone A, Topka H. Adaptation and skill learning: evidence for different neural substrates. In: Bloedel JR, Ebner TJ, Wise SP, eds. The acquisition of motor behavior in vertebrates. Cambridge, Mass: Massachusetts Institute of Technology Press, 1996:289-302.

59. Halsband U, Freund HJ. Motor learning. Curr Opin Neurobiol 1993;3:940-9.

60. Hanlon RE. Motor learning following unilateral stroke. Arch Phys Med Rehab 1996;77:811-5.

61. Hata Y, Stryker MP. Control of thalamocortical afferent rearrangement by postsynaptic activity in developing visual cortex. Science 1994;265:1731-5.

62. He SQ, Dum RP, Strick PL. Topographic organization of corticospinal projections from the frontal lobe: Motor areas on the medial surface of the hemisphere. J Neurosci 1995;15:3284-306.

63. Helgren ME, Goldberger ME. The recovery of postural reflexes and locomotion following low thoracic hemisection in adult cats involves compensation by undamaged primary afferent pathways [abstract]. Exp Neurol 1993;123:17-34.

64. Hongo T, Lundberg A, Phillips CG, Thompson RF. The pattern of monosynaptic Ia-connections to hindlimb motor nuclei in the baboon: a comparison with the cat. Proc R Soc Lond [Biol] 1984;221:261-89.

65. Horak FB, Diener HC. Cerebellar control of postural scaling and central set in stance. J Neurophysiol 1994;72:479-93.

66. Houk JC, Keifer J, Barto AG. Distributed motor commands in the limb premotor network. Trends Neurosci 1993;16:27-33.

67. Iriki A, Pavlides C, Keller A, Asanuma H. Long-term potentiation in the motor cortex. Science 1989;245:1385-8.

68. Ito M. Learning control mechanisms by the cerebellum: investigations in the flocculo-vestibular-ocular system. In: Tower DB, ed. The nervous system: basic neurosciences. New York: Raven, 1975:245-52.

69. Ito M. Movement and thought: identical control mechanisms by the cerebellum. Trends Neurosci 1993;16:448-50.

70. Jeannerod M. Mental imagery in the motor context. Neuropsychologia 1995;33:1419-32.

71. Jenkins IH, Brooks DJ, Nixon PD, Frackowiak RSJ, Passingham RE. Motor sequence learning: a study with

positron emission tomography [abstract]. J Neurosci 1994;14:3775-90.

72. Johansson BB, Grabowski M. Functional recovery after brain infarction—plasticity and neural transplantation. Brain Pathol 1994;4:85-95.

73. Kandel ER. Cellular mechanisms of learning and the biological basis of individuality. In: Kandel ER, Schwartz JH, Jessell TM, eds. Principles of neuroscience, 3rd ed. Norwalk, Conn: Appleton & Lange, 1991:1009-31.

74. Kandel ER, O'Dell TJ. Are adult learning mechanisms also used for development? Science 1992;258:243-5.

75. Karni A, Meyer G, Jezzard P, Adams MM, Turner R, . and Ungerleider LG. Functional MRI evidence for adult motor cortex plasticity during motor skill learning. Nature 1995;377:155-8.

76. Kass JH, Florence SL, Jain N. Reorganization of sensory systems of primates after injury. Neuroscientist 1997;3:123-30.

77. Kawato M. Learning internal models of the motor apparatus. In: Bloedel JR, Ebner TJ, Wise SP, eds. The acquisition of motor behavior in vertebrates. Cambridge, Mass: Massachusetts Institute of Technology Press, 1996:409-30.

78. Knowlton BJ, Mangels JA, Squire LR. A neostriatal habit learning system in humans [abstract]. Science 1996;273:1399-402.

79. Kocsis JD. Competition in the synaptic marketplace: activity is important. Neuroscientist 1995;1:185-7.

80. Kupfermann I. Learning and memory. In: Kandel ER, Schwartz JH, Jessell TM, eds. Principles of neural science, 3rd ed. Norwalk, Conn: Appleton & Lange, 1991:997-1008.

81. Le Vay S, Wiesel TN, Hubel DH. The development of ocular dominance columns in normal and visually deprived monkeys. J Comp Neurol 1980;191:1-51.

82. Leonard CT, Kane J, Perdaems J, Frank C, Graetzer DG, Moritani T. Neural modulation of muscle contractile properties during fatigue: afferent feedback dependence. Electroencephalogr Clin Neurophysiol 1994;93:209-17.

83. Llin'as R, Welsh JP. On the cerebellum and motor learning. Curr Opin Neurobiol 1993;3:958-65.

84. Merians A, Winstein CJ, Sullivan KJ, Pohl PS. Effects of feedback for motor skill learning in older healthy adults and individuals post-stroke. Neuroreport 1995;19:23-4.

85. Merzenich MM, Jenkins WM. Reorganization of cortical representations of the hand following alterations of skin inputs induced by nerve injury, skin island transfers, and experience. J Hand Ther 1993;6:89-104.

86. Merzenich MM, Kaas JH, Wall J, Nelson RJ, Sur M, Felleman D. Topographic reorganization of somatosensory cortical areas 3B and 1 in adult monkeys following restricted deafferentation. Neuroscience 1983:8:33-55.

87. Merzenich MM, Sameshima K. Cortical plasticity and memory. Curr Opin Neurobiol 1993;3:187-96.

88. Meunier S, Pierrot-Deseilligny E, Simonetta M. Pattern of monosynaptic heteronymous Ia connections in the human lower limb. Exp Brain Res 1993;96:534-44.

89. Milner B, Corkin S, Teuber HL. Further analysis of the hippocampal amnesic syndrome. Fourteen year follow-up study of H.M. Neuropsychologia 1968;6:215-34.

90. Moritani T. Muscle energetics and electromyography. In: Kumar S, Mital A, eds. Electromyography in ergonomics. London: Taylor and Francis, 1996:127-61.

91. Moritani T. Neuromuscular adaptations during the acquisition of muscle strength, power and motor tasks. J Biomech 1993;26:95-107.

92. Moritani T, Muro M, Nagata A. Intramuscular and surface electromyogram changes during muscle fatigue. J Appl Physiol 1986;60:1179-85.

93. Nelson PG, Yu C, Fields RD, Neale EA. Synaptic connections in vitro: modulation of number and efficacy by electrical activity. Science 1989;244:585-7.

94. Newman J, Rosenbach JH, Latimer BL, Matocha HR, Vost ER. An experimental test of the Mozart effect; does listening to his music improve spatial ability. Percept Mot Skills 1995;81:1379-87.

95. Niemann J, Winker T, Gerling J, Landwehrmeyer B, Jung R. Changes of slow cortical negative DC potentials during the acquisition of a complex finger motor task. Exp Brain Res 1991;85:417-22.

96. Nudo RJ, Milliken GW, Jenkins WM, Merzenich MM. Use-dependent alterations of movement representations in primary motor cortex of adult squirrel monkeys. J Neurosci 1996;16:785-807.

97. Nudo RJ, Wise BM, SiFuentes F, Milliken GW. Neural substrates for the effects of rehabilitative training on motor recovery after ischemic infarct. Science 1996;272:1791-4.

98. Nyland JJ, Brosky T, Currier D, Nitz A, Caborn D. Review of the afferent neural system of the knee and its contribution to motor learning. J Orthop Sports Phys Ther 1994;19:2-11.

99. Pierrot-Deseilligny E, Morin C, Bergego C, Tankov N. Pattern of group I fibre projections from ankle flexor and extensor muscles in man. Exp Brain Res 1981;42:337-50.

100. Porter R, Lemon R. Corticospinal function and voluntary movement, New York: Oxford University Press, 1993.

101. Prochazka A, Hulliger P, Trend P, Durmuller N. Dynamic and static fusimotor set in various behavioural contexts. In: Hnik P, Soukup T, Vejsada R, Zelena J, eds. Mechanoreceptors. New York: Plenum Press, 1988:417-30.

102. Purdie H, Baldwin S. Models of music therapy intervention in stroke rehabilitation. Int J Rehab Res 1995;18:341-50.

103. Purves D, Augustine GJ, Fitzpatrick D, Katz LC, LaMantia A, McNamara JO. Neuroscience. Sunderland: Sinauer Associates, 1997.

104. Purves D, Lichtman JW. Elimination of synapses in the developing nervous system. Science 1980;210:153-7.

105. Pysh JJ, Weiss GM. Exercise during development induces an increase in Purkinje cell dendritic tree size. Science 1979;206:230-2.

106. Rauscher FH, Shaw GL, Ky KN. Music and spatial task performance [abstract]. Nature 1993;365:611.

107. Raymond JL, Lisberger SG, Mauk MD. The cerebellum: a neuronal learning machine. Science 1996; 272:1126-31.

108. Rideout BE, Lauback CM. EEG correlates of enhanced spatial performance following exposure to music. Percept Mot Skills 1996;82:427-32.

109. Riedel G. Function of metabotropic glutamate receptors in learning and memory. Trends Neurosci 1996;19:219-23.

110. Rothstein E. Emblems of mind: the inner life of music and mathematics. New York: Avon, 1995.

111. Rothwell JC, Traub MM, Day BL, Obeso JA, Thomas PK, Marsden CD. Manual motor performance in a deafferented man. Brain 1982;105:515-42.

112. Roush W. The supple synapse: an affair that remembers. Science 1996;274:1102-3.

113. Ryding E, Decety J, Sjoholm H, Stenberg G, Ingvar DH. Motor imagery activates the cerebellum regionally. A SPECT rCBF study with 99mTc-HMPAO. Brain Res 1993;1:94-9.

114. Sabatini U, Toni D, Pantano P, et al. Motor recovery after early brain damage: a case of brain plasticity [abstract]. Stroke 1994;25:514-7.

115. Schacter DL. Searching for memory. New York: Basic Books, 1996.

116. Schauer M, Steingruber W, Mauritz KH. Effect of music on gait symmetry of stroke patients on a treadmill. Biomed Tech (Berl) 1996;41:291-6.

117. Scheibel AB, Conrad T, Perdue S, Tomiyasu U, Wechsler A. A quantitative study of dendrite complexity in selected areas of the human cerebral cortex. Brain Cogn 1990;12:85-101.

118. Schlaug G, Jancke L, Huang Y, Steinmetz H. In vivo evidence of structural brain asymmetry in musicians. Science 1995;267:699-701.

119. Schlaug G, Knorr U, Seitz RJ. Inter-subject variability of cerebral activations in acquiring a motor skill: a study with positron emission tomography. Exp Brain Res 1994;98:523-34.

120. Schmidt R. Motor control and learning. Champaign, Ill: Human Kinetics Publishing, 1988.

121. Seitz RJ, Roland PE. Learning of sequential finger movements in man: a combined kinematic and positron emission tomography (PET) study. Eur J Neurosci 1991;4:154-65.

122. Shumway-Cook A, Woollacott MH. Motor control: theory and applications. Baltimore: Williams & Wilkins, 1995.

123. Singer RN, Murphey M, Tennant LK. Handbook of research on sport psychology, New York: MacMillan Publishing Co, 1993.

124. Sirigu A, Duhamel J, Cohen L, Pillon B, Dubois B, Agid Y. The mental representation of hand movements after parietal cortex damage [abstract]. Science 1996;273:1564-8.

125. Smyrnis N, Taira M, Ashe J, Georgopoulos AP. Motor cortical activity in a memorized delay task. Exp Brain Res 1992;92:139-51.

126. Sossin WS. Mechanisms for the generation of synapse specificity in long-term memory: the implications of a requirement for transcription. Trends Neurosci 1996;19:215-8.

127. Thach WT. A cerebellar role in acquisition of novel static and dynamic muscle activities in holding, pointing, throwing, and reaching. In: Bloedel JR, Ebner TJ, Wise SP, eds. The acquisition of motor behavior in vertebrates. Cambridge, Mass: Massachusetts Institute of Technology Press, 1996:223-34.

128. Thorndike EL. The law of effect. Am J Psychol 1927;39:212-22.

129. Ungerleider LG. Functional brain imaging studies of cortical mechanisms for memory. Science 1995;270:769-75.

130. Vallbo AB, al Falahe NA. Human muscle spindle response in a motor learning task. J Physiol (Lond) 1990;421:553-68.

131. Walkerbatson D, Smith P, Curtis S, Unwin H, Greenlee R. Amphetamine paired with physical therapy accelerates motor recovery after stroke: further evidence. Stroke 1996;26:2254-9.

132. Wang X, Merzenich MM, Sameshima M, Jenkins WM. Remodelling of hand representation in adult cortex determined by timing of tactile stimulation. Nature 1995;378:13-4.

133. Weiller C, Chollet F, Friston KJ, Wise RJS, Frackowiak RSJ. Functional reorganization of the brain in recovery from striatocapsular infarction in man. Ann Neurol 1992;31:463-72.

134. Weiss T, Hansen E, Beyer L, et al. Activation processes during mental practice in stoke patients. Int J Psychophysiol 1994;17:91-100.

135. Weiss T, Hansen E, Rost R, et al. Mental practice of motor skills used in poststroke rehabilitation has own effects on central nervous activation. Int J Neurosci 1994;78:157-66.

136. Winstein CJ. Designing practice for motor learning: clinical implications. In: Lister M, ed. II step: contemporary management of motor control problems. Alexandria: Foundation for Physical Therapy, 1995:65-76.

137. Winstein CJ. Knowledge of results and motor learning—implications for physical therapy. Phys Ther 1991;71:140-9.

138. Winstein CJ, Pohl PS, Lewthwaite R. Effects of physical guidance and knowledge of results on motor learning: support for the guidance hypothesis. Res Q Exerc Sport 1994;65:316-23.

139. Winstein CJ, Schmidt RA. Reduced frequency of knowledge of results enhances motor skill learning. J Exp Psychol 1990;16:677-91.

140. Wolf SL, Segal RL. Reducing human biceps brachii spinal stretch reflex magnitude. J Neurophysiol 1996;75:1637-46.

141. Wolpaw JR, Herchenroder PA, Carp JS. Operant conditioning of the primate H-reflex: factors affecting the magnitude of change [abstract]. Exp Brain Res 1993;97:31-9.

142. Woods JJ, Furbush F, Bigland-Ritchie B. Evidence for a fatigue-induced reflex inhibition of motoneurone firing rates. J Neurophysiol 1987;50:125-37.

143. Zohary E, Celebrini S, Britten K, Newsome W. Neuronal plasticity that underlies improvement in perceptual performance. Science 1994;263:1289-92.

Acquisition of a motor skill: The execution and learning of a skill.

Action potential: An electric impulse consisting of a non-decremental propagation of polarizations or depolarizations transmitted across cell membranes during a nerve impulse.

Adaptation: Ability to modify a behavior in response to changing sensory input.

Afferent: Toward a center. With reference to nervous system, denotes nerve fibers transmitting information to spinal cord and higher brain centers

Agonist: The muscle(s) that are the prime movers of a joint during a movement.

Akinesia: Abnormal state of hypoactivity.

Alpha motor neuron: Large nerve cell located in the ventral horn of the spinal cord. Innervates skeletal (extrafusal) muscle.

Antagonist: The muscle(s) that oppose the action of the agonist muscles. Opposite of synergist.

Aphasia: A language disorder.

Apraxia: The loss of ability to perform familiar movements in the absence of motor or sensory impairment.

Ataxia: An inability to coordinate movement. Staggering gait and postural imbalances are common to this disorder, typically caused by damage or disease to the cerebellum, vestibular system, or spinal cord.

Athetosis: A neuromuscular condition characterized by slow, writhing, involuntary movements of the extremities. A motor disorder typically associated with damage or disease of the basal ganglia.

Augmented feedback: Provision of physical and verbal input in addition to one's own sensory feedback.

Autogenic inhibition (nonreciprocal inhibition): Golgi tendon organ and Ib afferent–mediated inhibition of agonist muscle and synergists concomitant with excitation of antagonists.

Autonomic nervous system: The "involuntary" component of the nervous system. Mainly responsible for metabolic activities of the body and for physiological adaptation based on situational need. Comprises the sympathetic and parasympathetic nervous systems.

Axon: The single one among a nerve cell's processes that conducts nervous impulses away from the cell body.

Basal ganglia: Gray matter structures located deep within the cerebral hemispheres. Composed of the caudate, putamen, amygdala, and globus pallidus.

Beta motor neurons: Spinal cord neurons that innervate intra- and extrafusal muscle fibers.

Bimanual coordination: The ability to use both hands acting in concert to achieve a common purpose.

Blocked practice: Practicing a skill repetitively during a practice session.

Bradykinesia: An abnormal condition of slowness of movement and speech.

Brain stem: Rostral extension of the spinal cord which includes the midbrain, pons, and medulla oblongata.

Bundling: Information processing mechanism hypothesized to combine multiple afferent signals into a single unit.

Caudal: Toward the tail end of an organism. Depending on context, synonymous with inferior or posterior.

Cell assembly: Cells that tend to fire synchronously during a movement.

Central nervous system (CNS): Includes the spinal cord, brain stem, cerebellum, and the cerebral cortex.

Central pattern generators (CPGs): Neural circuits that can generate coordinated, rhythmic movements autonomously.

Cerebellum: The large posterior brain mass lying above the pons and medulla and beneath the posterior portion of the cerebral cortex.

Cerebral cortex: Most accurately refers to the layer of gray matter covering the entire surface of the cerebral hemispheres of mammals. Typically refers to the brain located rostral to the brain stem. Includes two cerebral hemispheres.

Cervical: Relating to a neck, or cervix, in any sense (i.e., cervical spinal cord refers to that portion of the spinal cord located in the neck region).

Chorea: An abnormal motor disorder characterized by involuntary, purposeless, rapid movements and/or grimacing, e.g., Huntington's chorea.

Climbing fibers: Input from inferior olivary nucleus to Purkinje cells of cerebellum.

Contralateral: Relating to the opposite side, as when pain is felt or paralysis occurs on the side opposite to that of the lesion.

Concentric muscle contraction: Muscle fiber shortens as tension develops.

Conditioned-associative learning: Learning that is adaptive and automatic.

Convergence: Input arriving at a similar point.

Cortical columns: Groups of vertically linked cortical cells that have common response properties. They can expand and shrink (exhibit plasticity) depending on epigenetic factors.

Cortical field or cortical module: Often used synonymously with cortical column, but increasingly used to indicate any functional grouping within the brain.

Corticobulbar: Neural pathways originating in the cerebral cortex and terminating in the brain stem.

Corticofugal: Neural pathways originating in the cerebral cortex and terminating in subcortical structures such as the brain stem and spinal cord

Corticospinal: Neural pathways originating in the cerebral cortex and terminating in the spinal cord.

Critical periods: During ontogenetic development, different neural structures have varying periods of cell migration, projection growth, and membrane changes. Damage before or after critical periods will have different effects.

Cytoarchitectonics: Cellular organization within a structure.

Declarative learning: The type of learning that involves concepts and facts that can usually be communicated consciously.

Deep cerebellar nuclei: Three nuclei (fastigial, interposed, and dentate) that comprise the output of the cerebellum.

Dendrite: One of the two types of branching processes of the nerve cell (the axon being the other).

Depolarization: Reduction of a membrane potential to a less negative value (movement toward an action potential).

Diencephalon: Thalamus, epithalamus, hypothalamus, and subthalamus. Located between cerebrum and mesencephalon.

Disinhibition: The removal of inhibition; inhibition of an inhibitory input.

Disynaptic inhibition: Inhibition of antagonist muscle motor neuron pool mediated by an inhibitory interneuron.

Divergence: Separation of neural output to various locations.

Dorsal: Relating to the back; posterior.

Dorsal root ganglia (DRG): Ganglia containing sensory neuron cell bodies. Located on the dorsal root of a spinal nerve. Sensory neurons located here have a peripheral projection connected to a sensory receptor and a central projection to the spinal cord.

Dyskinesia: Impairment in the ability to initiate voluntary movement.

Dystonia: Any abnormal change in muscle tone.

Eccentric muscle contraction: Muscle fiber lengthens as tension develops. Common mode of muscle contraction to decelerate limb movement (e.g., hamstrings during terminal swing phase).

Efferent: Conducting a nerve impulse outward from the cell body.

Engram: A hypothetical alteration of living neural tissue, posed to explain memory.

Epigenetic: Factors (e.g., experience, learning, injury) other than genetics that influence the full phenotypic expression of the genome (e.g., activity and cerebral cortical cell column development).

Excitatory postsynaptic potential (EPSP): Change within a cell toward a more positive direction (toward an action potential) created by release of neurotransmitter and the presence of receptors on the postsynaptic membrane specific for that neurotransmitter.

Extrafusal muscle fiber: Skeletal muscle capable of voluntary contraction.

Exuberance: With respect to neural development, the presence of an abnormally large number of projections or neurons not normally found in the mature animal.

Feedback: Information sent back to a source that influences the output of the source.

Feed-forward: Operating independent of feedback (e.g., sending a neural message to cause stabilizing muscle contractions in anticipation of a destabilizing movement).

Flexor reflex afferents (FRAs): Common reflex action of flexion that can be caused by a variety of sensory inputs.

Frontal: Relating to the anterior part of the body.

Fusimotor system: Refers to muscle spindles and their gamma motor neuron innervation.

Gamma motor neuron: Nerve cell located in the ventral horn of the spinal cord that innervates muscle spindles.

Gaze: Looking in one direction or visually locating an object.

Generator potential: Graded potential that results from stimulating a peripheral receptor (e.g., touch, nociception, stretch).

Golgi tendon organs (GTOs): Receptors located primarily in musculotendinous junction that monitor force or tension.

Group Ib afferents: Sensory afferents that convey information from Golgi tendon organs.

Gyrencephalic: Referring to brains (e.g., human) that have convolutions, in contrast to smooth brains (*lissencephalic*) typical of rodents.

Habituation: A type of nonassociative learning that involves suppression of a response to a sensory stimulus.

Hemianopia: Blindness or ignoral of one half of a visual field.

Hemiplegia: Paralysis or paresis of one half of the body.

Heteronymous: Of a different type or name.

Homeostasis: The state of equilibrium in the body with respect to various physiological functions and to the chemical compositions of the fluids and tissues, e.g., temperature, heart rate, blood pressure, hormone levels, etc.

Homunculus: Drawing of human form draped over the motor area of the cerebral cortex with body parts accentuated proportional to areas that, when electrically stimulated, cause movement of that body part.

Homonymous: The same.

Hyperpolarization: Cell membrane changes toward a more negative direction (away from action potential).

Hypothalamus: Located on the ventral surface of the brain, it is a central nervous system structure that is involved with endocrine function, autonomic nervous system function, emotion, and motivational states.

Hypertonic: Elevated muscle tone.

Hypotonic: Decreased muscle tone.

Inferior: Below in relation to another structure; caudal.

Inhibitory postsynaptic potential (IPSP): Result of transmitter interaction on postsynaptic membrane that moves membrane potential in a more negative direction (away from action potential).

Internal capsule: Fibers traveling to and from the cerebral cortex. Located lateral to the thalamus.

Interneurons: Interconnecting neurons in a pathway. Typically they never project outside *their area of origin (e.g., spinal interneurons never project out of the spinal cord).*

Intrafusal muscle fiber: Muscle fibers associated with the muscle spindle.

Ipsilateral: On the same side.

Isocortex (neocortex): Six-layered cerebral cortex. A phylogenetically recent mammalian development.

Isometric muscle contraction: Fibers do not change length as tension develops during the contraction (e.g., pushing against an immovable object).

Kinesiology: The science or study of movement.

Kinesthesia: The sense perception of movement.

Labyrinthine system: Receptors of the inner ear that contribute to balance and head righting.

Lacunar infarcts: Small lesions in the central nervous system, typically of vascular origin. May or may not be detectable by scanning techniques.

Lateral (surround) inhibition: A mechanism that helps to localize sensory input (see Fig. 3-4).

Lenticular nucleus: Putamen and globus pallidus (part of the basal ganglia).

Limbic system: Anatomically indistinct collection of central nervous system structures collectively thought to be a center for emotion.

Lissencephalic: Smooth brain, no convolutions. Typical of rodents and small mammals.

Long-loop reflexes: Pathways that involve the cerebral cortex. They appear to integrate peripheral reflexes with willed intent of movement.

Long-term potentiation: Enhancement of synaptic transmission (increase in size of postsynaptic potential) after exposure to certain types of stimulation. It is thought to be one mechanism involved with learning and memory.

Lumbar: Relating to the part of the back or vertebral column located between the ribs and the pelvis.

Medial lemniscus: A tract system connecting the nucleus gracilis and nucleus cuneatus with the thalamus. The posterior columns of the spinal cord convey sensory information from the body and terminate in the nucleus gracilis and cuneatus. The medial lemniscus is thus a sensory pathway conveying sensory information from the head and body to the thalamus.

Medulla: Rostral extension of spinal cord just above foramen magnum and just caudal to pons. Part of the brain stem that contains vasomotor, cardiac, and respiratory centers.

Membrane potential: Electrical potential difference across the cell membrane as a result of the differences in electrical charges between the inside and outside of the cell.

Midbrain (mesencephalon): The part of the brain stem located rostral to the pons and caudal to the cerebral cortex. Contains the red nucleus and basis peduncles.

Monosynaptic: Referring to direct neural connections (those not involving an intermediary neuron); e.g., the direct connection between primary sensory nerve cells and motor neurons characterizing the monosynaptic reflex arc.

Mossy fibers: Afferent input arising from multiple sites within the brain stem and spinal cord and projecting to the cerebellum.

Motor equivalence: A motor control theory that proposes that movement is organized in relation to the desired goal and is guided by controlling degrees of freedom between joints. A typical example is handwriting—the style is the same regardless whether it is written in large or small letters. Different muscles are used, yet the output is the same.

Motor skill learning: Formation of new or novel movement sequences to gain speed, precision, accuracy, and efficiency in a task.

Motor unit: The alpha motor neuron and all the muscle fibers innervated by it.

Multimodal imaging: The use of electroencephalography with other scanning techniques such as positron emission tomography (PET) or magnetic resonance imaging (MRI). It is used to examine the global activity of cerebral cortex and underlying structures.

Muscle spindle: Encapsulated sensory organs located within skeletal muscle. They are responsive to the absolute length and the rate of the change in length of a muscle.

Neocortex (isocortex): See *isocortex*.

Neostriatum. See striatum.

Neuroglia: Nonneural cellular elements of the central and peripheral nervous systems. They are support cells and have important metabolic functions. Examples of neuroglial cells include astrocytes, oligodendroglia, ependymal cells, Schwann cells, and microglia.

Neuromodulators: Substances that alter the properties of a neuron. They can make a neuron more or less responsive to incoming stimuli and transmitters.

Neuromuscular junction: Referring to the point where a nerve meets and innervates muscle.

Neuron: Nerve cell; the morphologic and functional unit of the nervous system, consisting of the nerve cell body, the dendrites, and the axon.

Neurotransmitter: A chemical substance released from an axon that travels across the synaptic gap to either excite or inhibit the target cell.

Nonassociative learning: Conditioned responses that exhibit habituation or sensitization.

Nuclear bag: A type of spindle fiber. Dynamic nuclear bag fibers respond to the rate of change in muscle length. Static nuclear bag fibers detect the absolute length of a muscle.

Nuclear chain: A type of spindle fiber that responds to the absolute length of a muscle.

Nuclei: An anatomically distinct (either via topography or cell type) clustering of neurons that very often share similar functional characteristics.

Olfaction: Sense of smell.

Optokinetic reflexes: Reflex pathways that contribute to eye tracking during sustained movements.

Pallidotomy: The surgical production of lesions in the globus pallidus.

Parasympathetic nervous system: A component of the autonomic nervous system mainly responsible for vegetative functions of the body.

Paretic: Referring to a muscle that is partially paralyzed.

Part-task training: Breaking down a movement into its component parts.

Perinatal: Pertaining to period of time before, during, and after birth.

Peripheral nervous system (PNS): The motor and sensory nerves and ganglia located outside the cerebral cortex and spinal cord (CNS).

Plantigrade: Refers to striking with the heel first during the stance phase of bipedal gait and then transferring of weight to the forefoot. Unique to human species.

Plasticity: The ability of the central nervous system to change and modulate synaptic strength, dendritic arborization, and other processes as a result of experience or injury.

Plyometrics: Sport training technique that uses quick stretch to a muscle to enhance force production.

Polysynaptic: Multisynaptic; referring to neural conduction pathways formed by a chain of many, synaptically connected nerve cells.

Presynaptic inhibition: Inhibition caused by a decrease in the amount of neurotransmitter released by the presynaptic terminal.

Procedural learning: Learned behaviors or habits that are performed automatically and without excessive mental concentration (e.g., an acquired motor skill).

Proprioception: Sensory information regarding position sense and muscle static and dynamic tension resulting from stimuli originating from muscles, tendons, and joint capsules.

Purkinje cell: Cell located in cerebellar cortex that projects to deep cerebellar nuclei.

Random practice: Practicing various skills, rather than concentrating on the acquisition of a single skill, during a practice session.

Rate modulation: Refers to the motor neuron's ability to vary the number of action potentials it sends to the neuromuscular junction. The higher the rate, the greater the force production.

Receptor potential: Voltage change occurring in a sensory receptor in response to a stimulus.

Recurrent inhibition: Renshaw cell–mediated inhibition of its alpha motor neuron.

Reflex: A response elicited by a stimulus applied to peripheral receptors and conveyed to the nervous system by sensory afferents.

Renshaw cells: Spinal cord interneurons that mediate recurrent inhibition (see Fig. 3-10).

Retention of a motor skill: The memory of a skill and the ability to repeat it.

Reticular formation: A collection of neurons and nuclei located within the brain stem. It serves as a relay center for projections from higher brain centers and from the spinal cord.

Rostral: Directed toward the head of the organism. Can be synonymous with anterior or superior. Opposite of caudal.

Saccades: Rapid eye movements that occur during eye tracking tasks.

Sagittal: In an anteroposterior direction.

Sensitization: A form of nonassociative learning that typically results in accentuation of a response to a sensory stimulus (e.g., pain).

Size principle: General rule of motor unit recruitment that indicates that smaller motor units (typically innervating slower muscle fibers) are recruited first during a muscle contraction, followed by recruitment of larger motor units (innervate fast muscle fibers).

Smooth-pursuit: Eye movements that keep a moving object centered on the fovea.

Somatotopic: Refers to organization within central nervous system tracts and structures that compartmentalizes body parts (e.g., in the dorsal columns of the spinal cord, fibers conveying sensation from the leg are medial to those for the upper extremities).

Spasticity: A motor disorder characterized by velocity-dependent hypertonia, hyperactive tendon reflexes, and clonus. Abnormal patterns of muscular coordination and paresis are also associated with spasticity.

Spatial summation: Cumulative effect of multiple excitatory or inhibitory postsynaptic potentials arriving from multiple sources.

Spinal cord: Relating to the vertebral column.

Spinothalamic tract: Pathway originating in the spinal cord and terminating in the thalamus. Primarily conveys pain and temperature.

Stereognosis: The ability to perceive an object's nature through touch.

Striatum (neostriatum): A portion of the basal ganglia (caudate and putamen).

Superior: Above in relation to another structure; cephalic.

Supraspinal: Rostral to the spinal cord.

Sympathetic nervous system: A component of the autonomic nervous system. Responsible for visceral and glandular responses to stress. Often referred to as the "fight or flight" system.

Synapse: The functional contact between one nerve cell and another. The synapse subserves the transmission of nerve impulses. In most cases the impulse is transmitted by means of a chemical transmitter substance released from the synapse.

Synaptic potential: A graded change in the membrane potential that results from excitatory or inhibitory input. See *excitatory* or *inhibitory postsynaptic potentials*.

Synaptic threshold: Membrane potential at which an action potential or generator potential results (e.g., excitatory postsynaptic potentials summate to cause the postsynaptic membrane to reach a synaptic threshold, which results in an action potential).

Synergist: A muscle that aids in the action of another.

Synergistic: Pertaining to synergy; denoting a synergist.

Synergy: Coordinated or correlated action by two or more structures; coordination of muscles by the nervous system so that specific actions can be performed.

Temporal summation: The number of excitatory or inhibitory inputs per unit time.

Thalamic syndrome: Damage to the thalamus that results in pain, hemianesthesia, and sensory ataxia.

Thalamus: A large collection of nuclei located deep within the folds of the cerebral cortex. All sensory receptors send afferents to the thalamus, which, in turn, sends efferents to various locations within the cerebral cortex.

Theory of functional reorganization: Theory that a neural system can alter its function depending on need and secondary to damage to related areas.

Theory of mass action: Theory that various parts of the nervous system can mediate the same motor function.

Theory of substitution: Theory that a motor behavior can be performed by a different mechanism than that which originally controlled the behavior.

Theory of vicarious function: Theory that undamaged regions of the central nervous system have latent capabilities that can take over for damaged regions.

Thoracic: That part of the vertebral column lying between the cervical and lumbar segments. There are 12 thoracic vertebrae.

Tone (muscle): Background state of relative stiffness in a muscle. Clinically typically tested by assessing the resistance of the muscle to passive stretch. Neural and nonneural parameters contribute to tone.

Tract: A path, a grouping of axonal projections.

Transcortical loops: See *long-loop reflexes*.

Trigeminothalamic tract: Conveys pain and temperature from the face.

Trophic: Pertaining to a nutritive or supportive effect of cell activity.

Upper motor neuron: Typically refers to cortical or supraspinal neurons that contribute to descending pathways.

Ventral: Relating to the belly or the abdomen; opposite of dorsal or posterior.

Vestibulo-ocular reflexes: Reflexes subserved by neural circuitry connecting the vestibular system with eye musculature so that the eyes can remain fixated on an object during movements of the head.

INDEX

A

acetylcholine, 161

acquisition of a motor skill, 204, 212, 221-222, 227, 237

action potential, 19, 73-74, 91, 115, 227, 237

action potential threshold. *See* spike threshold

Adam's Closed Loop Model, 205, 207

adaptation, 203, 237

adaptive learning, 203, 211-212

afferent input, 54, 59, 61, 149, 154, 208, 225, 237

agonist muscle, 26, 58, 77-80, 82-83, 112, 156, 185, 209, 237

akinesia, 48, 135, 159, 237

alcohol, 10

Ali, Muhammed, 48, 58

alpha-gamma coactivation, 23

alpha motor neuron, 19-20, 24-25, 28, 32-33, 73, 77, 80-81, 83, 94-95, 112, 129, 131, 156, 161, 167, 225, 237

Alzheimer's disease, 161

amphetamine, 227

amygdala, 40, 42, 62, 161

Anderson's Act Model, 205

anencephaly, 147, 149

antagonist muscle, 23, 26, 28, 58, 80-85, 112, 156, 159, 185, 237

anterior, defined, 2

anterior falx, 108

anterior horn cell, 19

anterior nucleus of the thalamus, 62

aphasia, 137, 237

apraxia, 229, 237

archicortex, 121, 207

Ardipithecus ramidus, 146

arteries

anterior cerebral, 42

basilar, 41-42, 109

internal carotid, 42

middle cerebral, 42

posterior cerebral, 42

aspartate, 161

association areas, 59, 63, 193

association cortex, 45, 62

association neuron, 123

associativity, 216-217

ataxia, 58, 63, 237

athetosis, 159, 237

autogenic inhibition, 237. *See* nonreciprocal inhibition

auditory cortex, 62, 158

auditory input, 34, 36-37

augmented feedback, 223, 229, 237

autonomic nervous system, 4-5, 30, 33, 75, 161, 237

Australopithecus afarensis, 146-147

Australiopithecus anamensis, 146

axoaxonic synapse, 89-91

axodendritic synapse, 89-90

axon, 5-6, 9, 11, 89, 126-129, 220, 237

axosomatic synapse, 89-90

B

baclofen, 162

basal ganglia, 237

anatomy of, 3, 40-42, 44, 46, 106

connectivity of, 35-36, 45-46, 62-63, 88, 95-96, 116, 123, 157, 191, 212, 218